THE REVOLUTIONARY
7-WEEK
ANTI-AGING PLAN

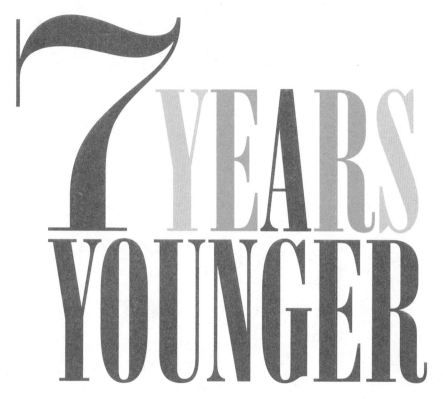

7 YEARS YOUNGER

BY THE EDITORS OF **GOOD HOUSEKEEPING**

7YY

An imprint of Hearst Magazines

Cont

ents

Acknowledgments

I am indebted to a multitasking, multitalented village of experts for bringing their insights, skills, and commitment to excellence to the *7 Years Younger* project. This endeavor involved multiple platforms, from print to digital to social media, and I'd like to thank all involved.

First and foremost, my deepest thanks go to Executive Editor Jennifer Cook. Jenny's enthusiastic and tireless work on the *7 Years Younger* project, from its inception until the last page was shipped to the printer, was unflagging. Her expertise, sound judgment, and graceful editing permeate every page of this book, and her excellent management skills in coordinating the small army that it takes to produce such a project were invaluable. The fact that she did all of this while still handling a full editorial load at the magazine is a testament to her dedication and drive. Thank you, Jenny.

Also, profound thanks to the tireless team at the Good Housekeeping Research Institute. Under the able leadership of Miriam Arond, GHRI's staff of discriminating scientists worked to research the best products to recommend for the 7YY plan. Her go-to gang includes Stacy Genovese; the beauty lab's Birnur Aral, Ph.D., Charmaine Rodriques, and Mary E. Clarke; and Samantha B. Cassetty, M.S., R.D., who developed the 7YY weight loss plan.

Equal and enormous thanks go to Susan Westmoreland and the Good Housekeeping Test Kitchen team: Genevieve Ko, Catherine Lo, Sherry Rujikarn, and Jessica Fox. The test kitchen is home base for every recipe on this project as well as in the magazine and on the website. Every recipe

Is tasted, perfected, and triple-tested by Susan and her team, so you can cook with confidence.

They say a picture is worth a thousand words. To that I'd add graphics and layout, which is why I'm so grateful to the design team behind this book. First, let me thank Creative Director Courtney Murphy, who guides the design of the magazine and the *Good Housekeeping* brand each month, as well as Joanna Williams, who worked on the book. Additionally, I want to recognize the dream team of GH, GH Art, and GH.com that puts together the *Good Housekeeping* presence each month and has been involved in this far-reaching project. On the edit side: Janet Siroto, Sarah Scrymser, Dana Levy, Nina Judar, Toni Gerber Hope, Benay Bubar, Rachel Bowie, Melanie Rud, Marnie Soman, Shelly Watson, Kathleen Corlett, and Kate Westervelt; in art: Trent Johnson, Laura Baer, Bill Swan, and Stephanie Green; online: Jennifer Barrett and Jennifer Fields. I'd also like to recognize the contribution of other editors from Hearst Magazines: Jill Herzig, editor in chief of *Redbook*; Sarah Gray Miller, editor in chief of *Country Living*; and Susan Spencer, editor in chief of *Woman's Day*.

And of course, this book would not exist without the masterminds behind Hearst Books, all of whom have supported the 7YY project from its start. Special thanks to the multi-talented Jacqueline Deval, who worked nonstop to make this project a success, as well as her brook-no-obstacles team, including Deede Dickson, Colleen Noonan, Laura Reid, David Schirmer, Stephan Wasserman, Deborah Burns, and TJ Mancini; and in production, Lynn Scaglione and Silvia Coppola.

The creative team behind the 7YY project deserves special singling out, from Jennifer Kinon and Bobby C. Martin, Jr., at OCD, who designed our beautiful logo and cover, to David Kang, Judith Bookbinder, and David Goffin and the video team at VIMBY.

This project would not exist in its multimedia form without the guidance of our marketing and digital teams. Thanks go out to Brian Carnahan, Kim Oscarson, Sharon Bailey Romano, Sarah Deem, Jennifer

Jenkins, Elyse Lindsey, Christina Dalton, Kerry Mazzacano, Brian Madden, Ross Geisel, Charlie Swift, Liberta Abbondante, Susan Allyn, Rachel Glickman, Elizabeth Shepard, Lauren Ruotolo, Amanda Brotherton, Jessica Brown, Hayley Kornbluh, and Erin Toland.

I also want to thank my partner at GH, publisher Pat Haegele, as well as Christine Rannazzisi, Sara Rad, Robbin Tick, and Orchid Burnside.

Backing this project all the way was the management team at Hearst. Thanks to the vision and enthusiasm of David Carey, president, Hearst Magazines; the tireless encouragement and support of John Loughlin, executive vice president and general manager; as well as Debi Chirichella, senior vice president, chief financial officer; Michael Clinton, president, marketing and publishing director; Duncan Edwards, executive vice president; Ellen Levine, editorial director; Debra Robinson, senior vice president, chief information officer; and Grant Whitmore, vice president, digital.

I am also indebted to those who helped hands-on with our 7YY panelists—Leesa Chalk Suzman, who worked with us to find them; Merle Taylor and his team at Hearst Towers–The Club, who weighed and measured; and those who created the eye-catching photographic results, including makeup artists Birgitte Philippides and Sandy Linter, from Lancôme. Kudus to master colorist Louis Licari and his cut-and-color team from the Louis Licari salon.

Last but not least, I am indebted to the talented writing team behind this project, intrepid researcher/reporter Daryn Eller and editor Stephanie Young, for collecting and presenting this vital anti-aging information in a clear, accessible, and vibrant way.

I hope you enjoy reading 7 *Years Younger*, but more important, I hope you look it!

Rosemary Ellis

Editor in Chief, *Good Housekeeping*

Get Ready to Turn Back the Clock

Imagine yourself suddenly 7 years younger—with beautiful, glowing skin, shiny hair, a flat belly, and feeling full of energy and life. This book gives you the tools and the plan you need to turn back the clock now—head to toe, body and mind. Perhaps you've noticed a few more wrinkles and gray hairs starting to appear. Maybe you don't feel as energetic as you once were, or you're frustrated by midlife pounds that crept on when you weren't looking. Or sometimes you find yourself so stressed and distracted you can hardly remember anything anymore. Whatever it is that's making you yearn to feel younger, get ready to reach your goal. Our research shows that by following our program—the right skin and hair care, appropriate cosmetics, consistent exercise, and strategic nutrition—you can look up to 7 Years Younger! And that's without resorting to surgery, injections, or other invasive procedures.

Here's the best part: It's satisfying, gratifying, and fun! You'll try out youth-restoring beauty products and get insider tips on everything from reviving limp hair to making fine lines and imperfections look less obvious. You'll sample satisfying snacks and delicious meals that also happen to be rich in anti-agers that fight disease (wrinkles, too). And you even get to play: We've got boredom-proof workouts for getting your body into shape and brainteasers for exercising your mind.

We *know* this program delivers proven results, because it was tested by women just like you. We auditioned 26 women to be testers by asking them why they wanted to look and feel 7 years younger. Twelve women submitted videos of themselves talking about everything from life challenges they've faced and the need for a fresh start to the dryness of their skin. We narrowed down the field and came up with a top-notch panel of testers: 10 women, ages 34 to 53, with busy lives just like yours. Throughout this book, you'll read their inspiring stories and see their amazing results.

Each panelist had her own reasons for wanting to look and feel younger, and many of them will sound familiar to you. Several women said they felt younger than their calendar age and wanted their looks to match their attitude and energy level. Many of them confessed to not having taken time to care for themselves in years. Almost all of the panelists wanted to lose weight, learn to eat more healthfully, master makeup application, and improve their hair and skin. More than one woman confessed to having started and stopped several other healthy-eating and skin-care routines, and hoping this one would stick.

Throughout the eight weeks, the 7 Years Younger panelists stayed connected to our experts—and each other—through Skype and Facebook. Their questions, quibbles, and creative solutions helped us fine-tune this program to suit real women's needs. And their successes proved that it really is possible to take years off your age in just a few short weeks. One woman lost 12 pounds, another lost 10 inches from her waist, another achieved turn-back-the-clock skin, and *all* of them reported feeling better than they'd felt in years. So get ready! With our beauty advice, your lines, wrinkles, and age spots will diminish and your skin will feel smoother. You'll learn expert makeup techniques to offset the changes that come with age. Your hair will gleam and be more manageable (even on humid days), and you'll eat your way to a younger, healthier body—our 7 Years Younger weight-loss plan will not only help you shed pounds, but ensure you get heaping helpings of age-fighting nutrients. The exercise you'll be doing will go a long way toward counteracting aging and disease, too, all the while making you fitter. You're also going to come through this program with long- and short-term tactics for sharpening your memory, getting a better night's sleep, and leading a life that's less stressed.

To develop the 7 Years Younger program, we drew on the latest scientific breakthroughs in anti-aging research as well as the advice of top experts in skin care, cosmetics, hair care, nutrition and diet, exercise, brain fitness, and emotional health. And for the lowdown on the products that promise youthfulness we needed to look no further than our own Good Housekeeping Research Institute, which put everything from eye creams and deep conditioners to wrinkle serums and teeth whiteners through scientific tests that reveal which products really work.

From this wealth of information, our experienced and discerning editors transformed the facts and findings into a workable, practical program. Our aim: to help you adopt new habits that will have a significant impact on how you look and feel—yet not overwhelm you. We know how incredibly busy you are, so rest assured that the changes you are about to embark upon are very doable. Each week, you'll add a few changes to your overall routine. That way you can ease into your new age-erasing lifestyle and increase your chances of success.

What makes this program one-of-a-kind is that it does as much to make you youthful on the inside as on the outside. Research shows that the right combination of healthy habits can make you physiologically younger than your chronological age—and, most important, help you live longer. The Baltimore Longitudinal Study on Aging, ongoing since 1959, has even determined that disease, often considered to be inevitable with time, is *not* a natural part of aging. By following our plan, you'll be putting yourself on the path to long-lasting good health.

THE 7 YEARS YOUNGER PROGRAM

The program starts with a written and signed pledge from you that highlights what you'd like to accomplish and learn from the plan. The chapters that follow are chock-full of age-erasing tips and tricks, each centered on the very practical philosophy that making small changes daily can yield significant results for the long term. Whether you've been eyeing a new way to apply makeup, wanting to understand what kinds of protein you should be eating as you get older, or getting concerned about memory lapses, we have the answers, detailed in the first seven chapters on skin care, makeup, hair, nutrition, fitness, brain health, and de-stressing.

So how do you put all those answers together in a plan that addresses your needs? The next three chapters, featuring the 7-Day Jumpstart Plan, the 7-Week Plan, and the Light and Delicious Recipes, walk you step-by-step into your new age-erasing lifestyle, integrating key anti-aging strategies into one manageable program. The Jumpstart Plan provides immediate gratification—you'll likely lose a pound or two in that week (one of our panelists lost four pounds!) and brighten your skin and hair. That takes you to the 7-Week Plan, which introduces something new to do every week and gives you time to get used to the changes.

One of our goals in creating this program was to make it possible for you to meet your own goals in the way that suits you best. You should make the 7 Years Younger plan your own. Not ready to commit to a week-by-week plan? Check out the "Activate Your Anti-Aging Plan Now!" tips at the end of each chapter. They'll recommend actions you can take to roll back the years that will introduce you to the program and let you focus on the areas where you'd most like to improve. You can also get more expert suggestions and learn from other readers' comments (and make some of your own) by logging on to the 7 Years Younger Facebook page at facebook.com/7yearsyounger.

GEARING UP FOR CHANGE

Even though the 7 Years Younger program is designed to help you make gradual changes you can stick with, it also helps to think about how you approach change before you take the plunge. If you've ever set out to make a big alteration in lifestyle before, you know that the first few days of a new routine can feel empowering: You set your mind to accomplishing something and prove to yourself that you can do it. Wow! But often your enthusiasm for this new style of living can begin to wane. For example, maybe you stop using a night cream or find you're too busy to bother with your hair. Or you find excuses to exercise less and eat more.

Don't feel guilty! It's not because you're weak or undisciplined. Researchers who study the process of change say that a temporary fallback into old habits or patterns is inevitable. It simply goes with the territory, because the pathway to your old behavior still exists in your brain. Yet our brains have enormous plasticity, meaning they can generate new cells and pathways to different behaviors. As long as you return to your new habits-in-the-making, you'll be able to make them stick and get the results you want.

So while you should expect some bumps along the way, here are seven things you should do *right now* to increase the likelihood that you'll stay on track and take temporary setbacks in stride.

1 **Make a promise to yourself** Call it a promise, a resolution, a vow, a pledge, a commitment. Whatever you name it, making it non-negotiable is a way to help keep you from backsliding after your initial enthusiasm fades. Writing down your intentions can favorably influence the outcome, according to researchers at Dominican University of California. They separated 267 people ages 23 to 72 into five groups. The groups were assigned different tasks—one group was to just think about goals they could achieve in four weeks, and the other four groups were to write down their four-week goals.

The groups who wrote down their goals were more likely to achieve them than those who merely made mental vows. Among the goal-writers, one group did best of all: people who also shared their commitments with a friend *and* sent a weekly progress report to that friend. Their success rate was 76 percent of goals accomplished as compared to a success rate of only 43 percent for the group that did no goal-writing. (See page 18 for the 7 Years Younger Pledge.)

2 **Visualize success** Find a photo of yourself taken seven (or more) years ago at a happy time in your life and put it someplace that will remind you every day of how you were when at your best.

3 **Write it down** Research shows that a written record of your actions helps you achieve your goals. See page 155 for information on keeping a food diary.

4 **Go public** Tell a friend or a group of buddies about your commitment, and then check in with the person or group regularly so you are accountable to someone other than yourself. Choose one or more people who will check in with you and who will support and encourage you along the way. Consider making this process a family affair as well. Whether you share your progress with your spouse, children, or other relatives, make sure those closest to you understand and appreciate that you've set a new goal for yourself and give you the time and space needed to accomplish it.

5 **Plan ahead to make time** Develop a schedule that allows for time to follow the program. Think of it the same way you think of your other important appointments, and make sure the people in your life understand and support the program. Whether it's scheduling "me time" on your calendar or instituting a "daddy-cooks-dinner night," developing a new schedule that builds in time for *you* will help you reach your goals and let everyone share in that success.

6 **Focus on the horizon** As you go through the plan—even as early as the second day on it—look back at how far you've come, not ahead at how much you still have left to do. Scientists call this the horizon effect. It creates encouragement ("I've done twice as much as a week ago!") and builds determination ("I've made it this far; I might as well keep going"). At the end of each week, take a moment to reflect on what you've accomplished, and use your success as the basis for ongoing inspiration.

7 **Stay positive** You'll do the best you can, but at some point you may mess up. And not just once. Don't feel guilty or ashamed (you're human!). Remember, making small changes consistently over time is the key to achieving and maintaining a younger you. Congratulate yourself for all that you have done already, and get back on the proverbial horse as soon as possible.

Simply setting out to learn how you can age beautifully and live longer is a step in the right direction, and when you see how far your age-erasing efforts go, we think you're going to want to stay on the path. Most of all, we think you'll be amazed at how much the rejuvenation of your body and mind reinvigorates your spirit. There's no better way to achieve a youthful zest for life than taking the time to pursue good health and happiness.

Want to be a test panelist for a future 7 Years Younger plan? Sign up today at 7yearsyounger.com/panelist to be considered—and get our free weekly e-newsletter, Your Anti-Aging Tip Sheet!

Meet the 7 Years Younger Team

All Good Housekeeping projects, from magazine articles and apps to books and television shows, are collaborative. That way we get to draw on the expertise of all our magazine editors and the Good Housekeeping Research Institute directors, who evaluate more than 2,000 products annually, to bring you the most concise, up-to-date advice and information. Here's the 7 *Years Younger* squad:

Birnur K. Aral, Ph.D.
Health, Beauty & Environmental Sciences Director, GHRI

Any product put to the test by Birnur and her team is in for a serious top-to-bottom analysis. That means the winners of the Anti-Aging Awards and other GHRI-sanctioned products mentioned throughout this book—74

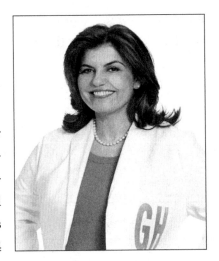

in all—are worthy of your hard-earned dollars. As leader of a group of scientists, Birnur, a chemical engineer, heads a lab filled with state-of-the-art machines like the Visia Complexion Analyzer, which counts wrinkles and detects UV damage, and the Instron, which tests hair strength. She also helps manage our volunteer testers, answers queries about formulations, and evaluates all the products for safety and potential efficacy before we test them.

Samantha B. Cassetty, M.S., R.D.

Nutrition Director, GHRI

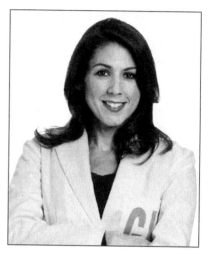

It's one thing to know which foods have the most antioxidants coupled with the fewest calories, but quite another to piece them all together into eight weeks of menus. Good thing we had Sam on the job. She not only developed the weight-loss plan for this book, but was our go-to expert on all the nutrition news and facts in Chapter Four. Sam was always on hand to answer our panelists' questions on specific foods and to help troubleshoot issues with the diet—how to make it work better, choose smart substitutions, and stave off hunger. Having her available to answer questions was, for the panelists, like having a personal nutritionist (and a cheerleader) on call.

Sam's nutrition and diet expertise is behind *Good Housekeeping*'s monthly *Nutrition News* and *Drop 5 lbs* columns as well as in all of GH's weight-loss plans. She has also shared her doable tips on Cooking Channel's *Drop 5 lbs with Good Housekeeping* show.

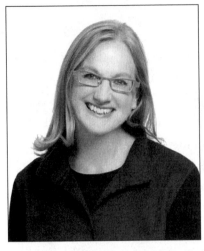

Jennifer Cook

Executive Editor,
Good Housekeeping

Jenny was involved with this project from the get-go, helping to formulate the concept and then bringing it to fruition. She also helped select our panel of testers, organized the 7 Years Younger Kickoff, and worked with the panelists as they navigated both the Jumpstart and 7-Week plans. During the writing and editing of the book, every title, every turn of phrase, and every punctuation mark was parsed by Jenny's watchful eye. Phew! There's a reason that she meditates as often as possible.

Jenny's anti-aging expertise predates *7 Years Younger.* She conceived of the Anti-Aging Awards and worked closely with the Good Housekeeping Research Institute as it investigated the products' youth-enhancing powers. She also has considerable knowledge about wellness and exercise, having been a top editor at several health magazines and co-author of a fitness book with exercise scientist Michael Wolf.

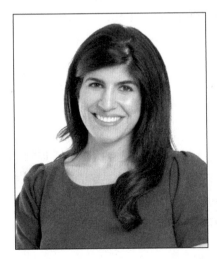

Nina Judar

Beauty Director,
Good Housekeeping

How do you use an eye primer? What hair color best complements fair skin? Is it OK to use more than one product with retinol? Any time our panelists had a beauty-related question, Nina had the answer. As *Good*

Housekeeping's Beauty Director, not only does Nina have an expansive knowledge of skin and hair care as well as makeup, but her electronic address book features the best dermatologists, makeup artists, hairstylists, and cosmetic scientists in the business. Her wide network of contacts allowed us to pack this book with great insider tips and up-to-the-minute anti-aging beauty news. Nina worked closely with GHRI on the Anti-Aging Awards for hair, so she understands which products do the job (and which don't).

Susan Westmoreland
Food Director, GHRI

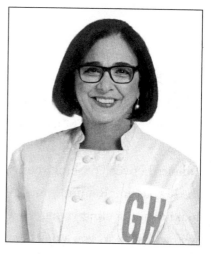

Recipes can't just *sound* healthy and delicious: To fit the 7 Years Younger standard they must also work and be reasonably simple to make. Susan and her team in the Good Housekeeping Test Kitchens tested all of the dinner recipes that appear in this book, tweaking them to ensure maximum flavor and minimum fuss—and every recipe passed the Triple-Test Promise, meaning that each one was tested at least three times to guarantee that it would work in anyone's home. She also helps develop special issues and our extensive line of cookbooks, and oversees a line of all-natural pantry products. If Susan's name is familiar, it may be because you've seen her on television—she appears regularly on Food Network and Cooking Channel and on shows like *Today* and *Good Morning America*—or heard her on radio shows like NPR's *All Things Considered*. Susan also has a video blog, *Susan to the Rescue*, and contributes regularly to the *In the Test Kitchen* blog on the *Good Housekeeping* website.

Your 7 Years Younger Pledge

There's no right or wrong way to write this pledge. In fact, your 7 Years Younger pledge should be personal, representing exactly what matters to you. The pledge may help you find a balance between pushing yourself and setting realistic goals. Think about the big picture: Remind yourself of all the ways that your ultimate goal—looking and feeling younger—will enhance your life. Also think about who will support you along the way, and perhaps even include a commitment to ask for help in your pledge. Before you boot up your computer (or pull out pen and paper), take a look at the sample pledge on the opposite page to give you ideas you can use when creating your own contract with yourself. (You can also turn to the color insert to read the pledges that our test panelists created for their 7 Years Younger journeys.) When you're finished, place your pledge where you'll be sure to see it—on your bathroom mirror, on your refrigerator door, or inside your journal.

Set aside at least 15 minutes to write your 7 Years Younger pledge. Be thoughtful, feel free to have fun and be creative, and remember to make it your own! It can be a motivating tool to remind you why you are taking this journey, especially when you slip up or feel tempted to quit. It's not set in stone; you can revise it as you go along through the upcoming eight weeks of the program and check it at the end to see how much you've accomplished.

Here's an example to get you started:

7 YEARS YOUNGER PLEDGE

I dedicate the next eight weeks to following the 7 Years Younger program.

My goal is to look and feel the very best that I possibly can.

I will invest the time and energy needed to follow the program.

I know that there will be challenging moments along the way, but with each new day I have another chance to continue the transformation that I have promised myself.

I will look to my family and friends to support me during these eight weeks and beyond, and I will support others making the same journey.

I am grateful for this opportunity to improve myself and to bring lasting, positive changes into my life.

_____ Day of _____ 20 _____

_____

(Signature)

Now, as you start your anti-aging program, is a great time to get even more expert advice and ongoing support. Sign up for our free weekly e-newsletter, Your Anti-Aging Tip Sheet, at 7yearsyounger.com/newsletter, and join us at facebook.com/7yearsyounger.

Age Eraser

1

Reclaim Your Beautiful Skin

A ppreciate how utterly alive skin is, and you'll have grasped the fundamental principle that allows you to turn back the clock on your complexion. As a living, breathing organ, your skin—like your heart or your lungs—is in a constant state of flux: dividing into new cells, repairing damaged cells, discarding old cells, and responding to changes in its internal and external environment 24/7. This natural repair and renewal system ensures that fresh skin cells are continually pushed to the surface, old ones sloughed off. And the cells responsible for structural support are constantly stimulated, keeping your skin fresh, intact, and resilient. The multistep nature of this cellular assembly line gives you plenty of opportunity to intervene at one, several, or all points during the process to create healthier, younger-looking skin.

You have more control over aging than you may think—and the time to take action is *now*. Surprisingly, genes have less to do with your skin's appearance through the years than your lifestyle. Lines, wrinkles, spots, uneven tone, and other signs of aging are primarily determined by factors like sun exposure, stress, a poor diet, and smoking. And if you have any doubt about the nature-nurture balance, consider this twin study conducted by researchers at Case Western Reserve University. Although each pair among the 186 identical twins assessed was genetically programmed to age at the same rate, some of the women might have been taken for their twin's older sister (ouch!). Based on professional ratings of photos of the subjects, the researchers calculated the following aging effects:

- **Smoking**—adds 2.5 years for every decade you puff.
- **Sun exposure (an extra 30 hours per week)**—makes you look 2 years older by age 40 and 3.5 years older by 70.
- **Stress**—divorce tacks on 1.7 years; being widowed, 2 years.

Most experts agree that one of the main reasons lifestyle factors can accelerate skin aging is that they create an abundance of free radicals. These unstable molecules damage cells, weakening their ability to repair themselves, and destroy skin's support fibers, collagen and elastin. Eventually, this excess injury takes its toll and shows up as skin aging. But as you'll see in this chapter, by fine-tuning your daily habits, lifestyle choices, and skin-care product selection as well as your body's internal and external environments, you can improve the appearance, feel, and health of your skin and look years younger than your actual age.

TOP 7 STRATEGIES FOR YOUNGER-LOOKING SKIN

Youth Booster #1: Develop Your Natural Dewiness

Your skin's appearance is a barometer of how hydrated your body is. Poor dietary choices, low water intake, stress, lack of sleep, sun exposure, and even slipshod daily care can all drain skin of its natural moisture content, making it look dull and feel rough. Here's how to balance your skin's hydration equation.

Achieve It By: Drinking Enough Water

Water inside cells is the medium in which every single chemical reaction occurs in your body. Keeping the right balance of internal H_2O levels means that vital repair and renewal processes proceed without a hitch, keeping skin looking plump and luscious. Internal hydration levels particularly affect the outermost layer of skin, the epidermis: Since skin has no blood vessels, it must rely on the underlying layers of the dermis to supply vital moisture. There's no specific rule for the amount of water to drink every day. Just be sure you're never thirsty. Nutritionists note that you can also "eat" water in the form of juicy fruits and vegetables.

Achieve It With: Regular Exfoliation

Twice a week, exfoliate your face first thing in the morning. (For "Your Younger-Skin Upkeep Schedule," see box, page 28.) A clean sweep for skin helps you face the day looking younger and dewier. During sleep, the rate of skin turnover slows, allowing old, dead cells to build up on the surface and leaving skin feeling rough and dry. But this is no simple cosmetic fix. Exfoliating not only removes dead cells, it encourages skin to increase production of new, healthy cells.

Your exfoliation options:

- **A scrub** These products contain a gentle physical exfoliating agent, such as jojoba beads. Avoid abrasive, rough-edged grains or granules like apricot kernels or walnut shells; these can cause micro tears in your skin, which up the odds of redness, irritation, and roughness.

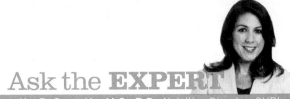

Ask the **EXPERT**

Samantha B. Cassetty, M.S., R.D., Nutrition Director, GHRI

Q *Does one piece of fruit equal a glass of water? And do coffee and tea count?*

Sam says: All three—fruit, coffee, and tea—count toward your fluid requirements, but the amount of fluid you get from each varies. Depending on the fruit, you'll get anywhere from one ounce (for an apricot) to five ounces (for a cup of pineapple, strawberries, or watermelon). Since coffee and tea both contain caffeine, which is a diuretic, you'll get less fluid from them. But don't get bogged down in the numbers. A scientific panel found that most of us do a good job of meeting our fluid needs by drinking with meals and when we're thirsty. Enjoying plenty of anti-aging produce—as outlined in our meal plan—will also go a long way toward helping you (and your skin) stay hydrated.

- **A brush** A natural-bristle brush can help you nudge away dead-cell buildup. If bristles don't appeal, try an electric-powered cleansing device, available at most drugstores. The brush heads rotate (as well as oscillate on some models), dislodging dirt from pores and sweeping away dead skin.
- **An exfoliating cleanser** Choose either a physical exfoliator, with scrubbing beads that let you remove dead cells and sebum (the waxy oil produced by the skin) with a little muscle, or a

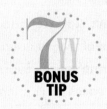

BONUS TIP

If you're using a retinol product (see page 41), forgo exfoliators with acids, since multiple sensitizing ingredients can be hard on facial skin.

chemical exfoliator, which works by dissolving the bonds between dead surface cells. The chemical exfoliating ingredients that many dermatologists recommend are salicylic and glycolic acids.

Achieve It With: Twice-Daily Cleansing

Wash your face with a skin-smoothing cleanser in the morning. Wonder how much anti-aging benefit you can get from something that spends so little time on skin? "Cleansers are yet another way to deliver active ingredients," explains Washington, DC, dermatologist Tina Alster, M.D. To defend against dryness, choose a creamy, non-foaming, hydrating formula. Repeat at night to rid skin of any dirt, sebum, or makeup that has accumulated during the day. Clean skin is more receptive to anti-aging ingredients.

Achieve It By: Minding Your Moisturizer, Day and Night

Smoothing on a moisturizer after cleansing makes skin look and feel good. These products are formulated to attract water and keep it in the top layers of your skin, creating a dewier look. For day use, choose a moisturizer that has anti-aging ingredients (see "Your Younger-Looking Skin Repair Kit," page 58), and if you like, one that also has a sunscreen. Look for a product with a sun-protection factor (SPF) of 15 or above. If you opt for a moisturizer that doesn't contain a sunscreen, apply a regular sunscreen first, then your moisturizer. At night, choose a moisturizing anti-aging night cream either with retinol or with collagen-building peptides. Nighttime is also a good time to apply a serum, a concentrated special-effects treatment product that contains a blend of vitamins, peptides, antioxidants, and/or botanicals. You'll find formulas for specific areas, such as eyes, or conditions, such as fine lines, wrinkles, and sagging skin.

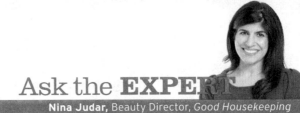

Ask the EXPERT

Nina Judar, Beauty Director, *Good Housekeeping*

Q *I've never exfoliated before. Can you give me some tips on getting started?*

Nina says: As you get older, dead cells stick together and stay on skin longer than they did when you were 20. Sloughing off this dead layer is a quick way to turn back the clock. There are lots of ways to accomplish this, which means you're sure to find one that works with your lifestyle. One method we don't recommend: using a washcloth. It exfoliates unevenly, and a damp cloth can gather bacteria, which you wouldn't want to put on your face. If you're concerned about sensitivity, start slowly and see how your skin reacts. You may want to try a new product at night on the off chance that your skin has a reaction; any redness or irritation should subside by morning.

Achieve It By: Trying Fruit Acids

Alpha hydroxy acids (AHAs) are fruit acids derived from edibles like grapes, apples, oranges, milk, and cane sugar. These gentle acids dissolve clumps of dead cells, clearing them away. Some researchers also speculate that AHAs may stimulate collagen production. The bottom line: AHAs make skin more luminous. On an ingredients list, look for glycolic, lactic, citric, malic, or tartaric acid. There are a variety of ways to work an AHA product into your routine; pick one of the following:

- **Try an AHA cleanser** A cleanser that contains a cell-sloughing AHA lets you exfoliate and cleanse at the same time.
- **Use a moisturizer with an AHA** This double-duty product locks moisture into skin while also whisking away dead cells. Glycolic acid is one of the most popular AHAs found in moisturizers; most over-the-counter products have between 5 and 10 percent. While these concentrations are suitable for most people, take care not

to over-exfoliate. It you mix and match too many AHA products—say, an acid-based cleanser and AHA moisturizer in the morning and an exfoliating cream at night—you run the risk of inflaming your skin. A gentler option than glycolic acid is lactic acid, which is also a moisturizer.

- **Test-drive an at-home peel** Do-it-yourself peels improve radiance and smoothness. "It's one of the best ways to see a quick difference," says Miami-based dermatologist Leslie Baumann, M.D. When you slough those dead cells with a peel, it enhances the functioning of your skin, and active ingredients in your skin care—like antioxidants and retinoids—penetrate better.

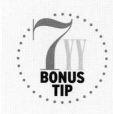

BONUS TIP If you give yourself an at-home peel, be extra cautious about sun exposure afterward. **AHAs may leave skin extra sensitive to sunlight.** Also avoid using either exfoliators (such as scrubs) or retinol products until a week after you finish treatment.

Youth Booster #2: Even Out Complexion Color

Evenness of tone is the hallmark of youthful skin. Although your tanning days may be long past, incidental UV exposure (running out to get the mail, walking from the car to your office) etches itself on your skin. "Unfortunately, sun damage on your face and body begins to show up as brown spots, redness, blotchiness, or even sallowness as early as in your 30s," says David Bank, M.D., a dermatologist in Mount Kisco, NY. Here's how to roll back the years.

Achieve It By: Wearing Sunscreen Daily

Sun exposure, no surprise, is the top culprit behind uneven skin tone, no matter what your ethnic background. Over time, UV rays thin the skin

Your Younger-Skin Upkeep Schedule

This easy daily routine involves just a few steps: weekly exfoliation, cleansing, moisturization, and protection. It's called a routine for a reason: Consistent care is what makes the difference between so-so and sensational skin. Nothing takes more than a few minutes, but the gains—younger-looking skin now and fewer wrinkles and lines in the future—will be considerable.

In the morning:

1. **Twice a week, exfoliate to wake up skin,** using your choice of a scrub, a brush, or an exfoliating cleanser.
2. **Cleanse your skin with an anti-aging formula;** think of it as another dose of rejuvenating goodies for your face.
3. **Moisturize to plump the outer layer of cells,** so skin looks firmer, dewier, and more luminous. Choose an anti-aging formula or one that contains sunscreen. If you opt for a moisturizer that doesn't have a sunscreen, apply a regular sunscreen first, then your moisturizer.
4. **Protect** Smooth on sunscreen if your moisturizer doesn't contain one. Another time to apply sunscreen solo: if you're headed for all-day sun exposure. (See "Sunscreen Smarts," page 33.)

In the evening:

1. **Cleanse** to wash off the day's accumulation of oil, dirt, sunscreen, and makeup.
2. **Treat** Put all that downtime in bed to work for your face. Apply a serum (see "Achieve It By: Using Nighttime Treatments," page 30) and follow up with a moisturizing night cream.

and dilate superficial blood vessels. UV exposure throws dark-pigment-producing melanocyte cells into overdrive, and the melanin they produce can cluster into brown spots, creating a mottled or pebbled appearance in Caucasian and Asian complexions. In Hispanic, African-American, and

East Asian skin, the opposite is the case: More baseline melanin protects against superficial sun damage, but may give rise to light spots or blotchiness. No matter what your skin type, use sunscreen on a daily basis—it protects cells from additional damage while giving skin a chance to make visible repairs on previously damaged cells.

Just like brushing your teeth, applying sunscreen every morning should be an automatic habit, even when you won't be outside much. UVA rays can penetrate windshield and window glass and can beam through clouds and fog. If you prefer wearing a moisturizer with sunscreen, scrutinize the ingredients before you buy (see "Sunscreen Smarts," page 33): A recent analysis of 29 top-selling SPF moisturizers at Memorial Sloan-Kettering Cancer Center in Basking Ridge, NJ, revealed that six of them—including the most expensive, at $64 an ounce—had no UVA filters at all. Six had acceptable levels, and the others contained some filters, but not in adequate doses or effective combinations.

Whether you choose a facial moisturizer with SPF or a regular sunscreen, make it your first layer of the day. When the sun-protection factor of any product is determined, it's tested by application of the product directly to the skin, not over other skin-care

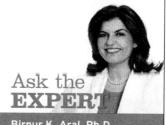

Ask the EXPERT

Birnur K. Aral, Ph.D.
Health, Beauty & Environmental Sciences Director, GHRI

Q *You are recommending lots of anti-aging ingredients. Is it OK to combine so many on my skin?*

Birnur says: Certain top-notch anti-agers, such as retinoids and alpha hydroxy acids (AHAs), can increase skin sensitivity. To minimize the risk of irritation, try introducing one such product into your routine for a period of weeks to see how your skin adjusts. If there's no sign of sensitivity, you can add another. However, if your skin reacts with redness, flaking, or irritation, dial back. Sometimes using a product only every second or third night can solve the problem. Or you can opt to use less sensitizing anti-agers, like peptides.

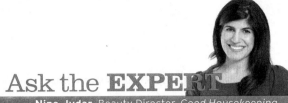

Ask the **EXPERT**

Nina Judar, Beauty Director, *Good Housekeeping*

Q *I'm confused about what should go on first, second, etc. Do you have any general tips about layering skin-care products so I know they'll work?*

Nina says: In general, you should put on the lighter layers first—serum, then moisturizer, because a serum won't be able to penetrate through the thicker moisturizer. One way to keep things simple is to use fewer products. In the morning, use a moisturizer with SPF; if you'd like to step it up, first apply a serum with antioxidants and then put on the moisturizer. At night, after cleansing, apply a night cream or nighttime treatment (see below). Again, if you'd like to step it up, first use a serum. You can add an eye cream at night, if needed.

products and makeup. "The most common mistake I see among my patients is putting on moisturizer before sunscreen," says New York City dermatologist Neal Schultz, M.D. The only exception: If you're using an antioxidant serum for daytime use, smooth on the serum first, then sunscreen.

Achieve It By: Addressing Redness

You see patchy splotches in the mirror, but do you know what causes them? Consult your dermatologist to pinpoint the culprit. Certain dermatologic conditions, such as rosacea, seborrheic dermatitis, psoriasis, and atopic dermatitis, can cause facial redness in lighter skin. In more pigmented complexions, redness actually appears as darker spots. Topical treatments and even laser treatments can help diminish redness and dark spots.

Achieve It By: Using Nighttime Treatments

Doctors recommend treating skin in the evening, when it's free of sun-protection products and treatments can be in contact with your skin for an uninterrupted block of time.

- **Smooth on a serum** These concentrated blends of vitamins, peptides, antioxidants, and botanicals are formulated to avert or minimize uneven tone as well as fine lines, wrinkles, and sagging skin.
- **Restore evenness with retinol creams** Follow the serum with a light application of a retinol night cream, which speeds cell renewal and skin-tone evening. (For more on retinols, see page 41.)

Achieve It By: Fading Age Spots

The most effective skin lightener is hydroquinone, which has long been used to bleach age spots or dark spots. Hydroquinone can be found at up to 2 percent concentrations in over-the-counter products; higher concentrations are usually in prescription creams. There has been some concern over links between hydroquinone and cancer, but the American Academy of Dermatology holds that levels of up to 4 percent are safe. Dermatologists recommend that you spot treat with hydroquinone products, applying them only to dark areas and discontinuing use once those areas lighten. Dabbed on daily, hydroquinone products could take four to eight months to fade spots, and sometimes up to a year. Using a bleaching cream together with a glycolic acid exfoliator can help speed up the sloughing of pigmented cells. Make sure to use sunscreen daily, too, so spots don't return. There are also other cosmetic ways to treat spots. Products containing retinol, niacinamide, kojic acid, and glucosamine may also lighten (but not completely eliminate) dark spots.

Achieve It By: Lightening Up Via Laser

If you're willing to pay more, doctor's-office laser or intense pulsed light (IPL) treatments can give you a faster result than a cream. It takes just seconds to break up melanin on individual spots with the Nd:YAG laser. (A scab may form, but should fall off within a few days.) For larger patches of pigmentation, fractional lasers (Fraxel; there are three levels, from least to most skin-renewing) have begun replacing IPL treatments

Who Should Handle Your Skin Care?

Skin-care procedures are best done in the office of a **board-certified dermatologist** (board certification verifies that a doctor has had special training). Some treatments may be administered by a nurse, but make sure the doctor does the initial consultation and oversees the procedure. To find a board-certified dermatologist in your area, log on to the American Academy of Dermatology's website at aad.org/findaderm.

as derms' go-to treatments. Both will even out skin tone—and smooth wrinkles!—but lasers direct more heat, yielding dramatic clearing in three or four sessions versus IPL's six, says Ariel Ostad, M.D., a dermatologist in New York City. The catch: Fraxel:Restore, the type that's right for the job, leaves skin red for a few days, while IPL is a true "lunchtime" procedure. Costs can range from $300 to $500 for one IPL treatment to $750 to $2,500 for one Fraxel treatment.

Achieve It By: Opting for an In-Office Peel Treatment

Talk to your dermatologist about an in-office peel. Peels reduce skin discoloration, freckles, and age spots as well as other agers. Lighter peels— ones that only penetrate the outer layer of the skin—are generally alpha hydroxy acid solutions, but many dermatologists also offer peels that reach into the deeper layers of the skin to remove damaged cells. Peels of all varieties require some commitment (including financial: $100 to $300 for a light one, and up to $1,000 for the deepest) on your part. Your skin will be only slightly red after a light peel (called a "lunchtime peel," not only because it takes 30 minutes to an hour but also because you can return to work afterward). Deeper peels require healing time and necessitate follow-up visits.

Sunscreen Smarts

Short of staying out of the sun completely, you can save your skin from UV damage by wearing sunglasses plus UV-ray-deflecting clothes and a hat, avoiding peak hours of intensity (10 A.M. to 4 P.M.), and seeking shade whenever possible, even if you're just waiting for the streetlight to change. (Did you know that walking on the shady side of the street can reduce your UV exposure by 30 percent? It pays to cross the street!) Whenever you go outside and wherever your skin is exposed, slather on the sunscreen.

Here's what you need to know to get the best protection from a sunscreen:

Look for "broad spectrum"

You need a sunscreen that guards against both UVA *and* UVB rays. Sunlight emits up to 95 percent UVA rays (those that cause wrinkles, spots, and skin cancer) and around 5 percent UVB rays (the more energetic ones that cause sunburn and can also contribute to skin cancer). You'll know you're covered on both fronts if the label says "broad-spectrum SPF" followed by a number that's 15 or higher. (Under new FDA rules, products that lack adequate UVA protection are now required to carry a warning.)

Choose a high SPF

The SPF number on sunscreens is a lab measure of the time it takes skin to burn when exposed to UVB light. With an SPF of 15, for example, your skin takes 15 times longer to redden versus unprotected skin. Most dermatologists suggest using an SPF of 30.

Higher is not necessarily better. "SPFs higher than 30 don't offer that much more protection," emphasizes Santa Monica, CA, dermatologist Ava Shamban, M.D. An SPF of 30 absorbs about 97 percent of UVB rays, but an SPF 45 is only about one percentage point better. Still, you should probably go for a higher SPF if you have very fair skin or have already had skin cancer.

Julie Ann Raab
"Lightening my dark circles and spots was like an instant age makeover!"

"Julie Ann Raab, 40, already took very good care of her skin when she started the 7 Years Younger program. But she still had a lot of recalcitrant dark spots from sun exposure and hoped that a new routine might help. When Julie Ann tried the GHRI-approved anti-aging products, she could see the difference immediately. "I had no trouble adjusting to the new products, and after the first two weeks my skin looked noticeably better," she says. The skin-care program was eye-opening in another way, too. "I learned that you don't necessarily have to spend a lot of money on skin-care products to get good, noticeable results," she says. "Some of the drugstore products worked the best."

A cut above The younger, more layered haircut Julie Ann got at the end of the program looked terrific. She booked a session with her

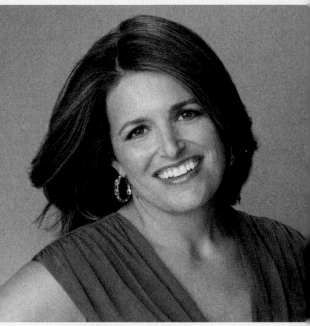

Pounds shed
1

Body-fat decrease
3%

Total inches lost
2.5

Skin's overall appearance: dark circles looked lighter; Visia* score— pores improved by 13%, skin discolorations were reduced by 7%, and texture improved by 45%

regular stylist, who taught her how to handle the layers. Julie Ann's color change was also a great success. "My hair had gotten brassier over the last few years," she says. "The colorist toned that down and warmed it up with highlights. This is a look I'm going to keep." Her new color also helped balance her complexion.

Working in more workouts Since she's an avid tennis player who hits the courts about four times a week, Julie Ann was already very fit when she started the program. Even so, she realized she needed to do more cardiovascular workouts (tennis is a stop-and-start game, so it doesn't strengthen your heart in the same way continuous aerobic exercise does). She also needed to work on her core strength, which not only flattened her belly but also improved her game. Julie Ann loved the band exercises, and the changes, she says, "have helped my body look and feel more balanced."

Personalized pound paring Julie Ann worked in 7 Years Younger menu suggestions when she could—"I already cook separate meals for my kids," says the mother of two, "so it was hard for me to have the bandwidth to follow new recipes." Her solution was to tweak her usual diet to fit the calorie and nutrition guidelines GHRI nutritionist Sam Cassetty outlined. Julie Ann's weight loss put her on the path. "I'm committed to continuing to work on it," she says.

For more about Julie Ann Raab, see color insert.

Want to be a test panelist for a future 7 Years Younger plan? Sign up today at 7yearsyounger.com/panelist to be considered—and get our free weekly e-newsletter, Your Anti-Aging Tip Sheet!

* The Visia Complexion Analyzer electronically counts wrinkles and age spots, examines skin's texture, and exposes UV damage before it appears on skin's surface.

Match Your Sunscreen to You

The best sunscreen is one you'll actually wear. Find a formula that fits your life and lifestyle. If it's too heavy, drippy, gummy, smelly, or expensive, you're not going to want to put it on. Also important: Pick a product that works with, not against, your skin type. Here's how to purchase the one that's just right for you.

If your skin is...	LOOK FOR
Sensitive	A brand that's labeled hypoallergenic and fragrance-free. Scan the ingredients list for titanium dioxide and zinc oxide—these minerals are less sensitizing and deflect both UVA and UVB rays. "In general, zinc is better for everyday wear because it's lighter and won't show through makeup. Titanium has stronger photo protection for beach days," says Zoe Diana Draelos, M.D., a dermatologist in High Point, NC. However, these physical blockers are strongest when paired up.
Acne-prone	A light, oil-free lotion. Ingredients to avoid: physical sunblocks, such as zinc oxide or titanium dioxide. These can be too heavy and sticky for your skin type, and may exacerbate breakouts. Instead, look for lighter, chemical sunscreens such as avobenzone and oxybenzone.
Dry	A lotion or cream formula that contains added hydrating ingredients like glycerin and aloe. Avoid sprays and gels laden with alcohol; you'll feel their drying effects with repeated use.
Oily	Avoid products containing mineral oil; these will only add more shine to your skin.

Pick protective ingredients

Scan the "active ingredients" section of the label to see what's actually doing the protecting. Top picks: physical sunblocks, titanium dioxide and zinc oxide (they sit on top of skin and physically deflect UV rays; look for 5 percent zinc oxide), as well as the chemical sunscreens avobenzone (a.k.a. Parsol 1789—ideally, more than 2 percent) and octocrylene (more than 3.6 percent) or another chemical sunscreen called ecamsule (brand name Mexoryl).

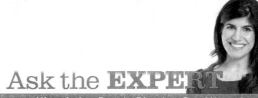

Ask the **EXPERT**

Nina Judar, Beauty Director, *Good Housekeeping*

Q *If I go out for a walk in the middle of the day, should I apply sunscreen over my makeup?*

Nina says: If you're going for a stroll on an overcast day, your morning moisturizer with SPF 15 or higher will provide enough skin protection. However, if it's sunny and you're going for a hardcore workout walk (there will be sweat!), you'll want to apply a sunscreen with an SPF of at least 30 that has some water (and sweat) resistance. Check skincancer .org for a list of sunscreens the organization recommends for "active" use. Ideally, you'd apply these directly to clean skin. And if you are going to be sweating, it's best if you don't have makeup on. But it's preferable to apply extra sunscreen over makeup than to not use it at all; look for one with a physical ingredient like titanium dioxide or zinc oxide that doesn't need to be absorbed into skin to be effective.

Apply it properly

A sunscreen is only as good as its application, and research shows that skimping is virtually the norm: Most of us apply only 25 to 50 percent of the recommended amount. Half the proper amount of sunscreen equals half the skin protection.

- **Put on enough** An ounce (a shot glass–full) of sunscreen is the recommendation for full-body coverage from the American Academy of Dermatology. Devote at least a teaspoon of that ounce to your face, ears, and neck. For non-lotion sunscreens such as spray-ons and mists, apply enough to give skin an even sheen. Use a heavy hand with wipes, brush-on powders, and sunscreen sticks, too.
- **Plan ahead** Apply sunscreen at least 15 or, ideally, 30 minutes before you head outdoors, so your skin has a chance to absorb

the protective ingredients. Apply sunscreen before you get dressed for the most complete coverage.

- **Reapply regularly** Renew your sunscreen every two hours, or after every sweaty sporting activity or water submersion. Under the new FDA rules, sunscreens can no longer be called waterproof (since they eventually wash off); however, they can be called water-resistant. How long they resist water must now be clearly stated on their labels. "Water resistant (80 minutes)" protects you through four 20-minute swims, with drying time between each. For a quick dip, a 40-minute lotion is OK (and less sticky).

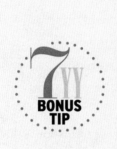

BONUS TIP

Don't forget your lips. They don't tan like the rest of your skin, so they're **defenseless against the sun.** Plus, you actually *increase* light penetration through the lip surface by applying something clear and shiny, says Christine Brown, M.D., a dermatologist at Baylor University Medical Center at Dallas. That can increase your risk of skin cancer, and cancer on the lower lip can be particularly aggressive. **Instead of gloss, opt for a lip balm with SPF 30** and apply it before putting on your lipstick. Reapply throughout the day.

Youth Booster #3: Radiate a Healthy Glow

Recapturing a youthful luminosity is easier than you think. Take these steps to get your glow going.

Achieve It With: Regular Exfoliation

This skin-care move translates into near-immediate gratification. Simply by removing the accumulations of dead cells via exfoliation (see exfoliation basics, page 23), your skin will look brighter, smoother, healthier, and (need we add?) younger.

Achieve It By: Ditching Known Skin Dullers

Your skin is a reflection of what you eat and drink, both good and bad. So if you want to improve the look of your skin, take a look at what you consume on a daily basis. First, count the cups of coffee (or caffeinated soft drinks). Too much caffeine can be dehydrating, dulling skin. Instead, drink green tea. Although it contains caffeine (in smaller amounts), it also has polyphenols, plant nutrients that are anti-inflammatory. "Regular consumption—two to three cups a day—will result in better skin texture and inhibit wrinkling," says Santosh K. Katiyar, Ph.D., a professor of dermatology at the University of Alabama at Birmingham. The polyphenols in green tea also help sun-exposed cells repair themselves more rapidly.

A diet full of refined carbohydrates (white sugar, white flour, white pasta) can also dull skin. It turns out that these carbs disturb the body's insulin-glucose levels, leading to an accumulation of advanced glycation end products (AGEs), which impair the skin's normal repair of collagen and elastin.

Achieve It With: Daily Sunscreen Use

Sun damage results in a dull, discolored complexion. By applying sunscreen daily, you'll protect against this aging aftereffect of UV radiation. Remember, sun damage is cumulative—your skin is storing the damage from all those times you dashed out without sunscreen. The harmful results can take anywhere from five to 20-plus years to surface on the skin, depending on how fair or dark your skin is and the extent of your sun exposure, so start using sunscreen today for your skin's future.

Achieve It By: Eating Your Antioxidants

Good-for-you foods give skin the nutrients it needs to look and stay healthy. Take antioxidants, for example. Think of them as an active ingredient in most colorful fruits and vegetables. Antioxidants fight free radicals, which can dull skin and pummel collagen, leading to visible signs of aging. (Check out "The Younger-Skin Food Guide," page 61.)

Achieve It By: Self-Tanning

A sun-kissed glow without UV damage? That's the beauty of a self-tanner. You don't necessarily have to buy a face-specific formula; most body self-tanners work just as well on your face, so check the product instructions. (For more application tips, see "Sunless Tanning," page 50.) To prevent a horizontal line across the top of your forehead, rub the self-tanner up and down into your hairline—unless you're blonde: Tanners can alter blonde hair. Rub any residual self-tanner on your hands onto your ears and the back of your neck. If you have any dark spots on your face, finish by swiping them with a slightly damp cotton swab so they don't become darker.

Achieve It By: Eliminating Acne

Acne is the antithesis of a healthy glow, and it's surprisingly common. More than a quarter of 40-something women and 15 percent of those 50 and older report having had adult acne, according to a study in the *Journal of the American Academy of Dermatology*. East Asian skin is particularly prone to adult acne. To form, acne requires a perfect storm of clogged pores, bacteria, and inflammation. You'll get the best treatment results if you attack it on all fronts, says Audrey Kunin, M.D., a dermatologist in Kansas City, MO. A regimen to consider: Twice a day, unblock pores with a 1 to 2 percent salicylic acid cleanser, then kill bacteria and sop up oil with a 10 percent benzoyl peroxide spot treatment. And apply a sulfur mask a few times a week to draw out excess oil. Once skin calms down, maintain results by continuing to use a salicylic acid cleanser.

Adult acne can be persistent—and resistant to treatment. So if an at-home regimen doesn't clear up your skin within a few months, talk to a dermatologist about prescription retinoids (see below for more on retinoids). For breakouts seemingly immune to other therapies, oral antibiotics are another option. So is prescription Aldactone, which is typically used as a diuretic but has antitestosterone effects that prevent excess oil production.

Harnessing light to kill blemish-causing bacteria is another way some doctors treat acne, and there are now at-home devices that do the job, too. These handheld flashlight-like devices emit light from the blue spectrum to treat acne. Microorganisms inside bacteria absorb this light, which increases their energy, killing the bacteria, explains Dr. Draelos, consulting professor of dermatology at Duke University School of Medicine. The at-home devices are smaller, less powerful versions of the LED (light-emitting diode) machines doctors use to address inflamed-surface breakouts. But these gadgets must put out a sufficient amount of energy to work, so only those that have FDA clearance specifically for acne are worth the investment. Do-it-yourself treatments take about the same time as doctor's-office sessions (minus waiting-room and driving minutes). A dermatologist, however, can treat your entire face at once; the mini devices are better for smaller areas and must be used for several months for best results.

Youth Booster #4: Firm and Tighten Facial Skin

Over time, gravity eventually catches up with your skin. Add to that the slipping away of collagen, elastin, and fat, and your face (eyelids included) may look droopier. Here's how to turn back the clock.

Achieve It By: Adding a Retinoid to Your Routine

These tried-and-true skin repairers are derivatives of vitamin A and work by preventing collagen loss. They also signal skin to produce new collagen, helping to counteract the effects of gravity, and speed cell turnover, making skin tone more even. They help to heal and prevent acne, too, and can also reverse sun damage—although using a retinoid doesn't give you license to spend more time on the beach. In fact, retinoids make skin more sensitive to the sun, so when using one you have to be even more careful about UV exposure and all the more conscientious about using sunscreen.

Researchers at the University of Michigan Health System applied a 4 percent retinol solution on one arm of test subjects three times a week for 24 weeks. The other, untreated arm served as a control. Researchers attributed improvements to increased production of collagen and glycosaminoglycans (GAGs), gel-like substances that help the skin retain water. Retinoids not only fixed skin, they helped it function better and in a younger way.

You'll find retinoids in a variety of strengths and forms. The strongest are prescription-only creams, such as tretinoin (Retin-A), taxarotene, and adapalene. Retinoids also come in lower-strength, over-the-counter forms called retinol. Retinaldehyde, retinyl palmitate, and provitamin A are other retinoid variations you might see on an over-the-counter (OTC) label. Among them, retinol and retinaldehyde are the most effective wrinkle-fighters.

To renew your skin with retinoids:

- **Add a night cream with retinol to your arsenal** Start off using a retinol night cream two or three times a week in order to acclimate your skin to the ingredient, and apply a peptide-based night cream on your off nights. Retinols aren't as potent as prescription retinoids, but you should see some positive changes after a few months (stick with it!).
- **Ask your dermatologist for a sample** After a few months of trying OTC products, if you want more noticeable results, try out a

prescription retinoid. Take advantage of free samples. If you like what you see, your doctor can then give you a prescription and help you decide the best course of action. As with an OTC retinol, it's good to ease into prescription retinoid cream: Try a pea-size amount every second or third night. If your skin feels dry, smooth on a plain moisturizer (try CeraVe or Cetaphil) over the retinoid.

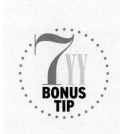

"Often when women try prescription Retin-A, their skin becomes so red and irritated that the tube is relegated to a bathroom drawer and never used again. **It's good to build up slowly,** over the course of a year or two, to Retin-A," explains dermatologist Karyn Grossman, M.D., who practices in Santa Monica, CA, and New York City.

Achieve It By: Getting a Lift from Topical Treatments

Some topical treatments can help in the short term by causing transient plumping of the skin. "Look for ingredients like hyaluronic acid, glycerin, or dimethicone," says Jeanine Downie, M.D., a dermatologist in Montclair, NJ. You can find them in moisturizers, masks, and wrinkle fillers. (See "Your Younger-Looking Skin Repair Kit," on page 58.)

Achieve It By: Looking Into High-Tech Heating

Ultrasound, radiofrequency, and laser treatments safely deliver heat deep into the skin to help shorten collagenous bands, tightening skin and giving it a lift. The technology is constantly improving; your doctor can fill you in on which treatment gives the best results. Note that these treatments are pricey and painful, but the results are visible and impressive.

Youth Booster #5: Smooth Your Skin's Surface

A smooth surface reflects light more evenly; lines (even expression lines), creases, and wrinkles disrupt that surface and create shadows, which can have an aging effect. Some smart steps to speed smoothness:

Achieve It By: Exfoliating Twice a Week

Give your skin a hand—literally. Regular exfoliation not only removes accumulated dead cells on the surface to smooth your skin, but stimulates deep-down layers to produce new, plumper cells and push them to the surface of your skin.

Achieve It By: Opting for Nighttime Treatments

Follow up your nighttime cleansing with a serum. For wrinkles, choose collagen-building ingredients like peptides and retinol or retinoic acid. These ingredients stimulate skin to produce new collagen, which can help smooth the surface of your skin.

Achieve It By: Trying Growth-Factor Products

Skin cells release growth factors, which signal cells to act—repair tissue, regenerate, stimulate protein production—in ways that make the skin look younger. There are more than 300 growth factors, but one in particular, transforming growth factor beta (TGF-beta for short), instructs cells to produce more collagen, helping to minimize wrinkles.

Dermatologists note that retinoids are still the most effective collagen-production stimulators, but lotions laced with TGF-beta are less drying and irritating to skin—plus, they don't require a prescription. And they seem to work. In a company-sponsored study, Citrix, maker of Citrix Cell Rejuvenation Serum 10% with Growth Factor, found that its product decreased wrinkles by an average of 22 percent in more than half the subjects after three months of twice-daily use. A growth-factor serum may be used as either an alternative or a complement to a regimen that includes retinoids.

How to get started with growth factors:

- **Smooth on a TGF-beta solution serum** Before you apply a moisturizer at night, try a product that features growth factors. If you use a prescription retinoid, alternate it with a TGF-beta solution. This approach might yield better or faster results, says Ronald Moy, M.D., a dermatologist in Beverly Hills, CA.

Achieve It By: Minimizing Pores

Pores don't really get bigger as you age, but they can look bigger as cell turnover lags and clinging cells draw the eye to the openings. In oily skin, excess sebum can also fill and stretch pores. Regular exfoliation is key to keeping pores clean. Although OTC products won't actually shrink pores, they may help them appear less noticeable. Try a serum or peel with salicylic acid—which chemically clears out dirt, oil, and cell buildup—and glycolic or lactic acid to slough and soften your skin's surface. Since it can take several weeks to see results from a pore-minimizing product, opt for a dermatologist-strength peel if you're in a hurry. One no-downtime glycolic acid treatment yields more even, toned skin, though you typically need several sessions with your doctor to see dramatic results.

Achieve It By: Trying OTC Fillers

Dozens of new nonprescription creams are claiming to mimic Botox, while others, housed in syringe-like dispensers, are billed as facial "fillers." While the benefits of these dermal doppelgängers don't come close to those of their injectable counterparts (see "Worth a Shot?", page 390), they may create some temporary superficial improvement, says Fredric Brandt, M.D., a dermatologist based in New York City and Miami.

How to finesse fillers:

- **Try a line "relaxer"** Ingredients like gamma-aminobutyric acid (GABA) and the peptide argireline have a cumulative, transient effect and may help modestly soften wrinkles for a youthful pick-me-up.
- **Give "fillers" a shot** Instant fillers are really just souped-up moisturizers, but they can smooth skin; those with hyaluronic acid bind water to skin so it looks plumper for the day. Another filler, dimethicone, is a form of silicone that sits on the surface of skin and literally fills in creases. Like makeup primers, these will help skin look and feel smoother and more youthful—temporarily.

Youth Booster #6: Improve Skin's Suppleness

The sign of suppleness: skin's ability to snap back when manipulated or pulled out of place. And that, in turn, is a measure of the health of your skin's collagen and elastin fibers. Here's how to make your skin more resistant to gravity.

Achieve It By: Shading Your Skin With Sunscreen

Use sunscreen every day, no matter what the weather. UV radiation penetrates clouds, so cover up even when it's overcast. If it's light enough to see, you're in the presence of UV. So, slather up.

Achieve It By: Upping Your Quota of Cosmetic Vitamin C

This free-radical quencher is one of the best-studied antioxidants. Research shows that C helps prevent water loss from the skin and plays a role in building collagen and elastin. Vitamin C has also been found to offer protection from both UVA and UVB rays when applied before sun exposure. These days many products, including sunscreens, contain C, but the vitamin can also be irritating to the skin. If your skin swells, try another formulation.

Achieve It By: Jumpstarting Collagen and Elastin Production

Your skin cells rely on a natural charge, called bioelectricity, to aid in healing and the production of collagen and elastin. You can stimulate this electrical repair system topically with products containing copper and zinc particles. Some serums now include these energized microparticles, which, when activated by a moisturizing component, appear to help speed up tissue renewal and collagen and elastin. Smoothing results are often visible within weeks, and are especially apparent around the eye because it's the thinnest skin on the face.

Achieve It By: Getting Enough Sleep

Long-standing fatigue causes cortisol, the stress hormone, to rise. "If cortisol is chronically high, it can age you by breaking down collagen in skin," says Amy Wechsler, M.D., dermatologist, psychiatrist, and author of *The Mind-Beauty Connection*. Just one nighttime sleep disruption can trigger the body's inflammation response and prompt your immune system to turn against healthy organs and tissue. It's no wonder that when you burn the midnight oil, your skin simply looks *blah*.

Achieve It By: Using Retinoids Routinely

Retinoids, in use since the 1980s, work by preventing collagen loss as well as helping the skin to produce new supportive collagen. (For more on these products, see page 41.)

Tessa Jean
"People told me I glowed!"

Tessa, our youngest tester, was thinking about looking and feeling 7 years younger—even though she's only 34 years old. "I was coming up on my 35th birthday and beginning to feel a little sluggish," she says. "Plus, I thought the program offered a great way to adopt some healthy habits that would help prolong my youthfulness. I'm a nurse, so I believe in prevention."

Lighter makeup dials back the years Tessa was happy to learn that she didn't have to layer on lots of makeup to achieve a youthful look. "Subtle has always been my thing when it comes to makeup," she says. But proper application of the right products is what makes a visible difference: She's now using a little foundation under her eyes, on the sides of her nose, and above her chin, then brushing a bronzer

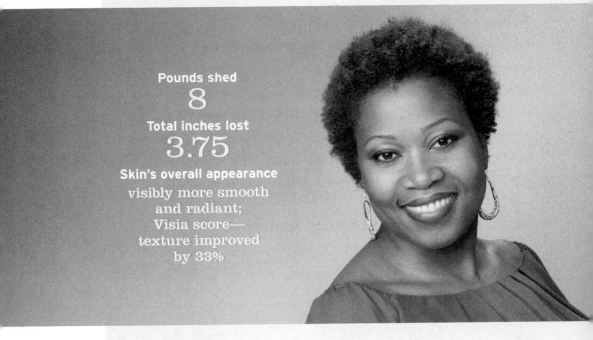

Pounds shed
8
Total inches lost
3.75
Skin's overall appearance
visibly more smooth
and radiant;
Visia score—
texture improved
by 33%

on the apples of her cheeks. And she dabs a light lip gloss on her mouth. "No more matte lipsticks," says Tessa. "I learned that they show the creases in your lips and make you look older."

Going deeper into deep conditioning For her very dry hair, Tessa found she needed more than just an off-the-shelf conditioner, so she created her own, made up of three different oils. She works them into her hair, puts on a shower cap, and lets the conditioners work in for 40 minutes. Then, after rinsing out and toweling dry, she applies a combination of coconut oil and shea butter for extra conditioning.

How she got her glow back Tessa was wildly happy about losing eight pounds on the program, but her biggest accomplishment, she says, was the change in her skin. Tessa diligently followed the 7 Years Younger skin-care recommendations morning and night. "People commented on how much I glowed," she says. "I was asked, 'Are you pregnant?' and 'Are you in love?' From my own perspective, I think my skin looks fresher, and I don't look as tired when I wake up."

Benefitting from her beauty sleep A consistent sleep schedule also helps Tessa wake up looking refreshed and ready to greet the day. She makes it a point to set her alarm for 6 A.M. five days a week so that she has time to exercise in the morning before work. "To do so means going to bed at 11:30 every night, no matter what I'm doing," she says.

For more about Tessa Jean, see color insert.

Want to be a test panelist for a future 7 Years Younger plan? Sign up today at 7yearsyounger.com/panelist to be considered—and get our free weekly e-newsletter, Your Anti-Aging Tip Sheet!

Sunless Tanning

To get a golden glow without the aging (and skin-cancer risks), reach for a self-tanner. While these products don't provide protection against UV rays, you're less likely to succumb to the urge to sit in the sun if you've already got a glow going.

Here's how to get the most believable color.

Prep Skin

- **Test it out** The day before, test a silver dollar–size area on the inside of your arm or inner thigh. If you get a rash, try another formulation.
- **Get your timing right** Wax at least 24 hours in advance; the same goes for any other kind of hair removal, such as threading or tweezing, that tears hair out of the follicle. Self-tanner can pool in open follicles, creating tiny dark spots. Plus, rubbing the active ingredient, DHA, on sensitized skin ups the odds of irritation.
- **Slough off old skin first** To turn golden, the active ingredient interacts with the proteins in the very outer layer of your skin. Any patches of old, dead skin will absorb more self-tanner, which can lead to spots and streaks. For an even start, dry-brush before your shower or use an exfoliating mitt with an oil-free body wash.
- **Be bare** Skip deodorant, antiperspirant, essential oils, perfume, or body lotion, all of which can cause skin to turn a funny green-gray color when used with a tanner.

Self-Tan Head to Toe

- **Start light** If you're a newbie, start with a light formulation. Once you've gotten the application down pat, you can graduate to medium or dark (these last longer but streak more easily).
- **Begin at your thighs** and rub the self-tanner down the length of your legs. Then rub self-tanner on the front of your torso fol-

lowed by your arms (starting with your shoulders). When you reach your wrists, the product should have thinned out.

- **Spritz hard-to-reach spots** Your feet, too; a lotion, gel, or mousse will tend to lay on too much color.
- **Go easy on your hands** Orange nail beds and dark hands are telltale signs of a bad self-tan. Once you've finished the rest of your application, wash your hands thoroughly with soap and dry them; now you're ready to apply self-tanner there. Curl your hand into a claw so the tanner will be less likely to pool in the creases of your knuckles. If you're using a lotion or mousse, rub a bit on the back of your hand and then feather out any residue onto your fingers. (And, of course, avoid your palm.)
- **Buff trouble spots** Finish by wiping cuticles with a tissue. Then take a dry washcloth and buff knuckles, elbows, knees, the insides of your wrists, and the backs of your heels with a few back-and-forth swipes.

Optimize the Glow

- **Catch streaks early** If streaks do appear, scrub down the color (ideally within four hours) with a strong exfoliator. Or, tan again. Simply rub self-tanner on any areas that have turned out lighter, buffing or feathering it out so as not to create more lines.
- **Fend off odor** Showering eight hours after you've put on self-tanner will minimize the smell by washing away any excess product.
- **Skip long swims (and showers)** A self-tan lasts between four and 10 days, till the outer layer of your skin sheds—and your self-tan goes with it.
- **Keep skin hydrated** The drier your skin, the faster your self-tan will flake off. Moisturize daily, and you'll get more mileage out of your tan.

Youth Booster #7: Revitalize Your Eyes

The skin around your eyes is some of the thinnest and most fragile of your body; that's why signs of age surface here first. And if your eyes look tired, the rest of your face does, too. These tips can help you put the twinkle back in your eyes.

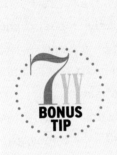

BONUS TIP

Relax about wrinkles–at least around your eyes: A study published in *Plastic and Reconstructive Surgery* found that **crow's feet on a woman's face are a sign of happiness.** When 20 people were shown an image of a young woman's face with crow's feet digitally added, viewers perceived the woman as nearly twice as happy. "Fine lines in the corners of the eyes indicate a broader, more natural smile," explains Eva Ritvo, M.D., vice chair of the department of psychiatry and behavioral sciences at the University of Miami. "People associate this type of smile with greater happiness."

Achieve It By: Reducing Dark Circles

As your skin becomes more translucent with age, blood vessels begin to show through, giving the undereye area a bluish cast no matter how much sleep you're getting. A less common cause of darkness: post-inflammatory hyperpigmentation, an accumulation of brown pigment underneath the eyes due to heredity or chronic rubbing (often because of allergies or bothersome contact lenses). Daily use of an eye cream will temporarily plump skin so blood vessels are less visible. Eye creams have higher concentrations of plumping emollients than regular face creams. Their thicker texture also makes them adhere to the ever-mobile eye area so the plumping can continue long-term. If your circles are brown, try an eye cream with botanical skin lighteners like licorice and kojic acid.

Achieve It By: Diminishing Eye Puffiness

Some puffiness is genetic, and no eye cream will erase or reduce it. But if your bags come and go, fluid retention is probably the cause. Salty dinners, late nights, a cocktail or two—they can all make your body hold on to water. Thanks to gravity, morning facial puffiness is usually gone by lunchtime. To speed things up, try placing a chilled eye compress; cold, water-soaked tea bags; or chilled cucumber slices over lids for five minutes. Cold constricts blood vessels and reduces swelling. The caffeine in many eye creams is tightening, too. "Gently press on the bones around your eyes as you apply it," suggests Jody A. Levine, M.D., a dermatologist in New York City. "The pressure helps stimulate circulation and drain excess fluid."

Achieve It By: Smoothing Lines and Wrinkles

Every time you smile, frown, yawn, or squint, the skin around your eyes crinkles up. Eventually, as the collagen levels diminish, your skin literally stays scrunched, and deeper creases take the place of fine lines.

This is an instance when you might want to talk to your doctor about a prescription retinoid or try an eye cream with retinol. If you find that retinol is too harsh on your eye-area skin, you might want to swap those vitamin A–derived products for peptides, which also stimulate collagen growth.

Achieve It By: Using a Light Touch

The thinner your skin, the more likely it will register any impact. So treat it with TLC. After you've washed your face, pat around your eyes to dry the delicate skin—rubbing stretches it. Then, when you apply a moisturizer, use your ring finger; it's your weakest one and thus the least likely to cause damage or wrinkles. While you're being cautious, protect your eyes against infection, too, by trying roll-on eye depuffers and serums. There's less risk of bacterial growth when you don't dip your fingers into a jar.

The Body Parts That Make You Look Younger

Here's news you can use: A study of women ages 45 to 65 at the University of Göttingen in Germany found that skin exposure was an important indicator of attractiveness and youth. Researchers noted that when a woman's arms and chest were on view, she was perceived as younger than when just her face was visible.

Regular exfoliating and moisturizing coupled with sun protection will help your skin remain radiant. Two-in-one formulas (moisturizers with sunscreen, exfoliating moisturizers, or body scrubs) are a great way to save time and show off healthy, supple body skin. Here are additional tips, according to body part.

Chest

Treat Help fade spots with daily exfoliation. To skip an extra step, look for a body wash with niacinamide, a vitamin B derivative shown to help prevent dark spots. For a nighttime treatment, try a tone-improving 1.5 percent retinol serum.

Prevent Sun protection is the best way to avoid future brown spots. When you're applying sunscreen to your face and neck in the morning, extend it down to the exposed areas of your chest.

Doctor Rx In-office IPL treatments cause spots to darken and peel off within a few weeks. Typically, you'll need at least two sessions. "But if the whole chest area has uneven pigmentation and lots of freckling, the Fraxel laser—which can cover a wider area—is the best tool," says Dr. Bank. On average you'll need two to three Fraxel treatments. Expect skin to have some redness and flaking for about a week after each session.

Hands

Fast fix For the quickest results, moisturize. Over time, hands lose some of their fat cushioning and the skin gets less elastic. Applying a cream or ointment (vs. a lightweight lotion) will immediately plump up skin. Look for a formula with emollients, such as shea butter or petrolatum, and humectants like glycerin that attract moisture to the skin.

Treat Smooth on a retinoid treatment nightly to help diminish wrinkles, increase plumpness, remove dead cells, and bolster the thickness of thinning skin. The same prescription versions you'd use on your face (see page 41) make skin on the hands look firmer, fuller, and smoother, too. Also look for OTC overnight hand creams that feature retinol. (Tip: Always rub any extra anti-aging face cream on your hands once you're done applying it to your complexion.)

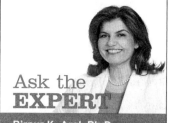

Ask the EXPERT

Birnur K. Aral, Ph.D.
Health, Beauty & Environmental Sciences Director, GHRI

Q *Should I use the same products on my body as on my face?*

Birnur says: The skin on your face is thinner than the skin on your body, so facial products are typically formulated to be gentler than body products. Note that the skin on the neck, décolletage, and hands is also relatively thin, and if you'd like, you can use your facial anti-agers (like retinols, spot-faders, and exfoliators, such as glycolics) on those areas, too. But there isn't much sense in using your pricey face products on the rest of your body, where they're likely to be less effective.

Using a sloughing cream with glycolic acid will also help speed cell turnover, yet both retinoids and AHAs can be irritating if your hands are very red and chapped. Instead, try slathering on a barrier cream with fat molecules called ceramides and hyaluronic acid, and wearing cotton gloves overnight. After your hands heal, you can treat the wrinkles.

Prevent Hands are sun-exposed nearly every day; that's the reason they're such giveaways of age. To prevent more dark spots and roughness, apply a hand cream with SPF several times daily. Keep tubes where you're likeliest to spot them—in your purse or desk, beside the sink—and, if possible, reapply every time you wash your hands. Not near a sink? Stash convenient sunscreen-infused wipes in your car, purse, or gym bag for on-the-go coverage.

Doctor Rx Laser treatments (such as DioLite, which heats and shrinks vessels in one or two sessions) can help reduce protruding back-of-hand veins. Injections of the filler Radiesse go at it from another direction, adding volume and hiding veins and tendons. "Results may last for more than a year," explains Linda K. Franks, M.D., a dermatologist in New York City. Finally, if brown spots are making you wish you could wear gloves in the summer, the best treatments are the same as for other parts of your body (see "Achieve It By: Fading Age Spots," page 31).

Legs

Treat About 40 percent of women develop varicose veins (women are two to three times more likely to get them than men), and the risk grows as you get older. Reticular veins, which are smaller than varicose veins, and spider veins—small dilated blood vessels—are additional hallmarks of time (they can occur on the face as well as the legs) but are more web-like in appearance. Exercises such as rolling up onto your toes to work your calf muscles and keep blood flowing (repeated throughout the day) help. Support hose can minimize the bulging of varicose veins; opaque legwear can hide spiders.

Prevent Pregnancy, obesity, and being on your feet for long periods increase the likelihood of varicose veins. Since there is a familial component, if you have a family history, take care to maintain a healthy body weight, put your feet up often, and exercise regularly. Margaret E. Parsons, M.D., assistant clinical professor of dermatology at the University of California, Davis, cautions against sitting with your legs crossed. "The pressure makes the body try to correct the cut-off circulation by creating new blood vessels—and those can become spider veins," she says.

Doctor Rx Veins bulge when valves that control blood flow weaken and blood pools in them. If you have bulging varicose veins, a vascular surgeon should evaluate you; they may be a sign of a medical condition. Spider veins, reticular veins, and small varicose veins can easily be treated by sclerotherapy, which dissolves veins with a quick injection of saline or glycerin. "The vessels then collapse and disappear within a month or so," says Dr. Parsons.

Feet

Treat Use pumice or a foot file regularly to prevent calluses from forming (foot files work best on dry skin). Also, rub olive or coconut oil onto rough spots, then put on a pair of socks and leave the treatment on for at least an hour a day to make feet sandal-worthy.

Prevent Regularly massage in an alpha hydroxy acid–containing cream to control the buildup of tough, dry skin. And whenever you can, choose supportive shoes (most lace-up athletic sneakers fit the bill) over zero-support alternatives such as flip-flops. Another smart strategy: Use insoles for a comfortable fit. When feet slip around inside shoes, calluses are frequently the result.

Doctor Rx "If calluses are uncomfortable and tough to file down, see a podiatrist to have the skin buildup safely removed," says Marlene Reid, D.P.M., a podiatrist who practices in Naperville, IL. (A pedicurist isn't licensed to use a blade to trim calluses.)

Your Younger-Looking Skin Repair Kit

When you have the right tool, the job is easy and gets done right. So think of the following products (all tested in the Good Housekeeping Research Institute beauty lab and by hundreds of women volunteers) as your look-younger skin tools.

Care category	Product	Why it's the top tool
Anti-aging serum	Boots No7 Protect & Perfect Intense Serum	This vitamin A- and E-enriched formula garnered high marks for its tone-evening and skin-firming properties; in the lab, it received a perfect firming score.
Anti-aging serum	Mary Kay TimeWise Replenishing Serum+C	Got high scores in the lab in terms of firmness, but panelists noted it was slightly more irritating than the Boots.
At-home peel	Boots No7 Glycolic Peel Kit	Evened skin tone and smoothed skin; consumers also reported that it minimized the look of creases while leaving skin soft and radiant.
Body bronzer	Victoria's Secret Beach Sexy Airbrush Instant Bronze Body Spray	Testers said the "quick-drying" spray produced "a natural glow" and "smelled like summer," while the lab gave it high marks for being transfer-proof—even in a room that was 80°F with 80 percent humidity.
Body moisturizer	Fresh Sugar Açai Age-Delay Body Cream	Earned top scores in the lab for moisturizing and firming and one of the highest consumer grades for its skin-tone-evening and radiance-enhancing properties. Panelists raved about the rich-but-not-too-greasy texture.

● Find these top anti-aging products at 7yearsyounger.com/shop.

Care category	Product	Why it's the top tool
Dark circle eraser	Biopelle Dark Circle Relief Cream	According to testers, this vitamin K oxide-infused treatment diminished darkness while moisturizing the eye area; lab tests showed a slight improvement.
Eye cream	Olay Pro-X Eye Restoration Complex	Soothing, nonirritating, and a standout hydrator. Testers noted it reduced their crow's feet, puffiness, and undereye bags.
Eye cream	Patricia Wexler M.D. Dermatology Intensive 3-in-1 Eye Cream	In the lab, this balm-like moisturizer excelled at reducing crow's feet, dark circles, and fine lines. Testers found it firmed the eye area well and did not irritate delicate skin.
Eye lifting treatment	Wrinkle MD	After one 40-minute treatment (undereye patches of moisturizer "helped" to penetrate skin via micro-current) the appearance of undereye lines and wrinkles was somewhat reduced.
Facial moisturizer (with SPF 15+)	Chanel Ultra Correction Lift Lifting Firming Day Cream SPF 15	Testers reported it as tops for firming, softening, smoothing, and adding radiance to skin. While pricey, it did result in a slight improvement in beneath-the-surface UV spots (which turn into splotchy skin over time).
Facial moisturizer (with SPF 15+)	Elizabeth Arden Ceramide Lift and Firm Day Cream Broad Spectrum Sunscreen SPF 30	The reliable sun-protective powers were a plus, said testers.
Facial skin firmer	Peter Thomas Roth Firmx Growth Factor Extreme Neuropeptide Serum	Lab tests showed that it toned and firmed the jawline, and more than half of testers agreed that it increased firmness. In the lab, the creamy serum also scored well for hydration.

Care category	Product	Why it's the top tool
Facial skin firmer	Kinerase Restructure Firming Cream	Came out on top in lab firmness measurements, and testers loved its tightening and smoothing effect.
Hand cream with SPF 15	Boots No7 Protect & Perfect Day Hand Cream	A favorite in almost every consumer category—from perceived wrinkle reduction to increasing smoothness. Testers gave it high marks for its low price.
Instant pore minimizer	Clinique Pore Refining Solutions Instant Perfector	Immediately reduced the appearance of pores, while instantly improving skin tone and radiance.
Instant pore minimizer	GoodSkin Labs Z-Pore Instant Pore Refiner	Minimized the look of pores, creating a smooth finish on skin without disturbing makeup.
Instant redness reducer	Clinique Redness Solutions Instant Relief Mineral Powder	Top scores for ease of use, consumer performance, and overall performance (a measure of lab and consumer results).
Instant wrinkle smoother	Olay Regenerist Filling + Sealing Wrinkle Treatment	Ranked highest in the lab for reducing forehead lines, and came in first with consumers for minimizing wrinkles all over the face.
Night cream	L'Oréal Paris Advanced RevitaLift Deep-Set Wrinkle Repair Night Creme	Budget-friendly and tops in minimizing forehead lines and wrinkles in lab results.
Night cream	Vichy LiftActiv Retinol HA Night	Best at evening out skin tone and addressing fine lines and wrinkles around the mouth and nose.

The Younger-Skin Food Guide

It's time to unveil what may be your new favorite beauty tool: a fork. Use it to eat the right foods, listed below, and you'll be delighted by the brighter, smoother, younger skin that will follow. (You'll see these foods in the Light and Delicious Recipes, too—see page 321.) Even if you don't want or need to lose weight, eating a mix of the right nutrients gives your skin what it needs to stay healthy and vital. Work the following beauty boosters into your diet, and your skin will glow.

Vitamin C-Rich Foods: Keep Skin Elastic and Wrinkle-Free

Anti-aging benefit Vitamin C is a powerful antioxidant that can quench free radicals. In a British study of 4,025 women ages 40 to 74, researchers found that those with higher intakes of vitamin C had fewer wrinkles and less dry skin.

What to put on your plate Aim to eat 75 mg a day: an orange for breakfast and five strips of a yellow pepper at lunch will get you there. So will a cup of broccoli with dinner and a bowl of strawberries for dessert. Citrus fruits, red pepper, tomatoes, kale, and melon are good sources of C. For an extra skin boost, try blackberries, raspberries, cranberries, and pomegranates—beyond vitamin C, they contain ellagic acid, which may counter the deleterious effects of UV rays.

Lean Protein: Plumps Skin, Pumps Up Collagen

Anti-aging benefit In the British study, women with lower protein intakes also had a more wrinkled appearance. "Protein provides the building blocks of collagen," says F. William Danby, M.D., adjunct assistant professor of surgery (dermatology) at Dartmouth Medical School. And collagen, of course, is critical to how plump and healthy your skin looks. Your skin will make collagen whether you dine on mar-

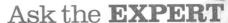

Ask the **EXPERT**

Birnur K. Aral, Ph.D., Health, Beauty & Environmental Sciences Director, GHRI

Should I take a skin supplement?

Birnur says: It may be tempting to try to get your skin-beautifying nutrients from a pill or specialty drink. Called nutricosmetics, these potions claim to supply you with many of the essential fatty acids, antioxidants, and other plant extracts associated with reducing lines and wrinkles. But when I consulted Diane L. McKay, Ph.D., of the Friedman School of Nutrition Science and Policy at Tufts, she confirmed that your daily servings of fruits and vegetables provide a lot more of the skin-enhancing vitamins and minerals. You also obtain a more complete dose of nutrients from a simple multivitamin.

bled steaks or skinless chicken breasts, but the leaner choice can help keep weight down.

What to put on your plate Skinless poultry, eggs (especially whites), and fish are good choices. For beef or pork, go for lower-fat cuts such as loin and round. Consider edamame and tofu, too: A small Japanese study found that women who consumed soy extract for 12 weeks showed improvement in fine lines around their eyes as well as greater elasticity in their skin.

Fatty Fish: Calms Inflammation

Anti-aging benefit Sea fare like tuna and salmon contains a hefty dose of omega-3 fatty acids, which may help guard against sun damage. In studies of mice, the fats significantly reduced inflammation and other immunological responses to sunlight that degrade collagen. And three British studies showed that omega-3s can protect against sunburn in humans, too.

Warning: 3 Foods That Make You Look Older

1. **Sugar** Sweets and other refined carbs raise blood-glucose levels, which in turn increases the creation of AGEs—advanced glycation end products. These take a toll on skin's appearance by interfering with the normal repair of collagen and elastin.

2. **Saturated Fat** Beyond its role in promoting heart disease, saturated fat—the type found in marbled meats and full-fat dairy products—induces skin-aging inflammation, notes Jane Grant-Kels, M.D., chair of dermatology at the University of Connecticut at Farmington. Chronic inflammation is an aging accelerator.

3. **Alcohol** Drinking alcohol makes skin dry, taut, and lined—all signs of dehydration. Also, as the liver metabolizes alcohol, it creates free radicals—that other enemy of firm, youthful skin.

What to put on your plate Aim for two four-ounce servings of omega-3-rich seafood a week. Besides tuna and salmon, try mackerel, herring, sardines, and lake trout. Walnuts, flaxseeds, canola oil, pumpkin seeds, and tofu contain the compound alpha linolenic acid (ALA), which the body converts into a similar type of beneficial omega fatty acid. If you're not partial to fish, however, an omega-3 supplement may be in order.

Whole Grains: Brighten Your Complexion

Anti-aging benefit "Refined grains can raise insulin levels, which in turn causes inflammation that damages the skin," says Adam Friedman, M.D., director of dermatologic research at Albert Einstein College of Medicine in New York City. Whole grains are also a good source of selenium—a mineral that helps protect against injury from UV rays.

Facelift on a Plate

Here is a delicious preview of the kinds of meals you'll find in the 7-Week Plan. These three incorporate the anti-aging foods mentioned here.

1. Salmon with braised red cabbage
   Whole wheat pita
   Cubed cantaloupe

2. Skinless chicken breast
   Roasted broccoli
   Couscous with chopped almonds and apricots
   Sliced strawberries

3. Tuna sandwich (made with water-packed tuna, low-fat mayo, and tomato slices on whole wheat bread)
   Cucumber and tomato salad with low-calorie vinaigrette
   Blueberries

What to put on your plate Grains rich in selenium include brown rice, oatmeal, barley, and whole wheat. Aim for three to four servings a day.

Colorful Produce: Discourages Wrinkling

Anti-aging benefit The yellow, orange, and red pigments found in fruits and vegetables are carotenoids, antioxidants that destroy free radicals, which can cause wrinkling. One carotenoid, beta-carotene, may help fight aging by increasing production of collagen and GAGs (glycosaminoglycans), which help your skin hold on to water. Lycopene is another carotenoid attracting attention. Researchers found that women who ate about two ounces of lycopene-rich tomato paste every day for 12 weeks sustained less skin damage when exposed to UV light than a control group that ate none.

What to put on your plate Load up on cooked tomato sauces and tomato paste for lycopene. Orange-tinted vegetables and fruits—carrots, cantaloupe, apricots, orange squash, and sweet potatoes—are all good sources of beta-carotene. So are leafy greens such as spinach, kale, chard, and collard greens. (These also supply lutein, another important carotenoid.) To increase your absorption of carotenoids, toss vegetables with avocado: One study found that eating salads including five ounces of avocado (about one medium) increased the absorption of another carotenoid, alpha-carotene (7.2 times) as well as beta-carotene (15.3 times) and lutein (5.1 times).

Activate Your Anti-Aging Plan Now!

Talk about instant gratification. Make these easy adjustments and see younger-looking skin in just days:

1 **Drink more water** Hydration is the key to clarity, radiance, and plumpness in skin cells. If you're not drinking enough (or if you're taking in lots of diuretics, such as caffeine), skin looks depleted and dull. The fix: Swap a cup of peppermint tea for your caffeinated beverage. It's a natural anti-inflammatory, and you'll notice its skin-brightening effects in a week or less! You can also eat juicy fruits or vegetables and get fluid as well as wrinkle-fighting antioxidants.

2 **Aim for consistent care** Cleansing, exfoliating, moisturizing, and treating skin on a regular basis are the keys to uncovering younger-looking (and -acting) skin. Hit-or-miss care shows up as signs of aging.

3 **Try an at-home peel** It's one of the quickest ways to improve the look of your skin. A peel is designed to dissolve accumulated dead cells on the surface of skin, leaving your complexion smoother and more luminous. When you shed those dead cells, active ingredients in your skin care—like antioxidants and retinoids—are better able to penetrate.

For more expert anti-aging beauty advice, get our free special report, 40 Best Anti-Aging Beauty Secrets, *at 7yearsyounger.com/antiagingsecrets.*

Age Eraser 2

Chapter Two

Your Makeup Makeover

Everything you've learned about caring for your skin in the previous chapter sets the stage for your next years-younger move: age-defying makeup. Good skin care gives you a smooth canvas to work on; otherwise it's like "having 10 layers of paint under your makeup," says Ellen Marmur, M.D., associate professor of dermatology at Mount Sinai School of Medicine in New York City. Makeup goes on more easily and colors and textures are more flattering on clean, healthy, well-moisturized skin. Clean, rejuvenated skin, coupled with the right makeup, can help you look years younger, starting today.

Like everything in life, makeup—color, product, and technique— doesn't stand still. Neither should you. When you're young, anything goes with makeup. You try new things, make bold changes, and move on to the next new trend. As years pass, experimentation tends to lead to complacency; it's easy to get into a rut. "But as your skin evolves, so should your makeup," says makeup artist Laura Geller. Changes in the tone, brightness, and texture of your skin may mean you need to update your palette of colors, opt for more moisturizing formulas, and freshen up your technique.

7 ESSENTIALS FOR YOUR 7 YEARS YOUNGER MAKEUP KIT

Youth Booster #1: A Freshening Foundation

It's not called foundation for nothing: The right base sets the stage for the rest of your makeup palette. The overall effect you want is dewy, to help compensate for any drier-looking or rough-textured skin. Check out "light reflecting" foundations, which deflect light from lines and crinkles, visually filling them in.

To find your perfect foundation:

Choose a fail-proof formula A hydrating or satin-finish liquid foundation is your best choice, especially as hormone levels dip and your skin gets drier. A product that contains the moisturizers glycerin or hyaluronic acid will help remedy dryness. You may be tempted to reach for a cream foundation, but these can actually be *more* drying, and that will make your skin's texture rougher and accentuate lines. Thicker, creamier formulas are usually made to provide fuller coverage for uneven skin tone, age spots, and more, which means they're packed with pigment. They may start out looking nice, but as your skin absorbs the hydrating ingredients the pigments can start to look cakey. However, if you like a creamy formula's coverage, try using it with a richer face moisturizer or a hydrating primer. You may also consider a foundation with added antioxidants and peptides, anti-agers that can boost your makeup's performance.

Pick a warmer shade The rule that says your foundation must exactly match your skin tone doesn't hold up any more. Your complexion grows paler with age, so a shade that replicates yours can leave you looking pasty, blotchy, or, in the case of brown skin tones, ashy: "Today, if I put on the ivory tone I wore in my 20s, I'd look like Bette Davis in *Whatever Happened to Baby Jane?*" says Sandy Linter, makeup artist and Lancôme's beauty-at-every-age expert. Plus, warmer base shades have fewer pink undertones, so they counteract ruddiness in light-skinned women. Linter keeps the life in her skin by using a slightly warmer tone a shade deeper than her old one. If you're wary of going up a full notch, mix your current shade with the next darkest on the back of your hand, and then apply with a foundation brush. Apply foundation over your entire face—including under the eyes, on the eyelids and brow-bones, along your jawline, and on your neck—with a damp sponge or brush.

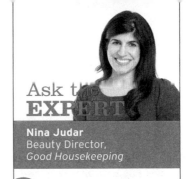

Ask the EXPERT

Nina Judar
Beauty Director,
Good Housekeeping

Q *Now that I'm in my 40s and beyond break-outs, do I still need to use an oil-free foundation?*

Nina says: If your skin feels a bit dryer and tighter now, a more emollient foundation is preferable; check for glycerin on the ingredients list. But also look for "non-comedogenic" on the label, which means the foundation has been tested and won't block pores. Clogged pores look more prominent—and can make you look older. And, of course, a clogged pore can lead to a pimple.

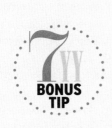

BONUS TIP

If your stock formula has been matte, trade it in for a tinted moisturizer to achieve a lighter, dewier look. Not enough coverage? You can **mix your foundation with a little moisturizer** to thin it out or even mix tinted moisturizer with your foundation. The sheer, less dense formulation prevents foundation from pooling and highlighting the lines, wrinkles, and pores you're trying to minimize, says Kimara Ahnert, a makeup artist in New York City.

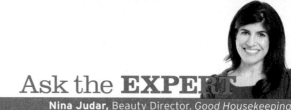

Nina Judar, Beauty Director, *Good Housekeeping*

Q *Help! No matter what concealer I use on my undereye circles, I always wind up with mascara and liner smudges, which make me look tired.*

Nina says: First, don't apply eye cream in the morning—doing so can contribute to smudging. And try using a waterproof mascara and liner *only* on your upper lashes, skipping your lower lashes and lashline. Those precautions should prevent smudging, but if you're ever in a pinch, keep a supply of Almay Oil-Free Makeup Eraser Sticks in your purse. One end of each swab houses eye makeup remover, so with a quick, gentle swipe, you're smudge-free.

Youth Booster #2: A Sheer Concealer

When it comes to using a concealer, now's the time to expand your horizons. Instead of saving it to disguise the occasional blemish or splotch, use it daily to smooth the look of your skin and add polish to your

Instant Anti-Ager

Get the Red Out

If your skin is looking more florid due to chronic irritation, thinning skin, dilated blood vessels, or skin conditions such as rosacea, be extra choosy about foundation. Skip sheer formulas, which just don't give you the coverage you need, reports Ahnert. Opt for a more opaque formula, and make sure it's oil-free so it won't trigger acne flare-ups. Apply base to your skin using a flat-bristle brush, so as to deliver more pigment to your red hot spots. Once you've covered your redness, blend with a damp makeup sponge to give skin a more lightweight look and feel. If redness affects only a few areas, invest in a foundation stick, which is easier to blend than most concealers. Apply a sheer foundation first and then warm the stick on the back of your hand. Dab on with a brush where you see discoloration.

appearance. Typically, you'll put on a concealer first and then a foundation on top.

Look for a water-based concealer formula that dries to a sheer finish. Creams have a stronger hold than liquids and won't settle into fine lines or be detectable at the thin-skinned inner eye, where most of us have shadows. Match the shade to your skin tone. Apply with a light hand: Concealer contains more pigment than foundation. You can use your finger—tapping gently until the makeup blends into your skin—but a small angled brush will give you the most precise coverage.

On-the-Spot Coverage

If you want to conceal...	Then use...	For best coverage
Undereye circles	Concealer	Stroke concealer from the inner corner of the eye to the midpoint beneath the pupil, then feather it out, blending away demarcation lines.
Age spots or freckles	A foundation stick in the same shade as your foundation (a lighter shade will make your face look like it has light dots on it)	Apply stick after you put on foundation, using a concealer or foundation brush. Finish by patting it in with your finger or a sponge.
Lines	A primer	Use fingertips to spread a tiny amount all over your face under foundation to keep your base from sinking into and accentuating lines.
Blemishes	A green-tinted concealer	Green tones cancel redness, so dot on with a concealer brush or cotton-tipped swab and then pat with your index finger to help set.

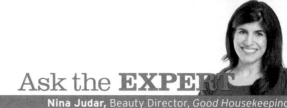

Ask the **EXPERT**

Nina Judar, Beauty Director, *Good Housekeeping*

Q *I have really dark circles under my eyes, and concealer doesn't seem to cover them. Is there anything else I can try?*

Nina says: It's frustrating, but stubborn "raccoon eyes" often show through concealer. That's because its pigments simply aren't the right tone to cancel out dark circles. First, you need to use a yellow- or orange-based corrector. Yellow cancels purple tones and orange minimizes blue tones; Bobbi Brown makes a wide range of correctors. Apply it with a brush—it's easy to glop on too much if you use your fingers. Then wear a thin layer of your usual concealer on top. If this sounds intimidating or complicated, it's worth a trip to the makeup counter for a demonstration. It can take some time to get the hang of it, but the results are so good, it's worth skimping on the rest of your routine (just curling your lashes and brushing on some blush) until you do.

Youth Booster #3: A Radiant Blush

A face that glows with good health is a rejuvenator at any age. The right blush offsets any paleness or color loss that accrues with the years; it has the added benefit of contouring and lifting your face. To attain your best blush:

● **Opt for powder over cream** Powder has a bad rap for aging the face, but it's time to backtrack: A cream blush can actually be more aging. If your skin's dehydrated and rough, cream blush sticks to dry patches and cakes, aging you. Look for a highly pigmented powder blush—that way you'll only need a touch and will avoid powdery buildup.

● **Apply with a light touch** Powder blush is quick and easy to apply. Swirl blush ever so slightly higher on the apples to lift your whole face; the mouth-to-ear stroke can leave you looking gaunt.

Youth Booster #4:
The Right Brow Tools

Brows not only frame your eyes, but are the backbone for your face. Fuller, extended brows can help lift your whole face, diverting attention from corner crinkles, dark circles, even undereye bags. Here are the key tools you'll need to make your brows work for, not against, you:

An appointment with a pro Unless you've got a good sense of the most flattering arch shape and brow thickness for your face, have a professional do it for you at least once. Then you can simply follow the line. "It's worth the expense," says Ahnert. "Clients have told me it made them look like they had their eyes lifted." Check in with your pro about

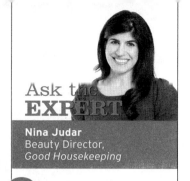

Ask the EXPERT

Nina Judar
Beauty Director,
Good Housekeeping

Q *Should I use bronzer only during the summer?*

Nina says: I love—and use—bronzer all year round. When skin becomes paler in winter, bronzer warms it up. Use a big fluffy brush to dust it lightly where the sun would normally hit: across the top of your forehead and cheekbones. Makeup artists also advise running it down the bridge of your nose and across the bottom of your chin.

Your Makeup at Ages 40, 50, 60+

Is your makeup age-appropriate? Use this decade-by-decade mini-guide to make sure your cosmetics flatter you, no matter what the calendar says.

Decade	Toss	Keep	Buy
40s	Anything with chunky glitter	Lengthening mascara	Eyelid primer
50s	Dark, harsh eye and lip liners	Rosy blush	Skin-illuminating foundation
60s and beyond	Chalky, drying face powder	Shimmery eye shadow	Hydrating lipstick

Revitalized Eyes

Eyes that sparkle freshen your whole face. To get the look on demand—to fake looking awake, bright-eyed and bushy-tailed—hundreds of morning news anchors rely on their makeup artists. Here, New York City makeup pro Deborah Bell shares the eye-enhancement tricks she deploys daily. These tips work just as well for an evening pick-me-up.

- **Use brightening eye drops** It's the easiest, quickest way to make eyes look more awake. "The drops zap redness and make your whites seem whiter," says Bell.
- **Skip dark eye shadows** They cast your whole lid in darkness. Instead, use a flesh-toned hue to even out skin tone and then top it with a sheer neutral shadow, such as gold, applied from lashline to crease.
- **Dust bronzer over blush** After applying blush, sweep bronzer along the cheekbones. Shimmer placed high on the cheeks brightens the whole face, including your eyes.

color, too. Brows may lighten with the years; a darker brow can rebalance your face.

Brow tweezers To maintain shape, use tweezers rather than an at-home waxing kit. They'll give you more precise control over the process.

A brow pencil Use it to fill in where nature has left gaps or where brows are sparse. "If you've been waxing your brows for years, the hairs may have simply stopped growing back," says Dr. Marmur. If you need to fill in a larger gap, like a missing tail, use a powder brow pencil instead. Unlike the usual brow pencil, which is designed to be hard and waxy and leave color on brow hairs, a powder pencil adheres to skin more easily. To replicate missing hairs, stroke pencils and powders so that you get fullness without that "filled-in" look.

Youth Booster #5: Eye-Enhancing Products

Perhaps more than any other feature, your eyes draw others in. And eyes are not just a window to your soul (as the saying goes); they can reveal

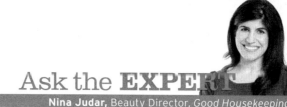

Ask the **EXPERT**

Nina Judar, Beauty Director, *Good Housekeeping*

Q *I've tried dabbing highlighter on my browbone, but it looks clownish. Any tips?*

Nina says: Strategic use of highlighter, a light-reflecting product, can visually reverse the effects of gravity, but you have to start with the right color. Look for a warmer tone like gold or champagne, and rub it in with your pinkie. The color should blend in with your skin tone, not stand out. Anything silver or too sparkly can look garish. Here's how to maximize its impact for:

- **Your brows** Dab a little bit of creamy or liquid highlighter just underneath your arch and blend to open and brighten eyes. If you use a gold-toned powder, apply it with a brush.
- **Your cheeks** Apply at the top of your cheekbones to make them more prominent and add a visual lift.
- **Your mouth** Apply to the top of your cupid's bow for fuller-looking lips.

your age, your health, and how well you care for yourself, too. Signs of age show up here first, requiring a delicate balance between maximizing the pluses of this feature and minimizing any minuses. Here, the fool-proof age-defying products you'll need:

Lid primer A neutral-shade eye primer smooths the surface of your lids so shadow adheres better and longer. In addition, a primer helps color stay put, preventing it from disappearing into the folds and forming unflattering creases. Using your fingers, glide the primer onto your entire top eyelid from the lashline up to the brow. Keep the layer very thin so it doesn't weigh lids down.

Liner Whether you prefer a pencil or a cake formula, the result is the same: an even, light outline opens up and enhances the shape of your eyes. Use a soft—but not too soft (or it will smudge)—pencil that doesn't tug at the skin, or wet the bristles of a liner brush and dip it into shadow.

Rachel Dorfman
"Getting my brows done really lifted my face"

"Committing to a plan like this alters your perspective on things. It pulls you out of your whole routine and makes you question mindless choices," says Rachel, 37. This year she needed some big, positive changes. She'd suffered through a breakup; helped care for her father, who has early-onset Alzheimer's; and seen her grandmother go into the hospital. On the bright side, she earned a promotion at work, but that added to her personal stress.

Taming tension, gaining calm Rachel had previously meditated, but her practice had lapsed. The 7 Years Younger program helped her rediscover it as an integral part of her life. "I was sometimes finding it easier to drink a glass of wine or bury myself in the computer, so the program served as a good reminder of how much meditation

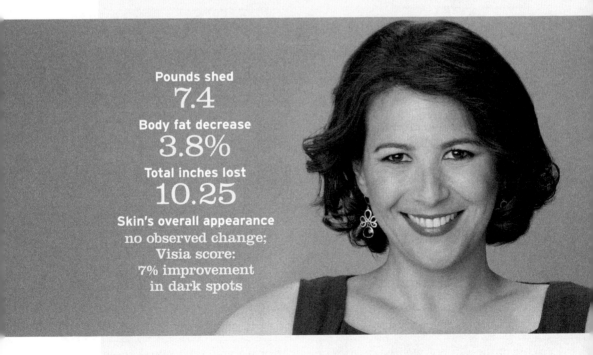

Pounds shed
7.4

Body fat decrease
3.8%

Total inches lost
10.25

Skin's overall appearance
no observed change;
Visia score:
7% improvement
in dark spots

helps," she says. She also took to heart the recommendation to turn off all electronics an hour before bed. "I found that it dramatically decreased the amount of time I watched TV. Instead, I do my nighttime skin-care routine, then do yoga, read a book, or listen to music. It's calmed me down."

The haircut and the two-minute face fix One of the biggest modifications she made during the program was to update her hairstyle, chopping her tresses to chin length. "My hair looks stylish, fuller, and healthier now," she says. "I'm still doing a double take whenever I look in the mirror." Wearing lip gloss and mascara was about the extent of Rachel's previous approach to makeup, but she was excited to do more. "The biggest difference came from getting my eyebrows shaped—it changed and lifted my face," she says. "I'm now using eyelid primer, shadow, liner, and blush. The whole process takes me about two minutes, and I look much more pulled together."

Found: more energy Another significant change Rachel made in her routine was to eliminate most of the added sugar in her diet. First to go were the couple of packets she automatically stirred into her coffee (she drinks two to three cups a day); once she acclimated to that change, she also stopped eating non-fruit desserts. "It's hard to deconstruct exactly why I feel different—I don't know if it was the diet, the exercise, the better sleep—but I think cutting out most sugar has given me more energy," she says. "I've been feeling a lot less tired in the afternoons."

For more about Rachel Dorfman, see color insert.

Want to be a test panelist for a future 7 Years Younger plan? Sign up today at 7yearsyounger.com/panelist to be considered—and get our free weekly e-newsletter, Your Anti-Aging Tip Sheet!

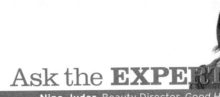

Ask the **EXPERT**

Nina Judar, Beauty Director, *Good Housekeeping*

Q *What's the difference between a "lengthening" and a "volumizing" mascara?*

Nina says: Two factors impact the effectiveness of mascara: the formula and the brush. A volumizing mascara has a thicker consistency and a fatter brush, designed to swipe the maximum amount of product onto each lash. It sounds good, but too much product can lead to clumping, especially if, like me, you have lashes that tend to overlap and clump anyway. A lengthening mascara, on the other hand, has a leaner brush, designed to separate lashes. If you can't decide which to use, do what makeup artists do and layer a volumizing formula over a lengthening one.

Then, point your chin up and look down, so your lids are half-closed but you can still see them. (Holding the lid taut by tugging at the outer corners can cause skin to crinkle, making the liner come out unevenly.) Start at the outer corner and draw inward, making the line as thin as possible; a thick band of liner will close up your eye area. On your bottom lashes, line with a color a shade or two lighter than the one you used on top (if you used dark brown on top, for instance, try a bronze or taupe on the bottom). And instead of using a pencil, use a *dry* liner brush and shadow.

True-to-you-toned shadow On pale skin tones, sheer, low-watt neutrals do for eyes what gloss does for lips: enhance size and provide a youthful, modern look. Plus, neutrals show off your eyes, not your lids. Your best bets: sage and jewel tones, which cancel red and yellow tones, making the whites of the eyes look brighter. Taupes are flattering, too, but avoid browns. "Brown has yellow or red pigments in it, either of which can actually make eyes look tired," says Geller. Also, browns are

the institute investigates

Eye Makeup Removers

Eye makeup removers are like snowflakes—no two are alike. That means you're sure to find one that works for you. A GHRI panel tested nine contenders on their ability to quickly remove makeup without requiring scrubbing, causing stinging or irritation, or leaving a greasy residue.

The product	Tester comments
Almay Moisturizing Eye Makeup Remover Pads	On the oily side: good for drier, aging skin (cleansing afterward helps dispel oiliness)
Clean & Clear Makeup Dissolving Facial Cleansing Wipes	Non-greasy; removed waterproof mascara speedily and easily
Andrea Eye Q's Ultra Quick Makeup Remover Pads	Most economical; most hydrating; effectively removed waterproof eye makeup
Neutrogena Night Calming Makeup Remover Cleansing Towelettes	Pleasant fragrance; good at removing makeup at home
Neutrogena Ultra-Soft Eye Makeup Remover Pads	Left no oily residue; good scores for ease of use and nonirritating formula
OleHenriksen's Purifying Eye Make-up Remover	Best for less sensitive skin; left a clean feeling behind; some irritation if product got into eye
Pond's Original Fresh Wet Cleansing Towelettes	Winner for "cleanest-feeling"
Rodan + Fields Anti-Age Eye Cloths	Oversized; left skin feeling clean and fresh

● Find these top anti-aging products at 7yearsyounger.com/shop.

often too light to give you even coverage. If you're Hispanic, jewel tones—especially vibrant plums—are a good choice, too (they complement the olive undertones of your skin). If you prefer something more neutral, go for grays and taupes.

Because dark skin rarely has a prominent or single color undertone, African-American women can really wear most makeup colors, "though brighter hues in particular look nice against this rich skin tone," says Ashunta Sheriff, lead makeup artist for Mary Kay. If you're Asian, avoid deep purples and blues, which aren't flattering to the yellow undertones typical of Asian skin. Instead, go for earth tones like browns and coppers, light minty greens, and dusty lilac shades.

For all women, shadows with subtle luminescence will also have an eye-brightening effect. In fact, adding a dot of light shimmer shadow to the inner corners of your eyes can open them up and make your whole face look brighter. Too much sparkle, on the other hand, can accentuate crepey skin. Sweep the color up to the crease; you can always add more depth by placing a deeper shade directly in the crease.

Lash curler Lash curlers can take eyelashes from droopy to drop-dead gorgeous. Eyes look more youthful and awake when lashes are curled because it reveals more of the whites and frames your eyes. Gently clamp the curler down on lashes and hold for a slow 15-second count. In our lab tests, we found that the compact Laura Mercier Eyelash Curler increased curl by 149 percent on average. Testers noted it curled lashes quickly and made them appear fuller and more defined.

Lengthening mascara Once you hit your 40s, you want your mascara to be more lengthening than volumizing, says Linter. "Longer lashes open up your eyes." Choose a formula that's also water-resistant to keep mascara from smudging and flaking. For flawless application, press the mascara wand against the base of your lashes for a few extra seconds and then jiggle the brush back and forth as you draw it out to the tips.

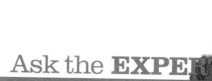

Ask the **EXPERT**

Nina Judar, Beauty Director, *Good Housekeeping*

Q *Are there any tricks to selecting a sheer lipstick?*

Nina says: It sounds obvious, but start by looking for the word "sheer" in the name or label. While a full-coverage lipstick hides your own lip color, a sheer one lets that natural hue show through a bit. Because the colors of sheer lipsticks are softer and more subtle, they don't require as much precision to apply. You can even go a little bit brighter than you normally would. Colored balms, if they have enough of a color boost, are similar to sheer lipsticks, and may be easier to find. If you'd like to give yourself a little tutorial, go to a Lancôme counter and swipe Lancôme L'Absolu Rouge, a full-coverage lipstick, and Lancôme L'Absolu Nu, the sheer version, side by side on your hands. You'll see the difference right away.

Youth Booster #6: Implements for Full, Attractive Lips

Together, lips plus teeth equal your smile. There's nothing like the flash of a healthy, dazzling grin to light up your face and make the years seem inconsequential. As with most of your features, lips evolve with age— their color may lighten or become more irregular, and their overall volume may dip. To plump up your pout, you'll need:

Concealer To prevent pigment from migrating into the lines just above your upper lip, pretreat the area with concealer. Using your fingertip, lightly dot on one that contains reflective particles; you'll block any color transfer, and the light-reflecting particles will minimize the appearance of lines.

Lip liner Using a clear or nude liner that's the same shade as your lips, carefully apply the liner around the perimeter of your lips to define your mouth. Nix the colored pencils; they can leave a telltale ring of liner after your lipstick is long gone.

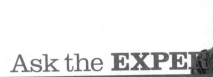

Ask the **EXPERT**

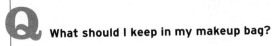

Nina Judar, Beauty Director, *Good Housekeeping*

Q **What should I keep in my makeup bag?**

Nina says: Essentials only. That way it'll be easy to remember your exact routine. And while the pros may give you a laundry list of what your essentials "should" be, this can definitely vary from person to person. If you're no-fuss, then powder, blush, and lipstick may be enough for you to feel put together. I require a *tad* more: I put on a pea-size amount of primer, which makes my tinted moisturizer easy to spread. I brush a concealer-highlighter, like Yves Saint Laurent's famous Touch Éclat, all around my eyes, and then dot on a tiny bit of concealer under each. To complete my eyes, I put on a neutral shadow, curl my lashes, swipe on mascara, and line my inner lower rims. (Most makeup artists say this last step makes eyes look smaller, but for me, it balances out my thick brows.) I swirl on blush and dust on bronzer where the sun would normally add color (across the cheekbones, forehead, and the bridge of the nose). I usually just wear balm or a neutral lipstick, since by mid-morning the color ends up on my coffee cup. Whatever your essentials, the key is to look natural, not overdone. (No one would ever guess my makeup routine takes 11 steps!)

A lip brush This tool gives you optimal precision as well as control over how much color you lay down near the lip border. Dip the brush into your lipstick and dab a little on the center of your lips, then spread it out to the corners.

A sheer, satiny lip color Matte finishes are opaque and drying, and can leave lips looking caked and crumbly. Instead, opt for a sheer shiny or satiny finish. Lip color containing the moisturizing ingredient hyaluronic acid can leave lips looking softer and fuller. Update your look by changing your lip color. If you've been wearing neutrals since the nineties, try red. And if you've been wedded to red, try a pink. Forget the color rules; the danger isn't in the shade, but in a heavy texture. "Anything that's

Smooth, Line-Free Lips

Give off-duty lips some pampering. If lip skin is dry or flaky, gently rub a warm, damp washcloth over lips to slough off dead skin once a week after removing makeup, then pat on a rich lip balm. It will smooth and soften your lips so that lipstick goes on more evenly the next day.

For times when you're not wearing lip color, make sure you use a daily protective lip balm. Lips, like all exposed skin, need a high-SPF, broad-spectrum sunscreen: "UV damage can manifest as inflammation of the lips, redness, and flaking, and, over time, can lead to wrinkling and even cancer," says New York City dermatologist Macrene Alexiades, Ph.D., M.D. Look for a lip balm with SPF 15 or higher.

severe—a lipstick or hairdo—will age you. So wear red, but a sheer one," says Linter. Roses, natural pinks, berry shades, and, if you like something dramatic, true red, can all be flattering.

Youth Booster #7: Dazzling-Smile Do's

Your teeth and jaw physically support your face, so good oral hygiene should be an ongoing priority. Keeping your gums healthy and your teeth free of decay prevents the gradual wearing down and shifting of your bite, which can contribute to the formation of frown lines, vertical lip lines, and even hollowing in the cheeks. Here are the basics:

Use a toothbrush and floss Brush your teeth at least twice a day and floss once a day. Use a soft-bristle brush and, to prevent gum erosion, clean teeth with a short, vertical sweeping motion, not a horizontal scrubbing one. Alternatively, many dentists recommend using an electric toothbrush. When you floss, slide the thread down under your gumline, not just between your teeth. Plaque and bacteria can get stuck in those hidden recesses, causing inflammation and decay.

Warning: Don't Try This at Home

According to cosmetic dentists, **at-home whitening is very safe in general,** but you shouldn't do your own whitening if you have:

- Teeth that are painfully sensitive to cold
- Crowns or fillings on your front teeth (these won't whiten and will end up looking much darker than surrounding teeth)
- Enamel that seems more gray than yellow (due to intrinsic stains from antibiotics such as tetracycline taken during childhood)

Rinse with water Simply rinsing your mouth after every meal is a small move that can make a big difference. And if you've had a glass of wine, it's essential: Wine has acids that penetrate the enamel, allowing staining and decaying food particles to penetrate more easily. But whatever you eat or drink, a subtle swishing and swallowing of water right away at the table or just afterward helps minimize residue, staining, and tooth decay (which also discolors teeth).

Eat a healthy diet You already know that sugar as well as anything that sticks to your teeth (from raisins to crackers) increases your risk of tooth decay, which can discolor—not to mention destroy—teeth. So you should eat less of the sweet and sticky stuff and more fruits and vegetables.

Instant Anti-Ager

Sugarless Gum

"As you age, your salivary glands shrink and produce less saliva, which is a natural antimicrobial that helps prevent decay," says New York City dentist and Supersmile creator Irwin Smigel, D.D.S. "But chewing sugarless gum restimulates the flow without increasing decay."

Research shows that the higher your consumption of folic acid from food (produce being a great source), the lower your risk of bleeding gums. Yogurt may help keep your smile healthy, too. One study found that people who consumed at least ¼ cup of yogurt every day were less than half as likely to have serious gum disease. Researchers believe the magic ingredients are probiotics, so-called "good" bacteria that may compete with cavity-causing oral bacteria.

Have regular checkups See your dentist regularly to make sure your fillings are in good shape (silver, or amalgam, lasts between 10 and 20 years). Also, ask to have the overall state of your mouth and bite assessed. Consider orthodontics if your teeth have shifted significantly. Your jaw shifts along with your teeth, and if left unchecked this can create a collapsed look.

Address your color concerns White teeth are a visual shorthand for youth. Fortunately, you can restore a younger look to your smile with options ranging from daily-use toothpastes to at-home kits to in-office treatments. Teeth naturally discolor over the years, because the outer enamel becomes thinner and more transparent, revealing the darker inner layer, or dentin, underneath. Teeth also absorb colored liquids (coffee, tea, cola, red wine) throughout your life, says Jeff Golub-Evans, D.D.S., a cosmetic dentist in New York City.

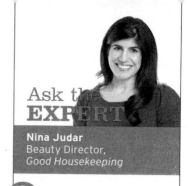

Ask the **EXPERT**

Nina Judar
Beauty Director,
Good Housekeeping

Q *Tooth whiteners make my teeth hurt. Is there anything that can help soothe them?*

Nina says: Sensitivity should be short-lived and subside within a few days. I checked with New York City dentist Brian Kantor, D.D.S., for ways to soothe pain in the meantime. He recommends using a desensitizing toothpaste like Sensodyne or taking an over-the-counter anti-inflammatory like ibuprofen (Advil) or naproxen (Aleve).

the institute investigates

At-Home Whitening Kits

The number of teeth-bleaching procedures performed in dentists' offices has increased by more than 300 percent in the last five years, reports the American Academy of Cosmetic Dentistry. Over-the-counter kits are less pricey than those, but which ones really deliver? GHRI tested three kits and found that all removed some degree of surface stain for most testers, leaving teeth noticeably whiter—though some were easier, better-tasting, and more effective than others.

The product	Tester comments
Aquafresh White Trays	These prefilled trays, worn 45 minutes a day for one week, ranked tops on whitening; on average, all teeth got two shades whiter. Some testers found trays messy or uncomfortable.
Paula's Choice Brighten Up 2-Minute Teeth Whitener	This tooth-whitening stick, which promises to lighten one shade in just two minutes (no rinsing required), visibly lightened the teeth of two-thirds of participants.
Go Smile Smile Whitening Light	The most expensive (about $200), this kit claims to lighten teeth up to six shades after just one 30-minute session. While some volunteers didn't like holding the light, at least half were satisfied with the degree and speed of the whitening.

● Find these top anti-aging products at 7yearsyounger.com/shop.

Most whiteners address the problem with the key ingredient peroxide. This safe-for-the-mouth bleaching agent forms bubbles on enamel that lift away stains. The higher the concentration of peroxide and the longer you leave it on your teeth, the whiter they'll get. The downside: Bleaching molecules can get trapped in nerve passageways, causing increased, though temporary, tooth sensitivity.

Get a Brush-Up

You don't need every brush in the book, but these top tools are ones you should have on hand when applying makeup:

Large flat brush–foundation   **Angled brush**–eyeliner
Small flat brush–concealer   **Spiral brush**–brows
Large fluffy brush–blush   **Small fluffy brush**–eye shadow

Other helpful tools: Cosmetic silk sponges, cotton-tipped swabs, makeup remover (see box, "The Institute Investigates: Eye Makeup Removers," page 81).

Whether you're considering a whitening toothpaste or an at-home kit, Golub-Evans says you can assess your brightening potential this way: Stand in front of a mirror in natural light and hold a piece of white printer paper next to your teeth. If they look yellow, the stains are probably just on the surface—teeth should turn at least a couple of shades lighter with at-home bleaching. If your teeth look grayish, the discoloration likely lies inside the teeth, and bleaching won't help much.

To help lighten or eliminate superficial staining, you've got choices: **At-home approaches** Trays and strips are the most effective at-home choices for dramatic whitening, say dentists. These "barrier method" whiteners keep the peroxide solution against the teeth for the longest time. Daily use can brighten teeth five or more shades. Most brands of trays and strips recommend you use them for around 30 minutes a day until you get the desired shade (usually at least a week). For the most dazzling results, look for higher concentrations of peroxide combined with longer application times. (See "The Institute Investigates: At-Home Whitening Kits," opposite.)

Other kinds of at-home whiteners—whitening toothpastes or rinses—use polishing and other nonbleach agents to either scrub off or chemically remove stains that are closer to the surface. Recently, in a study published in the *Journal of Clinical Dentistry*, researchers assessed a variety of whitening toothpastes. They found that many (especially those containing silica) were highly abrasive and potentially damaging to enamel. They concluded that, in general, these whitening products didn't remove stains much better than regular toothpaste.

Dental-office approaches Your dentist can make custom-bleaching trays for at-home use, and many dentists offer accelerated in-office bleaching options that lighten teeth up to 10 shades in a single visit. This option is pricey—the treatments start at about $400, and you may require more than one. Zoom! and BriteSmile are two of the most popular. They use light to pump up the effects of highly concentrated peroxide. However, any dramatic whitening can fade quickly without at-home maintenance (usually a tray, whitening strips, or toothpaste). Plus, you have to watch what you eat and drink for a couple of days afterward, since tooth enamel is very susceptible to staining for the first 48 hours after treatment. The higher concentration of peroxide also creates an increased risk of temporary sensitivity.

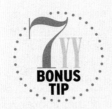

For easy, effective whitening, try Good Housekeeping Seal holder Crest 3D White Advanced Vivid White-strips with Advanced Vivid Technology. Wear them once per day for 30 minutes for two weeks—you should start to see a difference in three days.

Activate Your Anti-Aging Plan Now!

Get the most bang for your beauty buck and effort with this trio of instant-results turn-back-the-clock moves:

1. **Head to a makeup counter** As your skin evolves, so should your makeup. But when was the last time you experimented with a new product or shade? Take advantage of the pros from your favorite makeup manufacturer to get an update on the cosmetics you should consider to rejuvenate your looks. Changes in the tone, brightness, and texture of your skin may mean you need to freshen your palette of colors, opt for more moisturizing formulas, and polish your technique.

2. **Focus on your eyes** Concentrate your makeup efforts on your eyes; well-groomed eyes can lift your whole face. If you're pressed for time, you can skip the liner and shadow and just reach for the mascara. It gives eyes a wide-awake, fresh look that really perks up your face.

3. **Turn up the wattage on your smile** Try a whitening toothpaste or an at-home whitening kit for a few weeks to brighten your teeth. A whiter smile (and more smiling) telegraphs youthfulness.

For more expert anti-aging makeup advice, get our free special report, Best Anti-Aging Makeup, at 7yearsyounger.com/makeup.

Age Eraser 3

Chapter Three

Your Hair— Recapture Its Gloss, Bounce, and Body

Hair is fundamental to your self-image—its fullness, luster, and body telegraph youthful vigor and sexual appeal. No matter the state of your strands now, your hair can be its best— shinier, healthier, vibrant, and more manageable—thanks to our anti-aging techniques for care, cut, and color. In fact, there's never been a better time to recapture your hair's youthful bounce, shine, body, and fullness. Scientists as well as salon pros are much more attuned to age-related changes in hair, which has led not only to the development of better hair-care products, but to expert advice that specifically addresses the needs and issues of women 35 and up. In other words, getting gorgeous hair now is easier than ever.

7 TOP STEPS FOR YOUNGER-LOOKING HAIR

Youth Booster #1: Lather Right

Because it removes the debris and sebum that can weigh down your locks, shampooing is the starting point for creating voluminous hair. But a brush-up in basic technique may be in order, especially since your hair may have changed with the years. For instance, evidence suggests that the width of each hair gets smaller, probably due to hormonal changes. "At some point after 40, hair fibers get thinner and your overall ponytail diameter may shrink," says Wilma Fowler Bergfeld, M.D., senior dermatologist at the Cleveland Clinic in Ohio. In addition, the number of hairs you have on your head starts decreasing in your 20s and may shrink 30 to 35 percent by age 60. According to the American Academy of Dermatology, half of women will have some hair loss by age 50.

You want to maximize fullness while also minimizing damage—and the latter is especially important for keeping hair looking young. Shampoo's main purpose is to cleanse the scalp, preventing the buildup of flaky dandruff and oily sebum. Apply shampoo just to the roots; after you rub gently to work up a lather, allow the suds to run through your hair. No need to scrub the length of your strands; let the product lift away any surface debris. Downplay damage risk by skipping the repeat shampoo; you don't need to do it twice, no matter what the instructions say. Here, answers to key questions about product choice and usage so you don't sacrifice hair volume and health for cleanliness.

How frequently should I shampoo? Wash every day if you have oily hair, live in a polluted city or humid environment, or work out daily. Wash every other day if your hair is normal or combination (with dry ends and oily roots). Wash every few days if your scalp is on the dry side (this includes curly or color-treated hair, as well as most African-American hair).

The Right Shampoo for You

If your hair is...	Use...	And these pro/insider tips
Oily	An oil-free product or clarifying formula	Steer clear of any shampoo with silicone or lanolin on the ingredients list, and avoid two-in-one shampoo-and-conditioners.
Dry	Moisturizing shampoo alternating with a dry shampoo	Look for a brand that doesn't contain the common sudsing agent sodium lauryl sulfate, which can cause hair and scalp dryness.
Normal	Anti-aging or shine-enhancing formulas	Even normal hair can trend toward dullness with age. Choose shampoos that advertise themselves as softness, smoothness, and shine boosters.
Color-treated	Color-protecting formula	Be aware that color-care shampoos may have additional benefits, such as smoothing or volumizing. Choose according to your needs. Look for color-protecting styling products, too.

Can I overdo shampoo? Absolutely. Signs that you're shampooing too often are lots of flyaways and, possibly, little "baby hairs" at the crown. These may be not new growth, but full-grown strands that have broken. Dryness is evidence of overcleansing, too. If your hair is particularly dry, try alternating between dry shampoo and your usual formula. "Dry shampoo cleans and reinvigorates the scalp while sparing your strands the sapping that can come from a shampoo and blow-dry," says Oscar Blandi, owner of the eponymous salon in New York City. Dry shampoos come in spray and powdered forms; instead of washing away dirt, they soak it up. You then brush it out and enjoy fresh volume from the roots up.

Is it best to rinse with cold water? That idea has been around for a while, but there's no science to support it. When you do shampoo the traditional way, use a dollop the size of a quarter (you might need a little more if your hair is long), and don't allow the lather to sit on your hair for long—shampoo can deplete hair's natural oils, which give it luster and body. Work the product in using warm water, which will help dissolve the soap so that your hair rinses clean. Avoid superhot water, as it strips hair of the oils mentioned above, making hair dull and limp. But a cold-water rinse is no panacea—"we've all heard that cool water closes the cuticle and increases shine, but cuticles are not like shutters that open and close freely," says Jeni Thomas, principal scientist at P&G in Cincinnati. "Shampoos are formulated to work in temperatures between 90 and 105 degrees Fahrenheit—a warm to hot shower."

What's the best shampoo to use? Choose a product that meets the needs of your hair type, handles your hair issues, and fits your lifestyle. Don't assume, for example, that because you've always used an oily-hair formula you should continue with it. With age, your scalp tends to lose sebum (oil); by menopause, it may be producing only half as much sebum as it did in your 20s. All this adds up to hair that looks and behaves differently, so, yes, you may need to switch shampoos—because your hair has new needs. If you're not sure what direction to go in next, ask your stylist for a diagnosis.

Youth Booster #2: Maximize Softness and Manageability

Conditioner is the key to making your hair behave and feel soft when you run your fingers through it. Out-of-control hair is more likely to occur as your scalp's production of sebum wanes, leaving you looking flustered, a bit unkempt, and older. Conditioner can help fill in such gaps with moisturizing agents that attach to hair, decreasing flyaways by removing built-up static charge. These products make strands smoother by closing the cuticle so that hairs don't catch on one another; plus, they make hair plumper and more supple. Clear up conditioner conundrums with expert answers to these common queries.

Do I have to use the conditioner that matches its shampoo? The two products are usually sold in sets, and their ingredients do tend to complement one another, but that doesn't mean you have to use them that way. It's OK to use different brands as long as they share a common goal (like shine or curl enhancement). Don't use a shampoo formulated to attack one problem, such as volume, with a conditioner that has a contradictory goal, such as adding moisture; that type of conditioner will weigh hair down, deflating volume.

Can I use a two-in-one shampoo-and-conditioner to save time? Shampoo-conditioner combos don't provide as much conditioning as you'll find in stand-alone products. That can be a good thing if your hair is oily. And if you're seriously pressed for time or space (say, in a gym bag), they are better than skipping conditioner altogether.

How can I get the best results from my conditioner? Proper application is key. Start an inch or two away from your roots (you've already got natural conditioner—sebum—on your scalp) and work the conditioner down to the ends, using just enough to coat the strands. Gently detangle with your fingers or a wide-tooth comb, then rinse.

What if my hair is already thin and limp—won't conditioner make it look droopier? In fact, skipping conditioning will leave strands more

Instant Anti-Ager

On-the-Spot Smoother

Give your curly or textured hair instant youthful suppleness by keeping a travel-size spritzer of leave-in conditioner on hand.

Stash one in your purse or at your desk and treat any areas that start to feel crinkly. Restore the shine and bounce on the spot!

Ask the **EXPERT**

Birnur K. Aral, Ph.D., Health, Beauty & Environmental Sciences Director, GHRI

Q *What's the difference between a leave-in treatment and a serum?*

Birnur says: Use a leave-in treatment as you would a styling product: Put it in your hair and then blow-dry for the best-looking results. It has "treatment" in the name because it's designed to give hair an extra benefit, like adding shine or preventing frizz. The classic example is a leave-in conditioner, which has smoothers that improve the texture of hair. A serum is another kind of leave-in, named for its clear, glossy formula. Serums usually add shine or thicken hair. Like a styling product, a leave-in will wash out with your next shampoo.

vulnerable to breakage, and that can make your hair look even more lifeless. "The cuticles on hair are like shingles on a roof. Conditioner makes those shingles lie flat so they don't rub against one another," says Thom Priano, a hairstylist at Garren New York in New York City. "If you skip conditioner, you get more friction, which in turn further stresses damaged hair." One way to protect hair without adding unwanted weight is to apply conditioner *before* you shampoo. You'll wash out some of the conditioner when you shampoo, but not all of it. You will still have a little smoothing conditioner in your hair, but not enough to weigh it down.

Is using a leave-in conditioner a good idea? If your hair is thick, unruly, or particularly parched, then, yes, your hair will benefit from a leave-in treatment. When you use a leave-in conditioner or serum, start by applying a drop or two and gradually add more if needed. Too much can make strands greasy or limp.

Do I really need a deep conditioner? Masks, or deep conditioners, are designed to remedy dryness, roughness, and dullness with an intense dose of conditioners, including rich, plant-based oils. They're combed through hair, left on for anywhere from three to 15 minutes, and then rinsed out. If your hair is processed, colored, curly, coarse, thick, or damaged, you're a prime candidate for this treatment.

You may have to experiment to find the optimal frequency for your hair. Start by using a deep conditioner or mask every other week—if your hair is fine or thinning, apply it only from mid-shaft to ends to avoid weighing down strands. Or, if you already apply one every other week, see if weekly use leaves strands softer and healthier-feeling without weighing them down. If you already deep-condition once weekly, don't be afraid to up it to twice a week. If you have curly hair, you may want to use masks several times a week; scalp oil travels down ringlets more slowly than down straight strands and may never reach the very tips of your hair.

Youth Booster #3: Recapture Brightness

Nothing makes a more noticeable difference in how youthful hair looks than color. And it's not just because haircolor can cover grays. Even if you still have your natural color, that color gradually fades as the production of melanin (the pigment that gives hair its depth of color) declines. Once production of melanin decreases to a critical level, hair begins to turn gray. By age 50, half of us will be 50 percent gray. That fading comes with side effects: When melanin is present, it absorbs UV rays. In its absence, your hair's protein absorbs them, which damages and weakens strands. Melanin also boosts shine; less of it means duller hair.

The right haircolor can reinstate that natural vibrancy, taking years off your face. The wrong color, though, can have the opposite effect, so careful selection is key. "Really dramatic colors tend to look too severe," says Rita Hazan, owner of the eponymous New York City salon. "The contrast ages you by highlighting every flaw. Severe shades can also cast shadows on your skin so wrinkles look more pronounced." Darkness against a light scalp makes thinning more visible; plus, when grays make a sudden

Fern Richter
"I've got my red hair back— and it's spectacular!"

Fern began the 7 Years Younger program just as she was starting a new full-time job; she wanted to put her best face forward—literally. And in just a few weeks, she did: Once she began using our suggested skin-care steps, the transformation in her complexion was remarkable. "The computer told me that I had gone from 12 wrinkles on my face to five," says Fern, a 42-year-old married mother of a young daughter. The results made her toss out her old routine (just using a cleansing wipe). Fern now maintains a regular morning and nighttime regimen using targeted anti-aging products.

Makeup makeover A self-described cosmetics nut, Fern thought she wasn't going to need much schooling in colors and formulations. In fact, she ended up revamping everything. "I bought a foundation stick

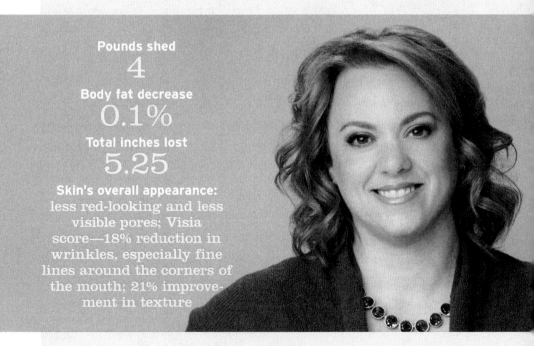

Pounds shed
4

Body fat decrease
0.1%

Total inches lost
5.25

Skin's overall appearance: less red-looking and less visible pores; Visia score—18% reduction in wrinkles, especially fine lines around the corners of the mouth; 21% improvement in texture

to use under my eyes, and started applying blush in a different place and using a shimmery pink eye shadow," she says. "That part was fun. It was my reward for keeping up with the skin care."

Red was right all along Fern had colored her hair red for years, but she had recently gone blonde. Turns out, she had it right the first time, at least according to renowned colorist Louis Licari. "He looked at me and said 'red' and he was right. He took me back to my old color, and it's spectacular." Fern kept her curly locks and followed the recommendation to deep-condition them to prevent dryness, discovering that she only needed to do it once in a while. "Too often, and my curls go limp."

A proven weight-loss meal plan The demands of her new job made it difficult for Fern to cook full meals, so the breakfasts were a lifesaver. "They were phenomenal," she says. "They kept me feeling full for such a long time that I would end up eating a later lunch, which would hold me over until dinner—and sometimes I wasn't even hungry for dinner." By the end of the eight weeks, she'd lost four pounds—and in the following month, she took off another six.

For more about Fern Richter, see color insert.

Want to be a test panelist for a future 7 Years Younger plan? Sign up today at 7yearsyounger.com/panelist to be considered—and get our free weekly e-newsletter, Your Anti-Aging Tip Sheet!

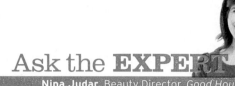

Ask the EXPERT

Nina Judar, Beauty Director, *Good Housekeeping*

Q **My hairstylist suggested that I use a clarifying shampoo. What will it do for my hair?**

Nina says: A clarifying shampoo is what I call a "sometimes" product. That means you should wash with it at most once a week. These shampoos contain a high level of detergents and are excellent for getting rid of buildup if you use a lot of styling and hair-care products. And since these formulas are designed to remove residue from hair, including its own smoothing and protective oils, always follow by using a conditioner. In general, you shouldn't use this type of formula if you color or highlight your hair; it will strip the color (see "How Can I Avoid Washout?", page 107). Clarifying formulas can also help clean an oily scalp, but be careful not to overdo it: Just as over-scrubbing oily skin can dry it out and stimulate oil production, over-cleansing your scalp can also lead to more oil. One I've used over the years is Fekkai Apple Cider Clarifying Shampoo, but just look for "clarifying" on the label of whatever you choose.

appearance, dark shades make them seem even more prominent. On the other end of the spectrum, it's possible to go too light. Light blonde shades can wash out your complexion, requiring more makeup to brighten your features.

If your hair has always been dark, now is the time to go two or three shades lighter with permanent color. And opt for a warm hue. For example, if you are naturally a cool, dark brown, choose a creamier chocolate instead. Adding in a few highlights around your face can help warm things up, too. If you are (or want to be) blonde, a bit of contrast can give your skin a healthier glow. Add in some deeper, caramel lowlights and choose a color that's brightening.

If you're going auburn, the same rules apply: Stay within a few tones of your natural shade. The only caveat: It may require more upkeep.

Red dye's small molecules leach out more quickly than those of any other hue.

How can I go gray gracefully? Some women, when they tire of coloring their hair, consider giving it up—only to march back into the salon or drugstore for color because the grow-out is just too painful. It's never going to be seamless, but there are a few ways to streamline going silver. And with these expert tips, going gray can be stunning.

One approach is to simply get a short cut (though not too short—see page 109) and just let your hair be. Alternatively, you can avoid the two-toned look by covering gray strands with demi-permanent color, which will blend in with grays to make them look like highlights. Once your grays reach critical mass (six months or longer), you can go cold turkey on the dye. The demi-permanent formula will wash out, revealing the gray.

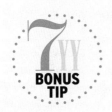

While some demi-permanents claim to cover up to 70 percent gray, in GHRI lab testing, the color looked most vibrant on 30 percent-gray swatches. On those that were 70 percent gray, the color looked more washed-out.

Childhood photos will help predict your future shade of silver: Black hair tends to turn steel-gray; redheads and brunettes often have more gold undertones mixed with their silver; and childhood blondes usually go white. Once the gray has come through, it doesn't have to add 10 years—as long as you keep the color vibrant and prevent yellowing. To do that, you'll need products with shine enhancers and UV filters. On hair that's more than half gray, use a shampoo with blue or violet undertones (look for shampoos with "anti yellow" on the label) to neutralize yellow. Tones in the yellow range tend to cling tenaciously, especially on 100 percent white hair, so consider coloring your hair a light shade of blonde to take the aging effect away.

Pro Tips for Perfect At-Home Color

Do-it-yourself haircolor can look impressively natural—even celebrity colorist Louis Licari, who has salons in New York City and Beverly Hills, thinks so. Here are his tips for healthy, gorgeous results.

Wash a day before This is important if you have a sensitive scalp. When you shampoo the same day, the chemicals are more likely to cause scalp irritation.

Select your shade If you're not sure, pick one that's a shade darker or lighter than your current color. If you make a mistake, you can always fix it, though it's easier to correct too-light mistakes by dyeing over them. **A too-dark slip-up may mean living with it until it fades or grows out.** If you can't commit to a color, try a demi-permanent shade that matches your natural color. You'll get brighter, smoother hair for about three months. Many at-home kits promise to color hair that's 50 to 70 percent gray to last through 28 shampoos.

Dye a test strand Even if you think you've got the right shade, test a length of hair on the back of your head. You can see how the color will turn out, and any "oops" results will be hidden. A test also lets you make sure a new dye doesn't cause an allergic reaction.

Protect your skin Hair dye can soak into your skin and leave a shadow that can last a couple of days—a dead giveaway of an at-home color job. **To stop staining, rub petroleum jelly as close as possible to your hairline, from ear to ear,** without actually touching your hair. This is especially important if you're using certain facial treatments like exfoliating alpha hydroxy acids, which make skin more likely to absorb pigment.

Avoid a one-color block The hair around your face is slightly lighter than that on the rest of your head, and hair becomes progressively darker as it reaches

Since gray hair can be coarser and wirier than your pigmented hair, it may need more conditioning to get it under control. A good choice: conditioners meant for curly or coarse hair, which tend to have softening and smoothing ingredients. Periodically, give your strands a deep cleaning

the nape. Salon colorists mimic this variation by applying a slightly lighter shade around the face. An at-home trick: In addition to your usual dye, purchase a box that's a shade softer and brush it on the first eighth of an inch around your face.

Watch the clock If you're going darker, start the dye at the roots and, in the last five minutes, work the color through to the ends. If you're lightening up, do the opposite: Start at the ends, which should look blonder than the rest of your hair, as they would naturally if they'd been bleached by the sun. Gray hairs can be dye-resistant, so leave the color on for the longest recommended time. Rinse out the color, of course, but wait 48 hours before shampooing so the pigment can soak in. When you do wash, avoid using very hot water, which can open the cuticle and release the dye.

Refresh your color When you touch up your roots, be careful not to overlap with what's already been dyed—you don't want to darken the color you currently have. After you let the dye process on your roots as instructed on the box, squirt on a bit of shampoo and work it through the rest of your hair for three to five minutes to help spread the color. (The shampoo also dilutes the power of the dye, which prevents the ends from absorbing too much color.)

Rethink gray coverage Certain shades, due to their chemistry, are better at covering gray. If you've got resistant grays, switch to a color with "neutral" or "natural" in its name (in other words, choose natural brown over ash brown): It will have the greatest spectrum of colors in the base and provide the most opaque result so grays won't show through.

with a clarifying shampoo to get rid of dulling residues. For upkeep, try a finishing mist that adds shine to your locks, and because gray hair has less natural sun protection (melanin deflects rays), use a hat and/or a UV spray if you're going to be in the sun.

Try a Hair Glaze

A glaze is a clear (rather than colored) semi-permanent salon process that does for hair what a topcoat does for nails or a gloss does for your lips—it adds instant shine. Blonde hair, in particular, dulls more quickly than other colors and can benefit from this boost. While the salon version lasts about four weeks, an at-home glaze, which you rub through hair like a conditioner in the shower, can add shine until your next shampoo, when it washes out. Try John Frieda Clear Shine Luminous Glaze.

Youth Booster #4: Maintain Lustrous, Silky Shine

As much as coloring can transform your hair from drab to dynamic, those same chemicals can leave it feeling dry and rough. Like the natural oils found on your skin, lipids make hair feel soft and smooth, and their loss has a cascade of negative effects. To give your colored hair the TLC it needs, take your cue from our pro answers:

How can I restore shine with haircolor? Cuticles, the outer layers of the hair, are like fish scales across each hair shaft. When they're lying flat, light bounces off them uniformly, and the even reflection produces shine. The active ingredients in haircolor (such as ammonia) lift those layers up so the dye can penetrate to where the permanent color molecules reside. Once your cuticles are roughed up, they scatter light, which makes hair look dull. To smooth down your cuticles (also key for protecting the color molecules once they're in the shafts) and get the shine back:

- **Patch up the cuticles** You can't completely reverse damage, but a repair product that delivers ceramides, hair's intercellular glue, can help replace what might be missing.

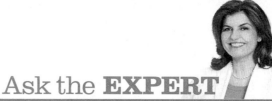

Ask the **EXPERT**

Birnur K. Aral, Ph.D., Health, Beauty & Environmental Sciences Director, GHRI

Q *I have never even heard of root touch-ups! What is the best way to use one?*

Birnur says: There are two kinds of root touch-up products, and these represent a smaller share of the haircolor market. Think of the first as a mini version of permanent haircolor. The package contains just enough to cover the roots. There are typically fewer shade variants in this category compared to the full-blown shade range of a permanent haircolor brand.

The second type, the instant root touch-up, is a temporary solution for visible roots at the temples and the part. These can be applied on the go, as they don't require mixing, and come in different types of delivery systems including mascara-like wands, markers, and sprays. They wash out completely with the next shampoo.

- **Add gloss with a serum or shine spray** They both reflect light for a shiny effect, but just a smidge will do: Too much of either leaves hair greasy. Many color extenders also contain UV filters to fend off sun-induced fading. Still, wear a hat for double protection when you're out in the sun.

How can I avoid washout? Color's worst enemy is water. In fact, the latest research shows as much as 80 percent of color-fade is caused by water alone, not shampooing or scrubbing. Colored hair is more porous, which is why in the shower it absorbs and releases water easily. As water exits, it steals some color molecules, sending your dye job, whether applied at home or in a salon, down the drain. To minimize this water-induced fading, take these precautions:

- **Reduce excessive rinsing** Once you've shampooed and conditioned, don't tilt your head back and just let the water run over it. And if you rely on the shower spray to wake you up in the morning, try to limit your hair's exposure to the water. Pay attention to temperature: Heat makes dye leach out faster, and the hotter the water is, the quicker the color loss.

- **Use a color-protecting shampoo** They're specifically formulated to be both gentle and protective. The exception: If you're using an at-home color, shampoo your hair with a clarifying formula the day before to remove silicone, wax, and hairspray resin. These residues can absorb dye and prevent color penetration into the hair shaft. The result: Less depth of color, so your color fades faster.
- **Shampoo less frequently** Refresh on your off days by flipping hair over and spraying a dry shampoo at the roots to soak up oil and restore volume.

Why does my colored hair feel like straw? Color treatments strip away the protective lipid layer that makes hair feel soft and supple. Your own scalp oils normally rely on hair's fatty layer as a transport system. Without it, they don't distribute themselves well down the length of the hair shaft, leaving strands feeling strawlike. What's more, conditioning ingredients like silicones won't adhere evenly if hair is depleted of its protective oils. So if you think you've been consistently conditioning with no results, it's not your imagination—most of that conditioner is getting rinsed out. Your new hair chemistry demands conditioners specifically for color-treated hair. Using them regularly creates a protective barrier that helps prevent dye molecules from washing out. To maximize the benefit:

- **Condition every time you shampoo,** even if you have fine hair; follow the techniques on page 97.
- **Use a mask once a week** and leave it in as you shower; its intense conditioners are activated by steam.

- **Guard against heat damage.** Flat irons generate heat up to 450°F. In essence, they cook your hair and evaporate its natural moisture. So before you reach for your flat iron, curling iron, or blow-dryer, spray on a heat-protective product.
- **Consider a leave-in conditioner.** Since you're not immediately rinsing it out, a leave-in stays put and does its job.

Youth Booster #5: Update Your Style

The best time machine for your looks? A great haircut. Not only does it help your locks maintain their youthful vitality, it helps compensate for changes in your face that surface as the birthdays add up. "The planes of the face shift and soften over the years," says Eva Scrivo, owner of the eponymously named salon in New York City, "so a haircut needs to provide a balance between structure and softness." When was the last time you refreshed your look? Most women find a style that suits them and never experiment with something different.

Your stylist is the key consultant when it comes to determining what will best complement your hair type, texture, and face shape, but go armed with some idea of what you want. Tear out photos of age-appropriate models and celebs as a visual aid. Here are the style do's (and don'ts) that will create the youthful look you crave:

Do: Shaggy short If you go short, keep it slightly shaggy. You'll look more modern, and the maintenance will be easier without blunt lines. You should soften things as you get older, says Jason Stanton, a hairstylist in Los Angeles and London. A take-seven-years-off option: a length somewhere between your collarbone and chin.

Don't: Too short At a certain point, gamine just looks too gaunt. But if your hair is healthy and plentiful, then go ahead and try a conservative crop.

Do: Choppy bob To keep some length, consider a choppy bob that sits just below the collarbone (unless you have fine hair—see below). Asymmetrical or less-than-perfect shapes deflect attention away from wrinkles.

Don't: Too long Excessive length can drag hair down, pulling your features along with it—the anti-facelift. The worst offender is long, parted-down-the-middle, shapeless locks, which simply date you.

Do: Well-considered bangs One way to bust out of a style rut (and hide forehead creases and eye crinkles at the same time) is to try bangs. But road test them first, suggests Gary Howse, creative director of the Gary Manuel salons in Seattle. Flip some hair from the side or the back of your head and then brush it away—which look do you prefer? Ask for bangs that are full, not wispy (which can make you look older), and that reach the center of your brows. Or opt for a longer, side-swept fringe. But skip both if you've got a stubborn cowlick or tight curls.

Don't: Too faddish Keep your style evolving without becoming a slave to trends. Look for photos of celebrities your age with great hair, and then show your favorites to your stylist.

Do: Blunt layers Longer, more bluntly cut layers add heft to hair and are less prone to frizz and flyaways.

Don't: Curly layers around the crown If you've got curly hair, layers way up top can create a mushroom-like effect (or, worse, a poodle look).

Do: Blunter cuts Fine hair looks best when it's chin- to shoulder-length, with either blunt ends or a few short layers.

Don't: Fine hair with choppy styles Too many tiny layer or razor cuts take away too much volume.

Do: A more subtle approach Minimize layers if you have highlights.

Don't: Multiple highlighted layers The overall effect may be too choppy.

Do: Layers around the face This will give you a soft frame and add volume to your hair.

Don't: Layers on the bottom When you remove thickness at the bottom of your hair, your locks can get stringy, the opposite of what you want.

Youth Booster #6: Build Boundless Body and Bounce

If you've reassessed your cut, it's a good idea to sync and rethink your styling routine, especially if you've noticed any age-related changes. Researchers in Japan have found that hair curvature changes as you age; texture becomes more wiry. The tiny kinks leave weak spots along the hair fiber, making individual strands more vulnerable. Consider, too, that as hair's natural oils are depleted with age, it's more susceptible to damage, so you need to be conscientious about the styling paces you put your locks through. Everything else you'll be doing—shampooing gently, conditioning diligently, coloring carefully, and getting a great cut—will help you get your hair's resiliency back, but it's still wise to avoid overworking those strands. Here's how to handle with care:

Opt for low-impact tools and techniques Combing and brushing are necessities, of course, but they can also injure hair if not done purposefully. Combing is ideal for wet hair, because hair is at its most fragile and prone to breakage when wet. Avoid tugging the comb; instead, smooth out knots, starting at the ends and working up in sections. Though the "100-strokes-a-night" rule is ubiquitous, brushing that much is way too hard on hair at any age. It not only pulls hairs out of their follicles, but it can weaken individual strands. Plus, anything beyond minimal brushing can create too much friction for hair that's turned wiry. Brush your hair only to style it, and if you can get away with using a wide-tooth comb instead, go for it. Otherwise, try a boar bristle–blend brush for detangling and getting your hair into place, and stop there.

Lauren Mintzer
"I can't believe how much healthier my hair is"

When a friend commented that her hair looked really healthy, Lauren, 44, ran her fingers through her strands: It *felt* nice and silky, too! Just a few weeks into the 7 Years Younger program, Lauren was seeing a difference, not only in her hair but in the way her skin looked as well. And to her relief, adopting new beauty habits was simple. "I was able to master the hair and skin routines very easily," she says.

Hair apparent Two of our hair-care tips worked particularly well for Lauren. She began deep-conditioning her previously very dry hair two times a week, leaving the product in for about five minutes. She also broke her habit of shampooing every day and now alternates days. "This involves some planning on my part," says Lauren. "If I'm

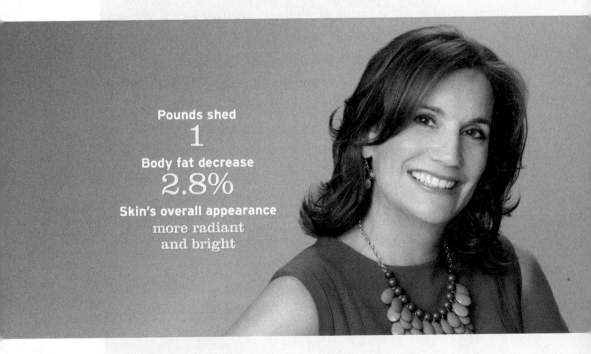

Pounds shed
1
Body fat decrease
2.8%
Skin's overall appearance
more radiant
and bright

going out on a Saturday night, I won't wash my hair on Friday so I can wash it on Saturday. I often end up putting it in a ponytail when I haven't washed it, but cutting back on shampooing is helping my color last longer."

Her makeup wake-up Lauren admits she was never a pro at applying makeup, so now she's taking more time with it. One new addition to her routine: wearing blush, which she had never used before. "I was always pretty good about washing my face and moisturizing, but the combination of wearing makeup and adding an anti-aging serum to my skin-care routine has gotten me a number of compliments," says Lauren.

Exercising more choice The fitness portion of the program was so exhilarating to Lauren, she ended up joining a gym. The variety of activities there has made working out fun, and she mixes it up with a combination of kickboxing, spinning, and Pilates mat classes. "I ended up doing similar exercises to the ones in the program," she says. "I look slimmer now, and I think it's mostly because of the exercise."

Weight loss her way "I really have a hard time with diets," Lauren confesses. Nonetheless, tips from the 7 Years Younger weight-loss plan did ultimately improve her eating habits. "Dinners were difficult for me—I don't love to cook—so I followed the healthy-breakfast and healthy-lunch suggestions," she says. "I found a happy medium."

For more on Lauren Mintzer, see color insert.

Want to be a test panelist for a future 7 Years Younger plan? Sign up today at 7yearsyounger.com/panelist to be considered—and get our free weekly e-newsletter, Your Anti-Aging Tip Sheet!

Protect hair from heat While we don't expect you to completely give up on blow-dryers and flat irons, go easy on the hot tools when possible. Not only does heat dry out hair, but it also picks away at its proteins, another cause of rough hair texture. If your hair isn't frizz-prone, let it air-dry till it's slightly damp and then, once you've spritzed on a heat-protection spray, use a blow-dryer and a big, round brush to smooth out your style. If air-drying increases your frizz, blow-dry straightaway, but avoid washing and styling every day.

Boost hair lift and volume Rollers and curling irons are often the go-to tools for making hair fuller, but they can also create an overly styled, matronly look, says Scrivo. You'll get a chicer look if you use a blow-dryer or flat iron. The exception: If your hair is curly or wavy, air-dry it, then use a small curling iron to define and enhance its natural shape.

If you've never quite mastered blow-drying, don't feel bad—stylists go to school to learn how to do it! One way to hone your skills is to consult a pro: Schedule an appointment and have her teach you how to do it by actually putting the brush in your hands. It's worth the investment. Scrivo's general volumizing blow-drying rule: Don't pull your hair down with a brush as you dry it. Instead, use the brush to raise your roots toward the ceiling so you get more lift at the crown.

If your hair is particularly fine (and thus more easily damaged), a root-lifting product or mousse can give your lank locks volume. And it's a lot easier on hair than another common volumizing trick: back-combing.

Coax curls and waves If your face is angular, soften the edges by wearing gentle waves or curls around your face. If a fuller, round face is your issue, do the opposite—a sleek, straight look is an easy way to instantly counteract heaviness. For shapely ringlets without product-induced stickiness, Ron King of the eponymous salon in Austin recommends a combination of conditioner and gel. Squirt a little of each product onto a

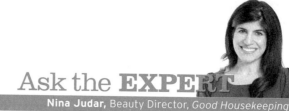

Ask the EXPERT

Nina Judar, Beauty Director, *Good Housekeeping*

Q *Which type of styling product is best for giving my hair a lift?*

Nina says: Your best choice is a root lifter. This product has an ingredient that coats hair, making roots firm so they stand up on end. And root lifters usually have a special nozzle to spritz the formula right on your roots. Apply while hair is damp and then massage it in with your fingertips before blow-drying. If you're looking for all-over fullness, then use a mousse; it's light, so it won't weigh down limp locks. Use a palm-size amount; work through damp hair, then comb through with a fine-tooth comb to distribute throughout hair. Blow out with a round brush to create lift. Quick trick: Flip your head upside down while blow-drying. The heat will set the root in that "upside down" position so once you flip your head back up, your hair will stay lifted.

paper towel, fold the sheet so they blend together, then scrunch wet hair with the product side. "Squeezing the paper towel into your hair keeps the curls clumped together," says King. "Using bare hands can end up unfurling the curls." Once hair dries, gently break up the curls so they're not too stiff. Finish with a dab of silicone serum on any frayed ends.

Weather bad-hair days If you go on the offensive, you can minimize the effects of barometric fluctuations. Try these tricks:

- **Humidity** Silicone-based products are better at locking out moisture than wax- or mineral-based formulas. Check the label to see if the first ingredients listed are words ending in "-one." If humidity is actually your friend (your hair lies flat otherwise), make the most of its plumping effects, but keep strands under control by spraying a volumizer at the roots of wet hair, then

Your Look-Younger Hair Repair Kit

When you have the right tool, the job is easy and gets done right. So think of the following products (all tested by our lab and more than 500 women volunteers) as your look-younger hair-care tools.

Care category	Product	Why it's the top tool
Shampoo and conditioner	Pureology Nano-works Shampoo and Conditioner	A pricey pair (though the concentrated formulas last for about 80 shampoos) took first place for its "rich, thick lather." The color-protecting formula made it popular among panelists with colored strands. Testers also noted that it improved softness and combability. And it got top marks for detangling and protecting strands from further damage.
Shampoo and conditioner	Biolage Rejuva-thérapie Age Rejuvenating Shampoo and Conditioner	More wallet-friendly than the winner; consumers loved how the "clean- and fresh-smelling" duo also helped boost smooth-ness and softness. It also got points for detangling and protecting wet strands from further damage.
Thickening shampoo and conditioner	Nexxus Diametress Luscious Volume Shampoo and Conditioner	In the lab, produced up to a 10 percent increase in strand diameter, especially in gray swatches; testers noted it made hair feel thicker.
Leave-in conditioner	L'Anza Healing Strength Neem Plant Silk Serum	In the lab, this serum increased shine on untreated hair swatches by 250 percent. Testers agreed, giving it the highest shine score and top marks for making their hair feel soft.

●Find these top anti-aging products at 7yearsyounger.com/shop.

Care category	Product	Why it's the top tool
Leave-in conditioner	Biolage Rejuva-thérapie Age Rejuvenating Leave-In Densifier	Notable for its ability to thicken and strengthen testers' hair. Lab testing showed it helped protect hair from breakage.
Deep conditioner	Biolage Rejuva-thérapie Age Rejuvenating Intensive Masque	Testers reported that it made their hair softer and easier to comb when wet. They also noted that it boosted smoothness and shine.
Permanent at-home color	Revlon ColorSilk With UV Defense	Tops at covering gray, both immediately and at four weeks. It also scored high marks for fade resistance. The lab simu-lated a month's worth of UVA exposure and checked the color retention at each one-week mark. The color stayed vibrant, especially the brown and blonde shades tested.
Permanent at-home color	Couture Colour	A panelist favorite for thorough gray coverage; rich, even color; fade resistance; and shine. Its shine-enhancing secret: a one-month supply of pequi oil treatment, derived from the Amazonian fruit, instead of the typical conditioner.
Demi-permanent at-home color	Clairol Natural Instincts	Top marks for both initial and final gray coverage as well as shine retention on hair swatches. Testers found that their hair color was the likeliest to match the labeled color swatch. This product had the least offensive smell and got raves from consumers for making hair smooth, soft, and silky.

Care category	Product	Why it's the top tool
Demi-permanent at-home color	Garnier HerbaShine Color Crème with Bamboo Extract	Kudos from panelists for covering grays and providing rich, even color; also praised for being the easiest to mix and apply.
Root touch-up	L'Oréal Paris Root Rescue 10 Minute Root Coloring Kit	Garnered top scores for seamless coverage and for the accuracy of the color's match with the swatch on the box.
Root touch-up	Clairol Nice 'n Easy Root Touch-Up	Testers reported it was less likely than the L'Oréal to fade over three weeks, and they liked the blue brush applicator.
Temporary root touch-up	Irene Gari Cover Your Gray Professional	Testers noted it covered gray the best and loved how well the shades matched their color, as well as the ease of application. Lab researchers noticed that it was especially popular with curly-haired testers; the lipstick-like stick was easy to maneuver and didn't get tangled in their hair.
Temporary root touch-up	QuickTint	This color-dispensing click pen and mini comb offers the widest range of shades (including six variations of brown). Testers particularly liked that it stayed put when they brushed their hair.
Frizz-taming styler	Remington Style Therapy Frizz Therapy Iron	In the lab and among testers, this flat iron earned high scores for keeping hair frizz-free and sleek—even in high humidity.

applying a dollop of mousse the size of a golf ball from an inch below your roots all the way to the ends. Once hair is dry, mist it with a humidity-resistant hairspray.

- **Sun and salt damage** A hat is imperative, but add a hair sunscreen to your arsenal, too. Hair sunscreens are formulated to protect your strands from the damaging, drying effects of UV radiation. And if you're going to the ocean or pool, tote along a conditioner and apply it often to keep hair hydrated.
- **Static** Mist hairspray onto a brush, then run it over your hair to smooth the strands. When you're on the go, rub a dab of hand cream into your hands and then run hands lightly through hair to tame flyaways.
- **Extreme cold or heat** Periodically change your part so that the same section of your hair isn't always exposed, says William George, owner of the James Joseph Salon in Boston. Otherwise you may end up seeing a lot of breakage.

Youth Booster #7: Bolster Thickness

It's normal to lose *some* hair, about 50 to 100 strands a day. But when you begin losing more, something else is going on. Illness, medication, fluctuating hormones, stress, and simply a genetic predisposition can all bring about hair loss. And unfortunately, by the time the deficiency becomes noticeable most women have already lost about 30 percent of their strands, according to Doris Day, M.D., a dermatologist in New York City. The more hair you've lost, the less likely you'll have regrowth.

Still, there are remedies that can help you keep the hair you have, and a few that can even bring about regrowth. It's important, though, to act fast, because the most effective treatments are for retaining hair rather than stimulating follicles that have been inactive for long periods. If you think something's amiss, get to a dermatologist, who can give you treat-

the bottom line

Are Keratin Hair-Straightening Treatments Safe?

This pricey but popular salon process leaves kinky hair straight, sleek, and frizz-free, but concerns have been raised that the formulas may contain formaldehyde, a known carcinogen. The Good Housekeeping Research Institute conducted its own analysis, testing four salon brands—Brazilian Blowout, Marcia Teixeira, Keratin Complex by Coppola, and Global Keratin Light Wave—at an outside lab for the presence of formaldehyde. We found the toxic chemical in all four products, at levels exceeding the Cosmetic Ingredient Review's 0.2 percent recommended threshold. The Oregon OSHA (Occupational Safety and Health Division) also tested hair-straightening salon treatments and found that many of those advertised as having no formaldehyde did in fact contain the chemical.

In separate tests of a new at-home version, Salon Favorite Do-It-Yourself Treatment Kit, GHRI found no formaldehyde, but discovered the presence of glutaraldehyde, a chemical from the same family. Glutaraldehyde is not currently on any restricted-chemical lists; however, exposure to it can still affect eyes, skin, and lungs.

No sooner had we sounded the alarm than members of Congress began calling on the FDA to issue a voluntary recall of two hair-straightening treatments in salons sold under the name Brazilian Blowout. The evidence is piling up: If you seek sleekness, use a flat iron instead.

---

ment options. There are also some things you can do to help hide hair loss. Here's a rundown on both.

How a Pro Can Help

Check your hormones Often the culprit behind hair loss (for both men and women) is a high level of testosterone. Getting a measurement of male hormones can determine if you have polycystic ovarian syndrome or other conditions tied to elevated testosterone. If you do, your doctor might prescribe birth control pills or hormone-replacement therapy as a remedy. Low thyroid hormones and anemia can also produce hair loss, so your doctor may test you for these, too.

Get the twice-a-day cure Only one hair-raising drug is FDA-approved for women: minoxidil (brand name: Rogaine). It works by turning fine hairs into thicker ones. "As hair follicles get older, some make shorter, finer hairs, called indeterminate hairs, similar to the ones we all normally have around our hairline," explains dermatologist Dr. Zoe Draelos. "Those hairs can be turned into thick ones by Rogaine." It happens to be more effective on the crown, where most women experience loss, than on the sides. Because the rate of hair growth is normally half an inch a month, you'll need three to six months to notice a difference; if you discontinue the drug, the results will subside.

Consider off-label use of a different drug The other hair-loss drug, finasteride (brand name: Propecia), is approved by the FDA for use on men only. While some doctors prescribe it off-label for women, it's only safe for women who are past childbearing age, because the drug acts on hormone receptors and can cause the feminization of a male fetus. As a result, it's only been studied in postmenopausal women, and in that group, Propecia did not lead to hair growth. "I think it didn't work because researchers picked older women whose hair loss, due to their age, was too advanced," says Dr. Draelos. Depending on the degree of your loss, your doctor may advise you to combine minoxidil and finasteride: Each drug acts on a different mechanism in the hair, and multiple approaches can maximize your results.

What You Can Do

Use styling camouflage Avoid heat, overstyling, and tight, pulled-back styles, such as ponytails—the constant pull weakens the hair follicles.

Whenever possible, let your hair air-dry. If you do blow-dry it, prep locks with a heat-protective primer, then turn the dryer to the low or medium setting, or use a diffuser on curls. Between washes, boost volume by spritzing dry shampoo at the roots. The powder formula adds texture.

Get help at a salon Often a hairdresser can do more for you than a doctor. Hair-thickening options include a layered or shaggy cut, deep bangs that mask sparse areas around your temples, or a "messy" style with an off-center part. Hair dye may be the best medicine, since adding color can rough up the cuticle, which makes hair drier but thicker (to reinstate moisture, try a once-weekly mask). Avoid extremely dark or light shades, which both draw attention to the scalp. And build depth with a few carefully placed highlights or lowlights around the face—but just a few, as too many highlights may weaken strands.

Activate Your Anti-Aging Plan Now!

Want an almost-instant way to look years younger? Here's your ticket:

1 **Brush up on your care basics and technique** Your hair is changing right under your fingers: Researchers have found that hair texture becomes more wiry with age, making individual strands more vulnerable to damage. Hormonal changes may also shrink the width of each hair with the years. That means you may need to readjust the way you shampoo, condition, and style your hair.

2 **Fast-forward your look** Updating your cut, color, or style is a sure-fire way to look and feel 7 years younger. Your stylist is a key consultant when it comes to determining what will best complement your hair type, texture, and face shape, but you should do some homework of your own. Tear out photos of age-appropriate models and celebs to bring to your appointment. You'll get the best results when you communicate your ideas clearly.

3 **Discover—and use—special-effects shortcuts** Take advantage of the plethora of products now available to recapture your hair's youthful bounce, shine, body, and fullness. Glazes, masks, color touch-ups, and even hair-protective styling products can help compensate for any current shortcomings in the look and feel of your hair.

For more expert anti-aging beauty advice, get our free special report, 40 Best Anti-Aging Beauty Secrets, at 7yearsyounger.com/antiagingsecrets.

Age Eraser 4

Chapter Four

Rejuvenate Your Diet (and Your Looks)

magine looking younger and feeling lighter, having boundless energy, and knowing that you're enjoying energy-packed, nutritious, and delicious foods that will help rejuvenate your looks and extend your life. Imagine all that *and* not feeling hungry! That's what this anti-aging weight-loss plan delivers.

First up, this chapter shows you how to fortify your meals and snacks with fabulous, nutrient-packed foods that slow down aging. These foods protect your body from visible signs of age, such as lines and wrinkles, and also make you healthier by keeping your bones strong and maintaining cholesterol and blood sugar at the right levels. Other foods on the plan help lower chronic, body-wide inflammation— a culprit in diseases like arthritis and diabetes (it's exacerbated by being overweight)—and many of them contain compounds that eliminate free radicals, those unstable molecules that damage or destroy cells.

Just as important as what you add to your eating plan is what you cut back on. The foods recommended here provide nutritious and satisfying alternatives to those loaded with unhealthy fats and refined carbohydrates (such as white sugar, white flour, and white pasta), which hasten the aging process and increase your risk for aging-related illnesses like diabetes, heart disease, and cancer.

What else you'll be paring down: calories. The 7 Years Younger nutrition strategy is your answer to addressing those pounds that may have crept on over the years. It's not unusual for women over 20 to gain up to 10 pounds per decade. By featuring a moderate calorie intake as well as plenty of delicious, appetite-thwarting foods, this plan will help you lose weight once and for all. (You can see how it all comes together in the 7-Week Plan, beginning on page 277.) Attaining a healthy weight is a critical part of age-proofing your body: Besides being linked to many diseases that can shorten your life, obesity is associated with age-accelerating inflammation. Plus, losing weight can not only make you more youthful, but also lessen the impact of some symptoms of menopause. Researchers at the University of California, San Francisco, for instance, found that women who lost weight through diet and exercise had fewer hot flashes. And finally, maintaining a healthy weight can make you feel lighter, more energetic, and more confident about your appearance—all of which are bound to put a youthful spring in your step!

YOUR 7 YEARS YOUNGER BLUEPRINT FOR A BETTER BODY

Youth-Boosting Step #1: Enjoy Foods That Fight Wrinkles

Study after study has shown that a diet high in antioxidants slows down the signs of aging and improves longevity. Antioxidants disarm free radicals, the rogue oxygen molecules that are created naturally by the body—as well as ingested and inhaled—and that damage cells. One family of antioxidants, the polyphenols, have been shown to inhibit the inflammation and tissue damage associated with aging, notes James L. Hargrove, Ph.D., of the University of Georgia in Athens. Vitamin C, another potent antioxidant, supplies the body with the active ingredient it needs to remodel and reconstruct skin's collagen.

In the Sister Study, a major National Institutes of Health research project following healthy sisters of breast cancer patients, women whose diets included lots of the antioxidant vitamins C and E had longer telomeres, the pieces of DNA that cap the ends of chromosomes, protecting them from damage. (Having shortened telomeres is associated with physical signs of aging.) A diet high in antioxidants is also linked with lowering the risks of cancer, heart disease, and diabetes.

Anti-wrinkle agents are easy to slip into your diet: Just think plant foods. Fruits and vegetables are among the foods richest in antioxidants. As part of your lunch, make a big spinach salad with two cups of greens. Throw in a half-cup each of tomatoes, sliced red pepper, and mushrooms, and you've already heightened your antioxidant intake for the day (and that's not even including a fruit dessert). There are other good sources of antioxidants—plant-based, but not ones you'd associate with produce—that deserve a spot in the antioxidant hall of fame, too. (Surprise! Coffee is one.) Here's how to make sure you get a good variety of antioxidant-rich foods:

Choose color-coded plants Typically, fruits and vegetables that are deeply colored have the most antioxidants. Two in particular to set your sights on are berries, which are full of vitamin C, and dark leafy greens—particularly kale, spinach, and collard greens—which are prime sources of the antioxidants lutein and zeaxanthin. These plant pigments (that's where the color connection comes in, as many pigments have antioxidant properties) help protect your eyes from the harmful effects of ultraviolet light. Dark, leafy greens are also rich in vitamin K, a nutrient that plays a role in reducing bone loss and preventing fractures. And these vibrant leaves are a source of zinc, a known anti-inflammatory. Zinc also helps break down damaged collagen, clearing the way for new collagen to form, smoothing surface lines in skin.

Reach for whole grains Not only are whole grains super sources of fiber (see page 138 for more on the other benefits of whole grains), but they're also particularly rich in polyphenols. You'll hit the gold mine for this wrinkle fighter by reaching for the right breakfast cereal. In 2009, University of Scranton chemistry professor Joe Vinson, Ph.D., measured the polyphenols in whole-grain flours, ready-to-eat whole-grain foods, and snacks. Breakfast cereals—especially whole-grain cold cereals—and popcorn came in on top, with antioxidant contents comparable to those of fruits and vegetables (for more on popcorn's healthy benefits, see page 153). Whole-grain flours, like those used to make whole wheat bread, scored high, too. Overall, whole-grain foods had significantly more antioxidants than processed grains.

Season it up Herbs and spices don't just make food taste better; they can help you look younger for longer periods of time. Spices are also loaded with polyphenols. Even a sprinkle can carry potent health benefits in addition to the anti-aging beauty bonus. Every shake helps, so sprinkle the following spices on your food liberally and often:

- Thyme, rosemary, parsley, sage, oregano, spearmint, and pep-permint all have been shown to contain anti-tumor properties that may reduce the risk of cancer. Both fresh and dried have benefits, although ounce for ounce, dried have a higher antioxidant count.

- Cinnamon is associated with preventing blood clots, improving circulation, and lowering the risk of heart attack and stroke. It may also help stabilize blood sugar, reducing the risk of type 2 diabetes.
- Turmeric shows promise in helping to curb diseases such as Alzheimer's, cancer, and arthritis.
- Red chili peppers are being probed for their potential to lower cholesterol and boost fat-burning.
- Cumin, thyme, and rosemary may cut the formation of heterocyclic amines (HCAs), the cancer-causing compounds found in meats cooked at high temperatures.

Some easy ways to work herbs and spices into your diet: Sprinkle cinnamon in your latte or on top of oatmeal (aim to get one-half to one teaspoon a day), or try a low-sugar cinnamon-flavored cold cereal—Vinson found that cinnamon boosts the antioxidant content of whole-grain cereal, so you get a double benefit if you pick a cinnamon-flavored whole-grain breakfast cereal. (Cinnamon would boost the antioxidant power of whole-grain toast, too.) Dust food with a quarter-teaspoon of turmeric or cumin, or use Indian-style recipes, which often call for these spices. Add cumin, dried thyme, rosemary, or sage to a marinade and then rub on more before cooking meat.

Youth-Boosting Step #2: Enjoy More Fat-Burning Foods

One of the best ways to combat aging is to develop a lean body—and eating lean protein can help you get it. Protein is more satisfying than fat or carbohydrates, so by bolstering your protein intake, you're going to feel fuller with less food, eat fewer calories, and lose weight as a result.

Muscle-boosting protein also becomes a key dietary component starting in your 40s, when muscle mass begins to decline by up to 1 percent a year. That drop in lean body tissue slows metabolism, which makes the pounds pile on more easily. The extra weight, in turn, puts your health at risk, and down the road, diminished muscle mass can throw off your balance (upping chances of a fall), sap your strength, and even threaten your ability to recover from an illness or accident. As part of the Framingham Osteoporosis Study, researchers looked at the protein intake of over 900 men and women with an average age of 75. Those who ate the most protein had a significantly lower risk of hip fracture. Since bone density didn't differ much, the researchers believe that the protein may have helped prevent breaks by increasing muscle mass and strength in the lower body.

Backed by this and other studies, the 7 Years Younger weight-loss plan calls for slightly more protein (five to seven ounces from seafood, poultry and pork, and plenty of additional protein from dairy, nuts, beans, and eggs). Eating more protein will help you keep your calorie intake lower, because the calories from protein do a better job filling you up and keeping you full than those from refined carbs. Plus, protein gives your body the nutrients to build and replace lean body tissue. And since lean tissue,

Instant Anti-Ager
Drink Your Vegetables

Sipping a glass of vegetable juice daily can help you attain your antioxidant quota, say researchers from the University of California, Davis. In their study, more than half of the participants who drank one glass of the juice a day were able to meet the goal of five daily veggie servings (eight ounces of vegetable juice counts as two servings), compared with less than a quarter of those who had no juice. Stash a six-pack of the mini cans in your desk or glove compartment for an on-the-go snack. One mini is a little more than a single serving.

such as muscle, is metabolically active (meaning it burns calories to maintain itself), the more muscle you build, the higher your overall metabolism. While higher in protein, this weight-loss plan is also low in saturated fat. This type of fat, which lurks in marbled cuts of meat, poultry skin, and full-fat dairy products, is known to raise cholesterol levels, increasing the risk of heart disease.

Lean proteins are what you should be shopping for, and those include skinless chicken and turkey breast, lean beef and pork (such as tenderloin), eggs, tofu, beans, and seafood. Nuts, although not lean, are another nutritious source of protein and a worthwhile addition to your diet in small amounts. You can get a picture of a perfect protein-rich day by flipping forward to the "Weight-Loss Meal Plan" in the 7-Week Plan on page 279.

Other ways to pack your diet with healthy protein: If you swap out red meat for poultry, fish, or legumes, you'll trim your saturated fat intake by 15 percent. One reason researchers believe the centenarians in Okinawa, Japan, home of some of the longest-living people in the world, have such youthfulness and vitality throughout their life spans is that they eat very little meat. Although they eat ample amounts of protein, it's mostly in the form of tofu, miso (a paste made of fermented

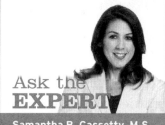

Ask the EXPERT

Samantha B. Cassetty, M.S., R.D., Nutrition Director, GHRI

Q *What about fruit juice? Can you drink your fruits, too?*

Sam says: While 100 percent fruit juices, like orange juice, have a wealth of good-for-you nutrients, drinking rather than eating the fruit will cost you in calories—there are 110 in an eight-ounce glass of OJ compared to 50 in a small orange. The juice also lacks fiber (a small orange has over two grams), so those additional calories don't do a good job of controlling your hunger. That's why I suggest reaching for a piece of fruit as a snack and using juice to add an element of flavor to a meal, as we've done with our Pomegranate-Glazed Salmon (see page 354).

soybeans), and fish. Following suit will help you get the same longevity benefits—and you can also add lean chicken and turkey to the list.

Consider, too, that when you replace meat with whole-food vegetarian substitutes like beans and tofu, you get not only protein, but antioxidants and age-erasing nutrients. The 7 Years Younger plan includes many vegetarian options. To work more vegetarian protein into your diet every day, think about instituting "meatless Mondays," and expand your repertoire with the vegetarian NBS—No Better Stuff—nuts, beans, and soy seeds. (For portion sizes, see the chart on page 134.)

Nuts

Nuts such as walnuts, almonds, cashews, peanuts, macadamia nuts, and pistachios are high in fiber and "good" monounsaturated and polyunsaturated fats, including heart-healthy omega-3 fatty acids. And, despite being a high-fat, high-cal food, nuts don't promote weight gain. The reason: People find nuts filling and, after eating them, offset some of the calories by eating less later on. Best of all, up to 20 percent of the calories in nuts don't get absorbed. Researchers aren't sure why, but people who eat nuts at least five days a week live longer than people who eat them infrequently. That effect seems to be independent of age, race, and whether the nut-eaters do or don't eat meat. Still, nuts are high in calories, so eat them sparingly.

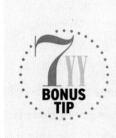
BONUS TIP

Sprinkle almonds or walnuts into cereal or top baked sweet potatoes with crushed peanuts. Nuts are also great mixed into salads, or paired with a piece of fruit or sliced veggies as a snack—the **fat in nuts helps increase the absorption of nutrients in produce.** Don't forget luscious nut butters, either. A serving of almond or peanut butter on whole-grain bread is a perfect lunch.

Beans and Lentils

These little protein powerhouses are nutritional fountains of youth. For starters, they're rich in fiber, including the soluble kind that research shows may help reduce belly fat (see page 140). Substituting beans for meat on a regular basis also slashes your intake of saturated fat, which can accelerate signs of aging. If you eat just half a cup of pinto beans a day, you can potentially slash your bad LDL cholesterol 8 percent or more in eight weeks. Considering that every 1 percent drop in LDL can lower heart disease risk by up to 3 percent, that's a strong case for eating more beans (other beans like white and black share most of pinto beans' healthy properties). Among the disease-fighting phytochemicals beans and lentils contain are saponins, which (in the lab, at least) inhibit cancer-cell reproduction.

To get more beans and lentils into your diet, add them to vegetable soups and salads, and pair them with rice or pasta. Make them the centerpiece of vegetarian chilis, spoon them into quesadillas made with low-fat cheese, or substitute them for beef in tacos.

Soy

Soy is an excellent source of isoflavones, powerful hormone blockers that researchers believe may play a role in the Okinawans' lower rates of breast cancer. Choose soy in whole rather than processed form: Tofu (add to soups or stir-fries), edamame (frozen whole soybeans can be microwaved for a quick snack), and miso (good for marinades and soups) are all healthy ways to get isoflavones. Other whole-soy sources include soy nuts (a convenient snack) and soy milk. For a quick smoothie, blend chocolate soy milk with a small banana and ice. Whole soy is better than the processed forms found in granola bars and veggie burgers; these foods contain soy isolates that don't have the same good-for-you properties.

How Vegetarian Sources of Protein Stack Up

When you think of protein, meat, fish, and poultry inevitably come to mind. But don't forget these vegetarian alternatives: nuts, beans, seeds, and soy. In addition to protein, they provide you with antioxidants and fiber.

Nuts, beans, seeds, and soy*	Calories
Almonds, 1 oz. (23 whole)	163
Cashews, 1 oz. (about 18 whole)	157
Macadamia nuts, 1 oz. (10 to 12)	204
Peanuts, 1 oz. (about 32 whole)	166
Pistachios, 1 oz. (49)	159
Walnuts, 1 oz. (14 halves)	185
Black beans, ½ c.	227
Chickpeas, ½ c.	269
Kidney beans, ½ c.	225
Lentils, ½ c.	227
Pinto beans, ½ c.	245
White (navy) beans, ½ c.	255
Chia seeds, 1 oz.	138
Flaxseeds, 1 oz. (ground)	74
Pumpkin seeds, 1 oz. (¼ c.)	158
Sunflower seeds, 1 oz. (¼ c.)	165
Edamame, ½ c.	127
Miso, 1 Tbsp.	34
Tofu, firm, 3 oz.	72
Tofu, silken, 3 oz.	40
Soy nuts, 1 oz. (⅓ c.)	97

* Without added oils
  Source: USDA Nutrient Database

Youth-Boosting Step #3: Enjoy Foods That Ease Inflammation

Omega-3 fatty acids, found primarily in cold-water fish, are anti-aging multitaskers. These essential fatty acids may help deflate inflamed pimples, calm red skin, battle free radicals, and smooth fine lines. Another years-younger bonus: Fatty fish also contain zinc, which spurs cell growth and renewal. And there are even more benefits: Omega-3s decrease disease-related inflammation, extend telomere length, improve cognitive function, and lower the risk of cancer and heart disease. Recall from Chapter 1 that consuming fatty fish helps guard against sun damage so skin stays beautiful. Omega-3s may also reduce blood pressure, and they have blood-thinning qualities that may prevent clot formation. Some of the longest-living people in the world—Icelanders, Swedes, and Europeans living on the Mediterranean diet—are big fish eaters, and researchers believe that's one reason for their longevity.

If you need more incentive, consider that in a European study of 2,031 elderly men and women, researchers found that those who regularly ate seafood performed significantly better on cognitive tests than those who ate little or none. The more fish the study subjects ate—top performers averaged 2.6 ounces a day—the better they did.

To ratchet up your omega-3 intake, get at least two three-ounce servings of omega-3–rich seafood a week. The best sources are wild salmon, various types of tuna (including albacore), mackerel, anchovies, herring, sardines, and lake trout. Think beyond fillets and steaks, too. Enjoy smoked salmon with your morning eggs (but go easy on the portion size—smoked salmon contains a lot of salt) or add canned tuna to a spicy tomato sauce and serve over pasta. You can also toss minced anchovies into your salad—they add zip without being too fishy.

If you don't like fish, non-seafood sources of omega-3s include walnuts, flaxseeds, canola oil, pumpkin seeds, chia seeds, and tofu. These all contain a compound (ALA) that the body converts into a similar benefi-

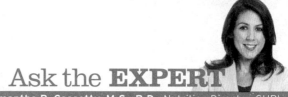
Samantha B. Cassetty, M.S., R.D., Nutrition Director, GHRI

 How much of every type of food do I need to eat?

Sam says: While following the 7 Years Younger weight-loss plan, you don't have to worry about daily servings and portion sizes—I've worked it all out for you. I designed the plan with an array of tastes and textures borrowed from different cuisines so that every time you sit down to eat, you'll discover delicious flavor in satisfying portions. I know you'll enjoy the results: If you follow the plan to a T, you can expect to lose the unwanted pounds that may have crept on over the years, and the diet will help you improve your overall looks and health. But even if you don't choose to follow my suggested menu, you can still get substantial improvements in how you look and feel. The following chart sets out your basic game plan.

If you're used to following government recommendations on nutrition, you may notice some differences here. I've included more produce—a wonderful source of anti-agers—and I advise that you stick with an assortment of easy-to-find, simple-to-prepare whole grains (rather than overly processed refined ones). The plan also ups your daily protein intake: Aim for a mix of animal and vegetarian protein foods even when you're devising your own menu. All that protein will really help you get a handle on hunger while also supplying crucial nutrients. Keep in mind that on any eating plan, amounts vary from day to day; just try to get it all in during the week. I also encourage you to treat your family to some of the meals and snacks suggested in this book. After all, everyone benefits from healthy eating—and somehow meals taste even more delicious when you're eating with people you love.

cial omega fatty acid—though it takes a lot more ALA to get adequate amounts of the other "good" omegas.

Another option: a daily supplement. Unlike broccoli pills, these are valid sources of omega-3s. Find one that contains 1,000 milligrams of the

Food	Number of daily servings	What's a serving?
Dairy	2 to 3	1 c. milk or yogurt; 1½ ounces cheese
Fruits	2 to 5	1 medium whole fruit, ½ c. cut-up fruit, or ¼ c. dried fruit
Protein	5 to 7 ounces from animal sources including pork, beef, seafood, eggs, and poultry, plus equivalent amounts from other sources such as nuts, beans, seeds, and soy	3 ounces meat or seafood; ½ c. cooked beans (= 2 ounces meat); 2 tablespoons peanut butter or 1 ounce nuts or seeds (= 2 ounces meat); ½ c. tofu (=2 ounces meat)
Vegetables	3 to 6	1 c. raw leafy vegetables, ½ c. cut-up raw or cooked vegetables, or ½ c. vegetable juice
Whole grains	3 to 5	1 slice bread; 1 c. ready-to-eat cereal; ½ c. cooked hot cereal; ½ c. cooked rice or other grains such as quinoa, faro, barley, bulgur, or polenta; ½ c. cooked pasta

fatty acids DHA and EPA. Both types of fatty acids are important, but DHA in particular is known to promote brain health. Be sure to read the fine print, too: The label may claim 1,000 mg, but it's often the case that only 30 percent of that comes from the right fish fats.

Youth-Boosting Step #4: Enjoy Foods That Brighten and Smooth Your Skin

Whole grains are rich in several B vitamins, which encourage the growth of fresh new skin cells, giving your skin new radiance. And switching to whole grains is a healthy move overall; a raft of research has shown that they offer protection against diabetes, heart disease, stroke, colon cancer, high blood pressure, and even gum disease. These benefits are tied not only to their vitamin content, but also to their minerals, plant chemicals, and fiber. That's why refined grains, which are stripped of these nutrients during manufacturing, don't offer the same advantages, even when some nutrients are added back later in the process.

Whole grains also have another asset that can roll back the clock: They promote weight loss. A research review of these diet-friendly foods—which include whole wheat, oats, brown rice, and the bread, cereal, and other products made from them—found that a menu loaded with whole grains helps you stay slim, thanks in part to fiber's role in appetite control. Their low rankings on the glycemic index (a system that rates the effect of different carbohydrates on blood-sugar levels) may also play a role. (See, too, "Enjoy the Belly-Flattening Power of Fiber" on page 140.) Here are some strategies for reaping the benefits of whole grains:

Bulk up your breakfast You can increase your consumption just by making over your morning meal. Surveys show that busy women tend to eat more or less the same breakfast on most days, so a simple whole-grain upgrade can make a big difference. Like toast in the morning? Make it with whole-grain bread (look for a loaf with at least three grams of fiber per slice and whole wheat at the top of the ingredients list). Cereal fans: Go for a whole-grain variety or an oat-based choice like Cheerios or oatmeal itself (even instant counts). Oats deliver heart-friendly soluble fiber. In one study that followed 9,776 women and men for 19 years, those who ate about six grams of soluble fiber a day (roughly the amount in a bowl

Time for an Oil Change

Changing what you slather on your toast and drizzle into the pan when you're cooking can add years to your life. **Your first step:** Put away the butter, a source of saturated fat, which can cause skin-aging inflammation (see page 63) as well as drive up cholesterol. **Next:** Start cooking with olive or canola oil, both of which are rich in monounsaturated fats. In one Norwegian study, **people who ate more unsaturated (and fewer saturated) fats had healthier levels of LDL** (so-called "bad" cholesterol) and heart-boosting HDL ("good" cholesterol). "As long as you're not overeating, having good fats instead of butter and even instead of some carbohydrates like bread, pasta, or other starches is a heart-healthy eating strategy," says Washington, DC, registered dietitian Mary Dickie, M.S., R.D., who counsels people at risk of heart disease.

Instead of butter for your toast, think margarine—but make certain you choose a trans-fat free "buttery" spread or stick, since regular stick margarine is a prime source of trans fats. Reviled by cardiologists as "Frankenfats" because they clog and inflame arteries, trans fats still show up in many processed foods, too—especially baked goods. You can't always go by the product label, since **foods that deliver under 0.5 grams of trans fats per serving are legally permitted to claim to have no trans fats.** Some non-dairy creamers, for example, are labeled "0 trans fats" because they're under the 0.5-grams-per-serving limit. But use several teaspoons of these to lighten your coffee, and you could get an unhealthy dose, says Dickie. The best strategy: Check the ingredients list and avoid anything that contains shortening or partially hydrogenated oil.

of oatmeal, a half-cup of barley, and a pear) had a 15 percent lower risk of heart disease than those who consumed less than a gram a day.

Work whole grains into the rest of your day Most markets now carry brown rice, whole wheat pasta (including whole wheat couscous), and even grains like quinoa, barley, bulgur, and polenta. Look for whole-

Lower Your Salt Intake

The fluid retention caused by sodium makes your entire face (including your undereyes) puffy. It doesn't stop there—fluid retained in the skin on your bottom and thighs can dimple them, making cellulite worse. For the salt-sensitive, high intake over time may also have a more serious health consequence: high blood pressure. Go easy on the shaker (the Daily Value for adults is 2,400 mg), and be vigilant when it comes to processed foods—they contribute 75 percent of the sodium in the typical diet. Depending on the food company, you may find surprising sodium counts in minestrone soup (690 mg per cup), salad dressing (340 mg and up per 2 tablespoons), pasta sauce (480 mg and up per ½ cup), frozen pancakes (580 mg per 3 pancakes), American cheese (277 mg per slice), baked beans (550 mg per ½ cup), and bagels (490 mg per bagel).

Look for breads, cereals, snacks, and condiments with no more than 400 mg sodium per serving (250 mg sodium per 2 tablespoons of salad dressing is ideal). Pizzas, frozen soups, and packaged meals, however, will range higher. Assess the nutrition facts, not just what the front label says. Even some products marked as lower in sodium can still be very salty: Reduced-sodium chicken noodle soup, for instance, can have up to 600 mg of sodium and still be considered "healthy" in terms of FDA labeling guidelines. You can also counterbalance the impact of sodium by increasing your intake of potassium and magnesium, which aid in lowering blood pressure (sources include bananas, broccoli, cantaloupe, lima beans, oranges, spinach, and sweet potatoes).

grain baguettes in the bread aisles. Replace regular pasta with the whole wheat kind, white rice with brown (it takes longer to cook, so plan accordingly or buy quick-cooking varieties)—the perfect base for a stir-fry with vegetables and lean protein. Use high-fiber faro, bulgur, and whole wheat couscous in grain salads or as side dishes.

Enjoy the belly-flattening power of fiber Increase your intake to 10 grams of soluble fiber a day, and you may lose the deep abdominal

How to Spot Whole Grains
In the Ingredients List

It's a whole grain if it's called...	It's refined grain if it's called...
Brown rice	Corn flour
Buckwheat	Cornmeal
Bulgur or cracked wheat	Degerminated cornmeal
Millet	Enriched flour
Quinoa	Multigrain (this simply means it's composed of various grains, not necessarily whole ones)
Sorghum	Pumpernickel
Triticale wheat berries	Rice
Whole-grain barley	Rice flour
Whole-grain corn	Rye flour or rye
Whole oats or oatmeal	Stone-ground wheat (though stone-ground *whole* wheat is a whole grain)
Wild rice	Wheat
Whole rye	Wheat flour
Whole spelt	Wheat germ (not a whole grain, but it's still good for you)
Whole wheat	Unbleached wheat flour

visceral fat, the kind that ruins your waistline. It's also considered a health threat, as it's associated with high blood pressure and higher rates of diabetes and liver disease. Researchers at Wake Forest University School of Medicine found that people who ate more than 10 grams of soluble fiber a day gained less dangerous belly fat during the course of the five-year study than those who ate less. Soluble fiber is the predominant component in oats and in many fruits and vegetables. One way to hit the 10-gram mark: Start your day with a cup of oatmeal topped with a

Diane Gurden
"Winning at weight loss taught me that I have control over my looks and my life"

Making lifestyle changes often requires overcoming life's many little obstacles and interruptions. But a five-day power outage? That's what Diane, 43, had to endure when a surprise October snowstorm struck during the middle of her 7 Years Younger program. She had to throw out everything in her refrigerator and freezer and basically lived on bagels for a few days. Instant diet disaster! "But when it was over, I stepped back and said to myself, 'My goals are important,' so I went right back and filled up my kitchen with the right food."

Diane's determination ultimately helped the married mother of two young girls lose a considerable amount of weight in just eight weeks. And the 7 Years Younger weight-loss plan, in particular, was a revelation. "There were certain foods that I always knew were good

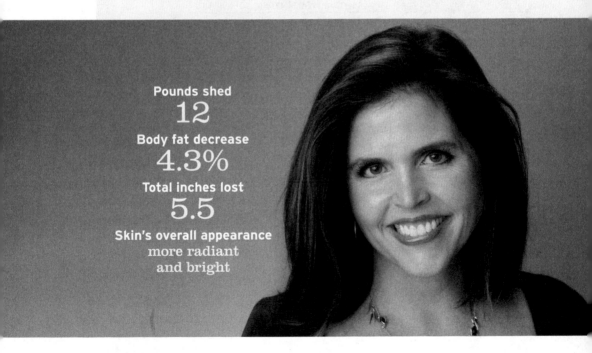

Pounds shed
12
Body fat decrease
4.3%
Total inches lost
5.5
Skin's overall appearance
more radiant
and bright

for me, but I couldn't figure out how to add them to my life," says Diane. "Suddenly, I'm putting Greek yogurt and guacamole and blueberries in my grocery cart and I know what to do with them. The weight-loss plan opened my eyes."

Her attitude adjustment Diane told us that if she was going to make the program work, she'd have to stop being a "mommy door-mat." She's asked the kids to take on more chores, and now the family calendar doesn't just have the girls' swim practices on it; it has Diane's Zumba class and other activities, too. "I don't have to be first on the list, but I now have to be *on* the list," she says.

A makeup update What little makeup Diane did wear wasn't helping her turn back the clock on her looks: "I'd been buying the same lipstick since high school." Advised to tone down her lips and play up her eyes to look younger, she relinquished her bright matte go-to in favor of a lighter, more sheer lipstick with a little gloss on top. ("It took me a while to figure out I had to blot the gloss—I was looking a little like Britney Spears in the beginning," she says.) She also practiced applying her makeup so that she was able to get her new routine—concealer on her lids and under her eyes to hide dark circles; a peachy, shimmery eye shadow; blush; and mascara—down to a convenient two minutes. Now she doesn't go out without doing it.

Biggest surprise "I found out that by taking better care of myself in every way, not only can I be a better mom," says Diane, "but I can do everything in my life better."

For more about Diane Gurden, see color insert.

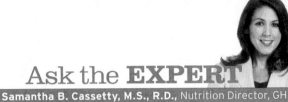

Ask the EXPERT

Samantha B. Cassetty, M.S., R.D., Nutrition Director, GHRI

Q *Do I need to take a multivitamin on this diet?*

Sam says: It's always better to get your nutrients through food—that's why the 7 Years Younger weight-loss plan is designed to help you meet all your vitamin and mineral recommendations.

At this point, whether taking a multivitamin extends life is debatable. In the Sister Study, the NIH research project following healthy sisters of breast cancer patients, women who took multis had longer telomeres, the protective caps on chromosomes that are an indicator of a cell's age. In this study, multis seemed to slow the aging process, but there's no other compelling evidence to suggest they lengthen life. We do know, though, that a multivitamin can't replace a nutritious diet. If you're not following the diet and are not meeting the recommendations for calcium and vitamin D, supplements for just those two nutrients might be in order (see page 146). Otherwise, stick to a nutrient-rich diet and forgo the multi.

chopped apple; have a sandwich on whole wheat bread for lunch, an orange for a snack, and a cup of cooked broccoli as a side with dinner. Other soluble fiber stars: dried beans, peas, and prunes.

Youth-Boosting Step #5: Enjoy Foods That Make You Taller and Thinner

Proper posture and body alignment go a long way toward helping you look slim and vital, so it pays to feed your bones. Calcium, of course, is key for a healthy, strong skeleton, especially as the years pass. Bone loss begins in your 30s and accelerates after menopause as levels of estrogen diminish (the hormone plays a role in protecting bone). Physical activity is critical for saving bone, but diet—especially dairy foods—also plays an essential role in keeping you independent, strong, and standing up straight.

Dairy products are not the only source of calcium, but they're particularly rich in the mineral. Many dairy products are also fortified with vitamin D, and they all provide protein—important because protein also contributes to your bone health. Calcium can't build bone if you're not getting enough protein, and current recommendations—about five ounces a day for a 145-pound woman—are too low, says Robert P. Heaney, M.D., professor of medicine at Creighton University in Omaha. That's one reason why the 7 Years Younger eating plan proposes heftier amounts of protein per day, from both animal and plant sources. And it's a key reason why this is a surefire way to help you lose weight once and for all.

Dietary calcium has other advantages, helping to reduce blood pressure and lower colon cancer risk. It's also critical to keeping your cardiovascular system young and vital. And dairy appears to have benefits of its own. A Japanese study found that eating a quarter-cup of yogurt a day led to a 50 percent reduction in tooth loss and a 60 percent lower risk of gum disease, possibly because of the probiotics in yogurt (probiotics are beneficial bacteria found in yogurt but not other forms of dairy).

Women need 1,000 mg of calcium a day (1,200 if they're postmenopausal), which translates to three (eight-ounce) servings of nonfat milk or yogurt, four and a half slices of reduced-fat cheese, or any combo of milk and cheese that equals the higher recommendation of three servings as outlined on page 137. Food is always a better source of nutrients, including calcium, than pills are.

The case for skinny versions The 7 Years Younger plan calls for low-fat or nonfat milk products exclusively—and for good reason. Full-fat dairy not only nearly doubles your calories, it ups your intake of age-accelerating saturated fat. If you're used to full-fat (about 3.25%) dairy, you can wean yourself off by starting with 2% milk, switching to 1% after a few weeks, and then either staying there (it's pretty low in sat fat) or making the move to fat-free (skim). Another option: use a protein-fortified ("plus")

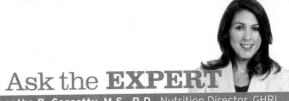

Ask the **EXPERT**

Samantha B. Cassetty, M.S., R.D., Nutrition Director, GHRI

Q *Is it OK to use two to three tablespoons of half-and-half in my coffee instead of skim or 1% milk?*

Sam says: At 20 calories per tablespoon, half-and-half actually has twice the calories of whole milk. If you're keeping calories steady by following our 7 Years Younger weight-loss plan, that amount once a day won't derail you. But more than two to three tablespoons a day and the calories will start to add up. I suggest you try to kick the half-and-half habit by mixing a tablespoon of the rich stuff with a tablespoon (or two) of 2% milk. Once your taste buds adjust to the blend, eliminate the half-and-half and try the same approach until you're using only 1% milk. Another option—and the one that I choose for my morning pick-me-up—is to go with an alternative to cow's milk. My favorite is soy milk, but almond milk can stand up to coffee, too. Just be sure to select something that has no more than 100 calories per cup—the same as 1% milk. The rich flavors in these beverages mean a couple of tablespoons go a long way.

variety of fat-free milk, which tastes creamier than regular fat-free. You'll be surprised how your palate adjusts to the lower-fat options. If you have milk with cereal, you'll hardly notice the difference, and you can jazz up plain low-fat or fat-free yogurt with flavorful fruits and other mix-ins, as you'll see in the plan.

The vitamin D anti-aging connection Vitamin D is turning out to be a nutrient that's vital in ways that we never knew before. For instance, in a British study of 2,160 women, researchers compared subjects' blood levels of vitamin D to changes in their telomeres. In the analysis, the difference between women with the highest and lowest levels of D was equivalent to *five years* of aging. Other studies have linked D to better heart health, lower blood pressure, reduced breast cancer risk, and a weight-loss boost.

With sun exposure, the skin converts an existing provitamin to vitamin D, though that ability diminishes somewhat with age. Not long ago, the Institute of Medicine, the health arm of the National Academy of Sciences, raised the Recommended Dietary Allowance for D to 600 IUs (up from 200 to 400) for adults. But many experts, including David L. Katz, M.D., M.P.H., director of the Yale-Griffin Prevention Research Center in Derby, CT, believe even the new figure is too low. "Considering that the likelihood of benefit is very high and the likelihood of any harm is remote, I think many people, particularly in more northern areas [where you get less D from the sun], could benefit from 1,000 to 2,000 IUs a day," says Dr. Katz. As one of the few whole-food sources of vitamin D, dairy can provide a chunk of that—eight ounces of milk has 100 IU (milk is fortified with D, but not all dairy products are). So can fatty fish (salmon has 310 IU per three ounces).

Look beyond dairy Statistics show that about two-thirds of Americans don't eat enough dairy products to supply the calcium and vitamin D their bodies need. If you eat little or no dairy—or you're lactose-intolerant—there are also other foods that can help you meet your daily goal. Kale, collard greens, Chinese mustard greens, broccoli, okra, and bok choy all contain calcium that is well-absorbed by the body (one cup of cooked kale, for instance, has 179 mg, and cooked collard greens are a star at 357 mg). Note that some greens like spinach, chard, and beet greens contain oxalic acid, which binds with calcium and reduces absorption. Other good sources of calcium: tofu processed with calcium sulfate (check labels); fortified soy, rice, and almond milks; almonds; and calcium-fortified orange juice. Beyond their calcium content, fruits and vegetables also promote a bone-strengthening acid-base balance in your bloodstream, which helps to keep the skeleton strong.

If you're not getting many (or any) calcium-rich foods into your diet, then taking two 500-mg or 600-mg calcium supplements, one in the morning and one in the afternoon or evening, is a good idea. (Your body

Ask the **EXPERT**

Susan Westmoreland, Food Director, GHRI

Q *I want to drink more water, but I find the taste pretty boring. How can I jazz up the flavor?*

Susan says: Try one or all of the following:

- Add a sprig of fresh mint or a slice of lemon, lime, or orange for flavor.
- Steal this spa secret: Each day, fill a pitcher with the amount of water you want to drink, then add cucumber slices or spears. Aim to empty the pitcher by day's end.
- If you're out and buying water, look for one of the no-calorie flavored waters on the market.
- Choose sparkling water, seltzer, or club soda, all of which have a little more pizzazz—and can potentially help you lose weight. According to a University of Ulster and University College Dublin report, the carbonation tricks your tummy into thinking it's full. Look into the home machines that add fizz to plain tap water.

only absorbs about 500 mg at a time, which is why two doses are usually better than one.) If your intake of calcium-rich foods falls somewhere between "lots" and "some," a single daily dose is OK. When supplement-shopping, read labels. Both calcium carbonate and calcium citrate are good sources of the mineral. The difference is that calcium carbonate is cheaper, but needs to be taken with food for effective absorption. The pricier calcium citrate can be taken at any time. Citracal has a 1,200-mg slow-release calcium citrate version that you take once a day.

Youth-Boosting Step #6: Drink to a Healthier, Fuller Life

Many beverages have anti-aging, lifespan-boosting benefits. There are a few exceptions, so when you reach for something to slake your thirst, keep this info in mind.

Water This should be your go-to drink. Every cell in your body needs water to operate effectively. So you need it daily, and plenty of it. The anti-aging effect? Water boosts your skin's moisture content; dehydrated skin has a gray cast. Plus, water can plump skin and make wrinkles less obvious. As if that weren't enough, water fills you up, with no calories! The question of how much is optimal has been kicked around a lot, but the Institute of Medicine, comes down on the side of letting thirst be your guide. In addition to the glassfuls you drink, you also get water from juicy fruits, vegetables, soups, and even caffeinated beverages. And keep in mind that if you drink water before a meal, research suggests that you'll consume fewer calories once you sit down to eat (see page 167).

Coffee The fact that coffee has anti-aging virtues may come as a surprise, because it's often considered a vice. But moderate amounts of coffee may lower the risk of type 2 diabetes, melanoma, and Parkinson's disease. Evidence also suggests that moderate coffee drinkers have better memories and a lower chance of dying from heart disease. Some of the benefit may come from caffeine, but coffee also contains chlorogenic acids, antioxidants that might play a protective role, too.

Tea Drinking tea may lower your risk of heart attack and stroke, strengthen your immune system, fight cancer, protect tooth enamel, and help fight memory loss associated with aging. Some research has shown that green tea can fight weight gain (only in mice so far—but worth trying, we say). But it's not just one type of tea that deters aging. Have at least two cups a day of green, black, white, or oolong tea—their leaves all come from the camellia sinensis, or tea plant. And their polyphenols, fluoride, and caffeine—which are thought to contribute to these health benefits—are largely missing from herbal brews. Still, don't count herbal tea out just yet. Research from the Jean Mayer USDA Human Nutrition Research Center on Aging at Tufts University shows that chamomile tea has significant blood-thinning activity, which may be heart-protective, and that peppermint tea has strong antioxidant and antitumor actions. One clinical trial also showed that drinking three cups of hibiscus tea daily for six weeks lowered high blood pressure in a group of adults.

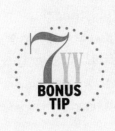

You'll get the most anti-aging benefits from tea if you brew your own: Testing done by the biotech company WellGen found that **bottled teas have fewer polyphenols than home-brewed.** Of the six brands analyzed, only half contained the disease-fighters, and amounts ranged from a measly 3 mg to 81 mg per 16-ounce bottle. Compare that with a cup of steeped green or black tea, which delivers 50 to 150 mg.

Alcohol More than 100 studies suggest that light to moderate drinkers have a lower risk of cardiovascular disease, and data from the Nurses' Health Study showed that middle-aged women who had a drink five to seven days a week had a 50 percent higher chance of aging successfully than teetotalers—that is, they were more likely to be free of illnesses like cancer and heart disease, cognitive decline, and physical impairments.

For all the good news about alcohol, there's still some question about whether drinking increases the likelihood of breast cancer. Research results have been mixed, although a recent study of over 1 million women in Britain found that those who drank the most (15 drinks or more a week) had a 2.6 percent risk of being diagnosed with breast cancer over seven years, compared with a 2 percent risk for those who had two or fewer drinks per week: not much of a difference in risk. Lighter drinking had even less impact.

Overused, alcohol can lower longevity—not to mention age your skin

Instant Anti-Ager

Improve Your Pour

It's fine, even healthy, to have a drink each day—as long as you stick to what constitutes "a drink." When we asked a group of wine fans to pour themselves a glass of red or white as they would at home, most of them did pretty well (five ounces) when using small (10-ounce and 12-ounce) glasses. But when testers were given a 28-ounce glass, nearly half of them overpoured by an average of two ounces. That's 40 percent more alcohol than a standard drink—a difference that tacks on 50 calories and can chip away at the one-a-day health payoffs. To get a just-right visual marker, fill a measuring cup with five ounces of water and pour it into your stemware. That's as far as you should go the next time you uncork—and keep that line in mind when you're sipping at a restaurant, where overly generous pours seem to have become the norm.

more rapidly—so moderation is key. Most experts agree women should limit themselves to one drink a day. Watch your portions: A "drink" is defined as five ounces of wine, 12 ounces of beer, or one and a half ounces of 80-proof distilled spirits. Some (but not all) research suggests wine may deliver the most benefits, thanks to being rich in grape antioxidants. As to the question of red or white, science hasn't shown that one type is clearly healthier than the other.

Youth-Boosting Step #7: Enjoy Healthy Snacks That Flatten Your Belly

It may seem virtuous to do without snacks and treats, but deprivation can lead to overindulging, adding pounds that age the body faster. One study found that women who put their favorite noshes on the verboten list actually ate 1.4 ounces more. More concrete terms may help you understand the extent of the potential diet damage: One ounce of potato chips contains about 160 calories, so eating 1.4 ounces hikes up your calorie intake to 224. The take-home: Labeling foods as off-limits may backfire on your weight-loss efforts.

It's key to find that happy medium: snacks and sweets that help deter excessive eating and even have some nutritious, anti-aging value of their own. Here are guidelines to help you nibble without a quibble.

Make smart switches Feel like a snack? Reach for something plant-based. Every time you have a fruit, vegetable, or whole grain as a snack or dessert, you're increasing your antioxidant intake as well as your disease-defending, age-thwarting power. Find dozens of snack-substitution ideas in the 7-Week Plan on page 277.

Shun the sweet stuff Sugar and other refined carbohydrates increase the creation of AGEs, which interfere with repair of collagen and elastin. But the age-accelerating effects of AGEs go even further, exposing cells in the body to more oxidative stress and inflammation (for more on AGEs as they relate to nutrition and skin, see pages 39 and 63). Research from Washington University in St. Louis also suggests that a diet over-loaded with fat and sugar may cause cell death, setting the stage for diabetes and even heart failure. Moderation is your ticket to staying young and healthy.

Instant Anti-Ager

Suss Out Where Sugar Lurks

Sugar by any name tastes as sweet—and ages you by increasing production of advanced glycation end products, or AGEs (not to mention your calorie intake). As you shop, check ingredients lists carefully. Sugar's aliases include glucose, fructose, sucrose, lactose, and maltose. High-fructose corn syrup, brown-rice syrup, agave syrup, maple syrup, evaporated cane juice, cane crystals, fruit-juice concentrate, honey, and molasses are all other names for sugar. Pass up products that list any of these among the first three ingredients.

Don't forget popcorn! Popcorn is a whole grain, rich in fiber and anti-oxidants—if you make it yourself. Even a small bag of movie-theater pop-corn can set you back 19 grams of saturated fat and 400 calories. Yet if you microwave your own 94-percent-fat-free butter-flavored popcorn (Jolly Time is one brand), you'll get all the whole-grain, high-fiber pluses of the snack—without the fat or extra calories. You can also cook popcorn on the stovetop with a hand-crank pot using surprisingly little oil—just a tablespoon per half-cup of kernels works well (get an additional payoff by using heart-healthy canola oil).

For added flavor, try one of these mix-ins:

- 2 teaspoons chili powder, 1 teaspoon cumin
- 2 teaspoons smoked paprika
- 3 tablespoons grated Parmesan cheese, $1/4$ teaspoon garlic powder, $1/2$ teaspoon red pepper flakes

Reach for the right chocolate Research shows that due to its antioxi-dant content, a little *dark* chocolate (milk chocolate doesn't have the same properties) keeps arteries functioning better, lowers bad LDL cholesterol and blood pressure, and helps improve blood flow to the skin and the brain. It can also lessen the odds of heart failure by 32 percent. To bite into its multitude of benefits, check out the low-calorie chocolatey snack options in our plan. You'll find them on page 335.

PUTTING THE PLAN INTO ACTION

Making the healthy choices outlined in the previous section can put you on the fast track to weight loss. Since so many of those foods fill you up with fewer calories, you can drop pounds simply by making these switches. But you can still have too much of a good thing, which is why your eating behavior has to come into play, too. The advice offered here will help you steer clear of obstacles that can make it harder to stay inspired and stick to a healthy way of eating. Up ahead, you'll learn how to manage your mindset, stress level, willpower, and schedule in ways that can keep you on the path to success.

Stick-To-It Strategy #1: KISS Away Failure

It's not enough to just look in the mirror and vehemently resolve that you're going to do something about your weight *right now*. The real key is to combine your emotional commitment with a clearheaded approach to setting up and achieving your weight-loss goal. And when it comes to formulating your goals, **K**eep **I**t **S**imple and **S**traightforward. Some guidelines:

Make realistic resolutions It's easier to get big results by making smaller, manageable changes rather than trying to do too much at one time. Only you know how much you can handle. Most diet-related resolutions actually require several simultaneous behavior changes: You not only have to shop and cook differently, you need to make different choices at restaurants and parties. Be honest with yourself about what you can accomplish and how much weight you can lose. When formulating your goals, avoid making draconian pledges. "Absolutes like 'I'm giving up all sweets' or 'I'll never eat butter again' set you up to try to get around your own overly strict rules," says Connie Stapleton, Ph.D., a psychologist in Augusta, GA. Instead, try drafting more limited restrictions like "I'll have dessert only when I'm in a fancy restaurant."

Compose a weight-loss contract In a study looking at predictors of success of goal-setters, researchers at Dominican University of California found that those who wrote down their aspirations were more likely to reach them than people who merely made mental vows. Commit your aspirations to paper, post them in places where you'll see them often (on the refrigerator, above your desk, on a bathroom mirror). Not only will it keep you accountable, but it just may (re)inspire you. "You want to be able to recapture again and again the intensity of that moment when you decided to change your life," says Marvin D. Seppala, M.D., chief medical officer at Hazelden, the addiction-treatment center.

Sweat the small stuff While it's helpful to have big-picture goals, also concentrate on the small stuff as you go along. Make resolutions that require small acts of will, not weeks of vigilance. For instance: "This week I'm going to work on drinking less soda and more water" or "This week is devoted to eating more whole grains." You'll feel good when you accomplish each goal, and your success will help bolster your resolve: The better you are at making small changes, the greater your sense of accomplishment will be, and the easier it will be for you to keep going. Write down your accomplishments as you go, and post them, too, to provide a visual reminder of your successes.

Keep track Once you've written down your new nutrition and pound-loss goals, don't stop recording. Keeping a food diary is another way to up the odds you'll successfully slim down. Nutrition experts have long advised dieters to log their meals and snacks (and any food eaten in between), and the advice was confirmed by researchers at Kaiser Permanente's Center for Health Research in Portland, OR. In a study of nearly 1,700 participants, those who kept daily food records lost twice as much weight as those who skipped the recording. And the more faithful they were about recording their meals each day, the more weight they lost.

Now it's easier than ever to keep track of what you're eating. There are many food diaries available, and any time you're out and don't have access to your diary, whether you use a hard-copy version or a virtual one, you can just jot down what you've consumed so you can add it to your diary later. Carry a little pad with you or, if you have a smartphone, simply text or e-mail yourself.

Stick-To-It Strategy #2: Work Up Your Willpower

Willpower isn't just a steady, steely resolve that some people are born with and others missed in the genetic lottery. It's comparable to a muscle: The more you use it, the stronger it gets.

When your willpower breaks down, that doesn't reflect a lack of self-discipline. Especially when it comes to food, there are strong biological factors we're all working against. As Joseph Shrand, M.D., an instructor of psychiatry at Harvard Medical School, explains, self-restraint is a rational desire, which means it lives in the front of the brain, the section that's most recently evolved and most vulnerable to being overruled by survival instincts. Pleasure, on the other hand, resides in the brain's most primitive portion, which has spent millions of years learning to reward us with a deeply satisfying jolt of dopamine when we give in to these kinds of urges. And while that brain circuitry evolved to encourage life-prolonging desires like eating and sex, says Dr. Shrand, we now get a rush from giving in to *anything* we want, whether it's an illicit drug, chocolate, or buying expensive purple peep-toe boots—even when the more evolved part of our brain tells us we'll quickly regret it. So you can see why getting the rational side of your brain to win out takes a little work.

Muscle up your willpower... The interesting thing about willpower is that it's transferable. If you can demonstrate determination in one area, you can often show it in another arena as well. In an experiment at the University at Albany–State University of New York, researchers asked 122 smokers who were trying to quit to exert extra self-control for two weeks, either by avoiding sweets or by squeezing on a grip-strengthener for as long as they could twice a day. Another group either did math problems or kept a diary. In the following month, 27 percent of those who were diligent about practicing their self-control exercise successfully kicked their cigarette habit, compared with just 12 percent of volunteers

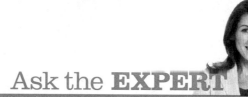

Ask the **EXPERT**

Samantha B. Cassetty, M.S., R.D., Nutrition Director, GHRI

Q *Should I weigh myself while I'm on the plan? If yes, how often?*

Sam says: When you're on the plan, research suggests that weighing yourself regularly is the way to go—as long as you keep it within reason—because it helps keep you on track.

Once you reach your goal weight, step on the scale regularly. The National Weight Control Registry (NWCR) is an ongoing project that collects data on people who have lost at least 30 pounds and kept them off for a year. Turns out that three-quarters of those losers hop on the scale once a week to keep those lost pounds in check; if the numbers go up, they take measures to lower them again.

Weighing yourself during maintenance is crucial. That way, you can spot when the scale starts to creep up and do something about it right away before five pounds turns into 25. As in everything, moderation is key. Weigh yourself just once or twice a week, often enough to remind you to keep your goals in sight, but not so much as to make yourself crazy.

who'd been given a task that didn't call for self-control. To try this at home, squeeze a grip-strengthener (available at sporting-goods stores for under $10) or a rubber ball till it becomes uncomfortable, then hold your grip as long as you can. Repeat at least twice a day and see if practicing self-control rubs off in other areas of your life, helping you to keep your hands off foods you normally can't resist.

...And visualize to boost it That primitive-cravings center in the brain is highly susceptible to visual cues, explains Tufts University psychologist Christopher Willard, Psy.D. Draw on the strength of images by putting a photo of a younger, thinner you on the fridge or mirror, or by hanging a pair of skinny jeans on the closet door to remind yourself of what you're working toward.

Give yourself a break occasionally As with a muscle, push too hard and you'll damage your willpower. "If you're very hungry, I can't imagine that any amount of willpower will keep you from eating a cupcake," says Mark Muraven, Ph.D., psychologist and author of the quit-smoking study. And even if you're not hungry, expecting too much of yourself can put you in the danger zone. Dieters who go cold turkey on everything often feel overwhelmed, and that can sabotage willpower.

Remember your accomplishments Whenever you feel your resolve waver, think about what you've accomplished in the past. "People beat themselves up about still needing to lose the baby weight or no longer going to yoga class. But they overlook the long list of things they have done that required major self-discipline, like building a nest egg or sticking with the computer training they needed in order to get a better job," says psychologist Elizabeth Lombardo, Ph.D. "Write down 100 things you're proud of, right down to 'I get out of bed when I don't want to.' It'll remind you how much willpower you really have."

Stick-To-It Strategy #3: Line Up Support From Family and Friends

You are your own best advocate. Just by picking up this book, you've shown that you're motivated to look and feel younger, and, ultimately, that's what's going to help you eat more healthfully and get a younger, leaner, more disease-resistant body. But you live among other people, some who can unintentionally thwart your anti-aging efforts (family members who plead for unhealthy favorite foods), and some who can help (the friend who wants to team up to lose weight). Focus for now on those who can help, because research shows that having a support system in place is an achievement enhancer.

For instance, in the Dominican University study on successfully meeting goals, the people who had the most success not only wrote down their

Can You Stick to a Diet?
You Can Bet on It

If you were to put your money where your mouth is, would it help you lose weight? The fact that bets on dieting have popped up everywhere—online, in gyms, at weight-loss classes, and as informal wagers among friends, spouses, and coworkers—suggests that a lot of people think a financial incentive works. Some research backs that up: A multicenter study of 57 dieters found that those who stood to lose money if they didn't shed weight were about five times more likely to reach their goal than those with no financial stake in the outcome. **Half of the bettors met a goal of losing 16 pounds in 16 weeks,** compared with just 10.5 percent of the no-wager group. And in a study of more than 200 dieters at the University of North Carolina at Chapel Hill, those who were told they'd pocket $14 for every 1 percent of body weight they shed were nearly five and a half times more likely to take off 5 percent of their body weight than participants not offered cash.

To some, putting money, ego, and bragging rights on the line is a potent formula for keeping motivation up. "If eating chocolate cake tonight means you'll lose $10 or $50 at your next weigh-in, dessert suddenly isn't very attractive," notes Dean Karlan, Ph.D., a Yale University behavioral economist. After losing 40 pounds in a personal bet with a friend, Karlan went on to found stickk.com, one of the first online habit-changing betting sites: **"When there's something big at stake, you can't say, 'Oh, I'll eat less next week.** I'll work out longer tomorrow.' You have to stay on track all the time, because doing the wrong thing would be very expensive." The trick, of course, is to be able to keep up the good work once the wager is over.

aspirations, but also shared them with a friend. In other words, they had someone who could hold them accountable if they were to stray from their course of action. Some participants in the study went even further by sending a weekly progress report to a friend—and they had the most success of all, reaching an average of 76 percent of their goals (the people who shared their commitments but didn't check in still realized an admirable 64 percent of their stated goals).

The study participants who sought out support might have done better because friends tend to give positive feedback. Social approval—as in "You look great!"—gives your brain a surge of soothing oxytocin, the neurochemical equivalent of a warm hug, explains Dr. Shrand.

Harnessing the power of others Sometimes it's not enough just to spread the word to close family or friends; you also need to let them know how they can help you, says Stefanie Barthmare, a psychotherapist with The Methodist Hospital's Weight Management Center in Houston. As you're assembling your support network, consider:

- **What do you need help with?** Start by making a list of what you need, which will help you be clearer and more organized as you ask for help. Maybe you need advice on grocery shopping or menu planning, someone who's a good listener, or a partner to help you stick to an exercise program. Perhaps it's inspiration or accountability that you need.

- **Who is best suited for what?** Match people you know to your needs. No one person may be able to handle your whole list, but most people can follow through with a request for something specific. If, for instance, you have a friend who cooks healthful food, she might be able to help you plan lower-calorie menus. If exercise is your Achilles' heel, find someone who can be a workout buddy or who'll check in with you to make sure you're on track. Maybe what you need is someone to let you vent when you're feeling stressed or angry, so you don't take it out on a piece of chocolate cake. On the home front, you may need to enlist the support and understanding of family members as you restock your kitchen cupboards and make more nutritious meals.

- **When will you need help?** Target certain times of the day when you'll need support (would a call from a friend on the way home from work be helpful in planning the evening?). It might be that too much alone time on a Sunday means boredom-eating. Maybe scheduling a yoga class at the local Y or a walk with a friend for the next three Sundays would be a good strategy for getting out of that pattern.

Try crowd power Joining a Web-based weight-loss program that includes expert counseling and access to chat rooms and message boards can be another beneficial form of support. Researchers from the University of North Carolina at Chapel Hill and Brown University found that people who followed these types of diet programs lost an average of 13 to 15 pounds in six months. In a similar study done in the U.K., the women who had the best outcomes from Web-based dieting were those who used the online forums, suggesting that the social support provided by the websites is key. "Getting to know others who are on the same path and who can relate to what you are doing will go a long way toward increasing motivation to stay on your plan," says Barthmare. "Additionally, online networks of weight-loss groups—or coworkers—can be an important way to check in with others about your progress. The trick is to make contact and stay connected with others who are doing the same thing." Start by joining the 7 Years Younger community on Facebook at facebook.com/7yearsyounger.

Stick-To-It Strategy #4: Schedule Your Calories

Simply rearranging your schedule can help you drop pounds and age-proof your body. It was long thought that a calorie was a calorie and it didn't matter when you ate it. But science is beginning to tell a different story, demonstrating that strategically scheduling when you eat can help you maintain and even lose weight. Here's a guide to getting your timing right.

Munch on more in the morning "Women often have one of two problems with breakfast," says Elisabetta Politi, R.D., nutrition director of the Duke Diet & Fitness Center in Durham, NC. "If they overindulge at night, they don't have much appetite in the morning. Or they're trying to cut calories early in the day, so they don't eat enough in the A.M." Others simply don't like to put something in their stomachs within the first few hours after getting up. But breakfast-skimpers ("Just coffee and dry toast, please") and -skippers commit the same faux pas: eating too little to fire up their metabolism. The rate at which you burn calories slows when you go hours without eating, making it harder to lose weight.

And studies show that rather than adding too many calories to your day, a substantial breakfast helps you eat fewer calories. When researchers at the University of Texas at El Paso analyzed 867 food diaries, study volunteers who ate a bigger meal in the morning went on to eat 100 to 200 fewer calories later in the day. Need more proof? Research from Michigan State University that tracked 4,218 people showed that women who skipped breakfast were 30 percent more likely to be overweight. The best A.M. filler-uppers: oatmeal, eggs, peanut butter on whole-grain toast, or anything with fiber and protein. If you're generally not a breakfast-eater, consider that you don't have to roll out of bed and into the kitchen to consume something right away. Just try to eat within three hours after getting up; you'll get the same benefits as eating an earlier breakfast.

Eat less at night The most recent research suggests that late-night eating may not be a great idea when it comes to weight. Animal studies show that rats who eat during sleeping hours gain more weight than those who eat the same amount during normal waking hours, possibly because night-eating puts them out of sync with their circadian rhythm, the biological clock that controls everything from energy expenditure to hormone release. Whether this is also true in humans is unknown. However, one study showed that people who stopped eating after 8 P.M. had more body fat than people with an earlier cutoff time.

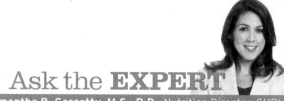

Ask the **EXPERT**

Samantha B. Cassetty, M.S., R.D., Nutrition Director, GHRI

Q *I'm nervous about adding snacks to the diet. I'm in a good groove, and it's hard to change. Plus, I lost four and a half pounds on the Jumpstart!*

Sam says: This is a very common concern. Even with two snacks a day, you should continue to lose weight, up to two pounds per week. Keep in mind that your goal is to develop healthy habits that will last a lifetime, and snacks play a key role. They help offset between-meals hunger, which will help you stick with the plan long-term. Also, since the program was designed to provide all of the key anti-aging nutrients, the produce- and dairy-rich snacks help on that front. If you're really concerned, you can stick with the Jumpstart plan for another week, but don't stay on it longer than that. Then, the following week, you can add one snack (instead of two) and see if the scale needle continues to move down.

Whether or not the body does metabolize late-night calories differently than calories eaten during the day, night calories are often *extra* calories eaten out of boredom. Stick to a regular snack and meal plan as outlined in the 7 Years Younger plan, and you'll keep your overall calorie intake in check.

Make time for snacks Our Jumpstart Plan helps you achieve a particular goal: Lose some weight quickly so you're inspired to continue changing your eating habits in ways that combat the aging process. For that reason, there are no snacks in the Jumpstart week, but as a general rule (and once the Jumpstart week is over), snacking is a great idea.

It may seem virtuous to go from meal to meal without eating anything in between, but it can leave you so hungry that by the time you get to lunch or dinner, you'll be famished. And the more famished you are, the more likely you will be to make poor choices or overeat. Plan for healthy snacks during the day, one in the morning and one in the afternoon, and even the occasional additional indulgence if you're feeling tempted by a favorite food. A group of dieters in a program developed by Susan Roberts, Ph.D., director of the Energy Metabolism Laboratory at Tufts University, not only gained more control over foods they typically craved by doing this, but also lost, on average, 22 pounds in 16 weeks on a 1,400-calorie diet. "Even people who thought they'd never be able to eat chocolate again lost 20 pounds while occasionally indulging," says Roberts.

Thinking ahead will also help you avoid unplanned, unhealthy snacking. Plan which snack you'll eat when. It's best to limit snacks to 100 to 150 calories and try to make sure most of them contain some fiber and/or protein—both are satisfying and will help stave off hunger later. See page 335 for good low-calorie snack choices.

Reach for a snack pack Those preportioned 100-calorie packs can really rein in calories. Brian Wansink, Ph.D., director of the Food and Brand Lab at Cornell University, gave 37 students either four 100-calorie packages of crackers or one 400-calorie package to eat while they watched TV. On average, the students who had the 100-calorie packs ate 25 percent less (about 75 calories) than those with the bulk packages. Overweight participants did best, eating 54 percent fewer calories from the smaller packages. All the students underestimated how much they actually consumed, which goes to show that you still have to pay attention to what you're eating if you hope to slim down. Individual sizes are more expensive (and create more paper waste), so consider buying in bulk, then measuring out your own single servings.

Stick-To-It Strategy #5: Outsmart Your Cravings and Hunger

Cravings and hunger have been the undoing of many a diet. To beat them, sometimes you have to pull out every trick in the book. And here they are: 15 tricks to help you keep hunger at bay and deal with cravings with as little diet damage as possible.

To suppress hunger

Commit *hara hachi bu* People living on the Okinawa Islands off Japan enjoy exceptionally long and healthy lives. One reason may be that the Okinawans practice a form of calorie moderation called *hara hachi bu*, which means, basically, "leave the table when you're 80 percent full." Okinawans eat plenty, but unlike many Westerners, they stop before their belts become tourniquets. And their cultural wisdom is scientifically on target, says Bradley J. Willcox, M.D., a Hawaii-based expert in geriatric medicine and co-investigator of the Okinawa Centenarian Study. When food enters your stomach, the internal stretch receptors help relay a message to your brain telling it you're full. But this is no instant message—it takes 20 minutes to arrive. "You actually feel fuller 20 minutes after you put down your fork," says Dr. Willcox. That means if you eat till you're 100 percent full at the dinner table, you go over capacity at each meal. Worse, because your stomach stretches every time you do this, you'll gradually have to eat more and more to feel satisfied.

Eat slowly and mindfully Slowing your pace can also help your brain catch up with your stomach. In one study, women who took half an hour to eat a pasta lunch consumed almost 70 fewer calories than those who scarfed it down in nine minutes. Take your time and notice what you're eating: Paying attention to the taste, texture, and smell of food will help your body register satisfaction.

Make noodles more satisfying By cooking pasta al dente, you can make it more filling. When you boil spaghetti for five minutes, its glycemic index (a measure of a food's effect on blood sugar) is 38; after 20 minutes, it shoots up to 61. The higher the glycemic index, the sooner you'll be hungry again.

Stop the music Turn off the tunes at mealtime. People linger at the dining table when there's background music—any tempo or volume. And the longer you spend at the table, the more likely you'll be tempted to have another serving or bite.

Watch out for sneak-eating "I just want a taste" (of pie, ice cream, pizza...) can add about 25 calories per mouthful. Taste enough times a day, and you'll undermine your efforts to cut calories.

Chew gum while cooking Not that it replaces exercise, but gum chewing actually burns 11 calories an hour (every little bit helps!). Plus, it can prevent you from taking "taste test" bites.

Remember your last meal Thinking about what you ate earlier in the day may make you inclined to eat less as the day wears on. When British researchers fed 47 women a midday meal, then three hours later asked them to write about their meal or their morning commute, those who savored the memory of their lunch ate a third less food later in the day than the women who reminisced about their A.M. travel.

To thwart cravings

Tap your forehead It may sound a little wacky, but there's science behind this five-second trick to displace your craving thoughts. Since the working memory is small, you can crowd out your food desires by placing all fingers of one hand on your forehead, spaced slightly apart, and then, at intervals of a second, tapping each finger while looking upward and watching it. You may need to do some reps "until your thoughts go elsewhere," says Dr. Roberts.

Have a whiff of mint A study at Wheeling Jesuit University in West Virginia found that people who sniffed peppermint periodically throughout the day ate 2,800 fewer calories during the week. "When you focus on the scent, your attention is driven away from cravings," says psychologist Bryan Raudenbush, Ph.D.

Call a friend Studies in rats suggest that eating comfort food reduces the stress response, which may explain why turmoil may send you looking for macaroni and cheese or chocolate chip cookies. But the fix is only temporary—better to vent to a friend. The relief lasts longer.

Sip some water Stanford researchers found that women who drank six glasses of water a day consumed about 200 fewer calories than women who skimped on H_2O. Let water fill you up, and see if your cravings pass.

To damage-proof your weight-loss plan

Limit yourself to the really good stuff Sometimes you may be more satisfied with a small amount of the real thing than with a lower-calorie substitute. "What can happen is that you say to yourself, 'I want chocolate, but I don't want the calories,'" says Joan Salge Blake, R.D., associate professor of nutrition at Boston University. "So you start with some cocoa, then go on to other foods that don't satisfy your craving, and you end up having the chocolate anyway."

Never eat a treat by itself Feed your yen for chips, but have only a few with a low-fat dip (like hummus or a yogurt-dill mix). Including something healthy and low-calorie, too, like red pepper strips and celery, will help you resist downing the whole bag of chips, suggests Roberts. The same holds true for dessert: Enjoy a square of dark chocolate or a small cookie with a bowlful of berries or a piece of fruit.

Go the distance Don't keep treats in the house. If you really want something special, go to the store and buy a snack-size amount—just one small pack of cookies or chips.

Clear your palate Once you've had your little taste, have a drink of water or brush your teeth, suggests weight-loss coach Janice Taylor: "If the taste of that food lingers in your mouth, it will trigger more eating."

(continued on page 171)

Binge Busters

16 Delicious Ways to Satisfy Your Cravings

If you crave...	Have this	You Save
Buffalo Wings 860 calories, 70 grams fat (7 pieces, served with celery sticks and ¼ c. blue-cheese dressing)	**Buffalo Tenders** 270 calories, 8 grams fat Heat 1 teaspoon canola oil in small skillet; add 5 ounces chicken-breast tenders, cut into 7 strips. Cook 5 minutes. Stir in 1 tablespoon cayenne-pepper sauce. Serve with celery sticks and ¼ cup low-fat blue-cheese dressing.	**590** calories **62** grams fat
Chinese Fried Rice 605 calories, 12 grams fat per 2 c.	**Rice with Steamed Veggies** 296 calories, 6 grams fat Combine 1 cup cooked brown rice, 1 cup steamed vegetables (frozen stir-fry variety works well), and a splash of soy sauce and Asian sesame oil; toss.	**309** calories **6** grams fat
Fast-Food Deluxe Hamburger 710 calories, 46 grams fat	**Veggie Burger** 253 calories, 5 grams fat Top with lettuce, tomato, pickles, ketchup, on sesame-seed bun.	**457** calories **41** grams fat
French Fries 450 calories, 22 grams fat per 5 ounces (large order of fries)	**Oven-Baked Fries** 148 calories, 5 grams fat Preheat oven to 425°F. Toss one unpeeled baking potato (about 5 ounces), cut into wedges, with 1 teaspoon oil. Arrange in single layer in shallow pan. Bake 25 minutes, turning once, until potatoes are golden.	**302** calories **17** grams fat
Four-Cheese Pizza 330 calories, 11 grams fat for ⅙ of an 11-inch pie	**Napoli Pita Pizza** 196 calories, 8 grams fat Use half of a 6½-inch whole wheat pita and top with ¼ cup chopped tomatoes (canned or fresh) and ¼ cup shredded light mozzarella cheese. Top with chopped fresh basil or oregano leaves, and sprinkle with 1 teaspoon Parmesan cheese and ¼ teaspoon olive oil. Bake to melt cheese.	**134** calories **3** grams fat

If you crave...	Have this	You Save
Deli-Style Potato Chips 105 calories, 7 grams fat for 12 chips	**Quick Chips** 16 calories, 0 grams fat On a microwave cooking rack (a small wire rack that fits into a microwave oven), arrange 12 very thin, unpeeled potato slices in a circle; sprinkle with salt. Microwave on High for 5½ to 6½ minutes until brown; rotate rack halfway through cooking. Let stand for one minute.	**89** calories **7** grams fat
Apple Pie 411 calories, 19 grams of fat for ⅛ of a 9-inch pie	**Cinnamon Apple Delight** 108 calories, 0 grams fat Core a cooking apple (about 6 ounces) and peel one-third of the way. Sprinkle the top with cinnamon, nutmeg, and 1 teaspoon of brown sugar. Microwave, covered, on Medium-High (70 percent power) for 2 to 3 minutes or until tender.	**303** calories **19** grams fat
Chocolate-Coated Ice Cream Bar 290 calories, 20 grams fat per 5-ounce bar	**Frozen Banana on a Stick** 78 calories, 1 gram fat Insert ice-cream stick into end of half a peeled banana. Roll in crumbs of one crushed reduced-fat chocolate wafer. Wrap, and freeze.	**212** calories **19** grams fat
Chunky Gourmet Ice Cream 240 to 370 calories, 14 to 26 grams fat for ½ c.	**Chocolate Dream Ice Cream** 157 to 203 calories, 4 to 5 grams fat Add one of the following to ½ cup low-fat ice cream: • 1 reduced-fat mini chocolate bar, cut up • 70 mini chocolate chips • ½ small chocolate-covered peppermint patty, cut up • 2 reduced-fat chocolate wafers, crumbled	**37–213** calories **9–22** grams fat
Custard-Filled Éclair 260 calories, 16 grams fat	**Vanilla Cream Bites** 72 calories, 1 gram fat Split a ladyfinger; spread 1 tablespoon low-fat vanilla pudding on each half.	**188** calories **15** grams fat

If you crave...	Have this	You Save
Chocolate Layer Cake 235 calories, 11 grams fat for ⅛ of a cake prepared from an 18-ounce box cake mix	**Angel-Devil Cake** 194 calories, 6 grams fat Take a 1-ounce piece of angel food cake and cut into 2 thin slices. Spread ¼ cup low-fat chocolate pudding between the slices. Sprinkle with some cocoa powder and garnish with 2 tablespoons light whipped topping.	**41** calories **5** grams fat
French Cruller 170 calories, 8 grams of fat	**Faux French Cruller** 95 calories, 3 grams fat Split 2 ladyfingers and coat on all sides with a butter-flavored cooking spray, then with a mixture of cinnamon and sugar.	**75** calories **5** grams fat
Ice Cream Sandwich 200 calories, 7 grams fat	**Ice Cream on Chocolate Wafers** 105 calories, 3 grams fat Spread two tablespoons low-fat ice cream between two reduced-fat chocolate wafers. Roll sides in 1 teaspoon chocolate sprinkles. Wrap, and freeze.	**95** calories **4** grams fat
Jelly Donut 290 calories, 16 grams fat	**Jelly-Jammed Ladyfinger** 84 calories, 1 gram fat Spread 2 teaspoons raspberry jam on a split ladyfinger.	**206** calories **15** grams fat
Lemon Meringue Pie 305 calories, 10 grams fat for ⅙ of an 8-inch pie	**Light Lemon Square** 81 calories, 1 gram fat Spread 1 graham cracker square with 1 tablespoon lemon curd (in the jelly aisle); sprinkle with confectioners' sugar.	**224** calories **9** grams fat
Strawberry Shortcake 420 calories, 21 grams fat for 3¼-inch by 3-inch piece	**Angel Berry Shortcake** 125 calories, 2 grams fat Take a 1-ounce piece of angel food cake and cut into 2 thin slices. Place 2 sliced strawberries between the slices. Top with ¼ cup light whipped topping and 1 sliced strawberry.	**295** calories **19** grams fat

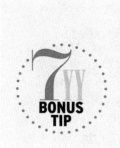

BONUS TIP

Any time you're in a gotta-have-a-candy-bar mood, hit the sidewalk for 15 minutes. That's how long it took for a group of 25 chocoholics to **exercise away their desire for a chocolate bar.** And their resistance was severely tested: In this University of Exeter study, the scientists had teased the subjects with mental challenges (stress triggers cravings) and **an actual chocolate bar**—which participants had to unwrap. The walk will not only curb your cravings, but burn calories as well.

Stick-To-It Strategy #6: Enjoy Food for the Right Reasons

Why eat? Because you're physically hungry. But emotions can often masquerade as hunger, and stress can kick off cravings. Managing your emotions and stress can really help you eat for the right reasons and stick to your weight-loss plan. These go-to strategies can help you weather any weakening.

Trip up your triggers Anger, depression, anxiety, sadness, ongoing stress, boredom—any one of them can make you turn to food. Whatever your triggers, part of breaking the emotional-eating habit is finding out what commonly makes you turn to food. That awareness may help you pause and, in that short time, make a conscious effort to find something else to comfort you.

In that moment, ask yourself if you are really, truly hungry. Physical hunger comes on gradually; emotional hunger is more immediate—you feel you *must* have something (and sometimes a very specific, highly indulgent thing) right now. Be prepared with an alternative. Calling a friend or family member to vent can help. Meditation or breathing techniques will give you a time-out (see page 242). Or busy your hands or mind with something else. Pick up knitting, do a crossword puzzle, go online, turn on music and sing. Test out various distractions until you find the one that works for you.

the bottom line

Can Yoga Help You Lose Weight?

Yoga is touted as a stress-buster, but does a regular practice help you curb emotional eating? A few years ago, scientists at the Fred Hutchinson Cancer Research Center in Seattle found that a regular yoga practice helped people avoid middle-age spread—over a 10-year period, practitioners gained less weight than non-practitioners. One reason for the difference, the researchers suspected, was that yoga makes people more aware of their bodies and more sensitive to hunger and satiety cues.

More recently, a follow-up study put even greater stock in yoga's ability to help people stay slim. The researchers administered questionnaires at yoga studios, gyms, and weight-loss programs that asked more than 300 participants about their eating and exercise habits. The results showed that people who did yoga regularly (but not necessarily those who did other types of exercise) were more mindful eaters. That is, they were more likely to stop when full, eat slowly, notice the flavors of foods, and be aware at restaurants when served portions that were too big. They also typically ate in response to hunger, versus anxiety or depression. And mindful eaters, the study found, weighed less than their counterparts who ate with less attention to their internal cues.

Create a feelings first-aid kit Food isn't the only thing that's soothing, a fact that sometimes gets lost when you're feeling that nothing except a double order of onion rings will help you cope. Susan Albers, Psy.D., a psychologist at the Cleveland Clinic who specializes in mindful eating, suggests filling a box with items that are comforting. You might toss in some individually wrapped tea bags, an old cozy sweater, warm socks, a bottle of lotion, a favorite book of short stories or poems, maybe a DVD. Before you succumb to a bag of M&Ms, open up the box and see if you can't find calorie-free relief first.

Scribble to de-stress Writing exercises can help create clarity and reduce anxiety, says Bruce Rabin, M.D., a professor of pathology and psychiatry at the University of Pittsburgh School of Medicine—and the lower your anxiety level, the greater your capacity for resilience and the lower the likelihood you'll self-soothe with food. Dr. Rabin's favorite technique: Find a quiet place where you won't be disturbed for 15 minutes. Write continuously about something that's bothering you. If you run out of things to say, repeat yourself. Don't worry about grammar, and don't stop to read what you've written. At the end of the 15 minutes, tear up the piece of paper and toss it out. "People feel calmer afterward," says Dr. Rabin. "Negative thoughts seem to float to the back of the brain."

Stick-To-It Strategy #7: Dine Out Wisely

Eating out at a restaurant can be one of life's great pleasures, but unfortunately most surveys show that the more meals you eat away from home, the more excess pounds you're likely to carry. Restaurant dishes are often more than double the size of a healthy single portion, and they can be loaded with hidden fat, salt, and sugar. Here's how to sidestep the biggest hazards of restaurant dining and travel.

Practice proactive eating More and more eateries (especially fast-food and chain restaurants) are posting calorie counts on their walls or making nutrition info available in brochures, letting you know what you're getting before you order. When you're going to a spot that doesn't provide information on-site, check online. If the restaurant doesn't post nutrition data, at least you'll have time to look over the menu in advance, find the healthiest choices, and go to the restaurant knowing what to order. Also check out the website healthydiningfinder.com, which is partly funded by the Centers for Disease Control and Prevention. You can type in your zip

Eating Internationally?
The Leanest Choices

Chinese
Now is your chance to get in more omega-3s and antioxidant-rich vegetables. Go for steamed (*zheng*) fish; stir-fries like white-meat chicken with carrots, broccoli, and pea pods in a light sauce; and dishes that are boiled (*gun*) or roasted (*kao*). Reduce the salt by asking for low-sodium soy sauce. And ask for brown rice, which is becoming as common as the white variety in Asian restaurants.

French
Choose fish dishes without sauces, or the classic simple roast chicken, and take advantage of the salads (with the dressing on the side, and hold the cheese).

Italian
Grilled chicken or fish is a great option, and most Italian restaurants serve vegetable sides like spinach or broccoli. If you have pasta, go for the red sauces and choose dishes that have vegetables mixed in. If no pastas on the menu fit the bill, order a side of vegetables and mix them in yourself.

Middle Eastern
Tabbouleh is made with whole-grain bulgur and has antioxidant-rich parsley. Choose chicken on a skewer, salads, and hummus.

code (and other criteria, like price) and the site will steer you toward restaurants with healthy options.

Order the "small" This may seem like a no-brainer, but when you consider that restaurants now supersize everything—and entice you to order it by making it a bargain to order big—it bears mentioning. And if you don't have a choice, rely on your body to tell you when to stop. As soon as you start to feel full, put down your fork, spoon, pastry, or sandwich and give yourself a few minutes to check your hunger level before you eat more. Cleaning your plate is not required in restaurants (and doggie bags are a girl's best friend).

Japanese

Naturally lean, Japanese food offers a lot of healthy choices: chicken or fish teriyaki, miso soup, and tofu. Soba noodles in soup with vegetables are a reasonable choice, too. Sushi can also be a good choice, but be careful: It's more caloric than you may realize (a piece of tuna sushi is about 50 calories, a spicy tuna roll about 380).

Mexican

You can't go wrong with rice and beans (all the better if the restaurant offers brown rice). Be certain, though, that you're not ordering refried beans: Most are cooked with lard, a source of saturated fat. (If you love refried beans, try them at home. There are several brands of vegetarian, fat-free refried beans on the market.) Salsa (without the chips) is a good source of vitamin C.

Grilled fish tacos in corn tortillas or chicken or bean tostadas on a non-fried tortilla will help you pack in more anti-aging nutrients, too.

Go for balance, not deprivation Eating out can be a treat; the trick is to balance good-for-you-foods with indulgences that have body-aging sugar and saturated fat. However, people who completely ban their favorite foods while trying to eat nutritiously tend to cycle between dieting and bingeing on the foods they restrict. So, compromise: If breakfast at a diner is just not the same without bacon, have a strip with a cup of oatmeal and some fresh fruit. If you can't live without the fries at your favorite bistro, order grilled fish and veggies as your entrée and split the fries with your dining companion. If you are craving a decadent dessert, share it with a friend.

Eat for the long term When faced with a basket of freshly baked bread, a bottle of wine on the table, that molten-chocolate-cake-that-you-can-only-get-here, or other temptations, it can be hard to say "No, thanks." If you occasionally say yes, simply neutralize the damage over the next few days. Choose lower-calorie options for your next few meals, and increase your activity level during that time. That way, your indulgence won't have a chance to stick to your hips (or backside or stomach).

Travel prepared When traveling, you don't always know where you're going to find healthy meals. But when you're going to a destination that's more predictable, plan ahead just as you would when dining out at a local restaurant. En route, look at your itinerary and map out a meal strategy for flight time and layovers. Take along healthy snacks and a brown-bag meal so you won't be susceptible to the scent of cinnamon buns wafting through the airport.

Activate Your Anti-Aging Plan Now!

1 **Enjoy more fabulous foods with fewer calories** Make colorful fruits and vegetables half of what you eat at any meal. Add two fruits to your breakfast cereal, start every lunch with a salad, dine on vegetable soup for a first course, and accessorize a dessert of berries with a small square of high-quality dark chocolate.

2 **Celebrate the power of small changes** Instead of sweeping all-or-nothing resolutions, set your sights on doable goals. Replace your daily soft drink with a large glass of water three times a week, or reduce by half the amount of cream you add to your coffee. The following week, add another mini-goal, and keep going.

3 **Crystalize your commitment** Write down your goals and the reason you want to accomplish them: "I want to lose weight to wow them at my reunion," "I'm losing weight to be happier and healthier." Then post them where you'll see them every day.

For more expert anti-aging diet advice, get our free special report, Eat to Look & Feel Younger, *at 7yearsyounger.com/eattolookyoung.*

Age Eraser 5

Chapter Five

Fitness That Feels Good

f you're turned off by the "work" in "workout," we've got game-changing news for you: Exercise can be so much more pleasant and accessible than you might think. It doesn't take a lot of equipment or even a lot of time or money to get fit, and fitness is truly the key to being 7 years younger. It makes everything—your sleep, your skin, even your sex life—better.

Exercise is simply the closest thing you've got to the fountain of youth, so drink deep. Physical activity has been consistently shown to help people who lose weight keep it from creeping back on, and body fat is a key cause of age-accelerating inflammation. The pounds you sweat off lower your risk of life-threatening conditions like diabetes, high blood pressure, and heart disease associated with being over-weight. Regular activity, in fact, cuts your heart-attack risk—by 50 percent, says one report—and just three 10-minute walks three days a week are enough to lower systolic blood pressure (the first number of your blood-pressure reading) an impressive five points. Exercise discourages the formation of blood clots, shrinks abdominal fat (the kind of fat linked to heart-attack risk), and raises heart-protective HDL cholesterol levels.

Exercise helps reverse age-related losses in muscle mass, bone strength, heart-lung capacity, and flexibility. Every hour you exercise results in measurable increases in bone density, and people who are physically active better retain the strength and size of their muscles. (The more muscle you have, the more calories you burn and the less body fat you're likely to store.) As you'll learn in Chapters 6 and 7 ("Your Brain—Only Better" and "Say Goodbye to Stress"), there's substantial evidence suggesting that exercise keeps your brain healthy and even helps improve scores on cognitive tests. And there's perhaps no better natural remedy for stress or a blue mood: Participants in exercise studies consistently show improvement in both areas when they move their bodies more. If there's one last thing we can say to inspire you to get moving, it's this: It's never too late to start. Even if you've never exercised a day in your adult life, you can make up for lost time. In a Swedish study that followed 2,205 men for 32 years (from age 50 to age 82), those who increased their physical activity from low/medium (casual walker) to high (at least three hours of sports or heavy gardening a week) cut their mortality rate to half that of those who stayed on the sofa. The researchers are confident the findings apply to women, too, and that if you keep it up over the years, your risk will eventually be as low as a lifelong exerciser's. And one thing you're sure to notice almost immediately: Exercise makes you feel and look younger, too—regular activity puts a bounce in your step, a twinkle in your eye, and color in your cheeks.

7 TOP ANTI-AGING FITNESS MOVES

Youth Booster #1: Keep It Moving!

Regular exercise can turn back the clock on your appearance and energy level, but what you do when you're *not* in your workout clothes is just as important for a younger, trimmer appearance. Several years ago, researchers examined whether lean women were more physically active during the day than obese women. They found that obese women sat two and a half hours more each day, stood two hours less, and spent half as much time moving compared with the lean women. Ultimately, they burned 300 fewer calories a day. Now newer research suggests that unplanned physical activity may have even greater benefits.

At the School of Kinesiology and Health Studies at Queen's University in Kingston, Ontario, researchers outfitted men and women with an accelerometer, a gadget that measured the duration and intensity of every move they made, then asked them to go about their usual daily activities. After a week, they looked at the participants' cardiorespiratory fitness, an important predictor of vitality, heart health, and longevity. Those who moved the most and had the most vigorous movements had better heart and lung

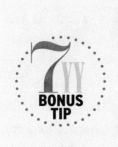

Whether you take formal ballroom dance classes, head out for a night of salsa, or just let loose in your living room, **dancing is a great calorie burner and stress reducer,** and it will up your daily activity quotient. Plus, the mental footwork of executing the choreography **increases blood flow to the brain,** boosting learning and memory. If you don't have a ballroom studio nearby, look for a Zumba class, a combination of aerobic exercise and Latin-style dancing.

Mini Moves Add Up to Major Body Benefits

Adopt a movement mantra: As you go about your day, think about all the chances you have to be active in both small and bigger ways. Here are 20 opportunities to get in more calorie-burning, age-resisting moves. (Calorie counts are calculated for a 150-pound woman.)

- Walk your dog daily (if you don't have one, borrow your sure-to-be-grateful neighbor's): 15 minutes, 74 calories
- Avoid drive-through banks, restaurants, mailboxes, and library-book drop-offs. Instead, **park and walk in:** 5 minutes and 22 calories per walk
- Park at the outer edge of parking lots and walk briskly to your destination: 2 minutes, 11 calories
- Take public transportation to work; **get off one stop before yours and walk** the rest of the way: 15 minutes, 74 calories
- When doing errands, park your car and walk between stops: 20 minutes, 99 calories
- Walk up the escalator rather than passively letting it carry you. **Trade elevators for the stairs:** for every minute climbing stairs, 9 calories
- Do a little bit of housecleaning daily and put some muscle into vacuuming, dusting, and sweeping (remember, in the Queen's University study, intensity of movement counted): 30 minutes, 99 calories
- Trade in your electric mower for a push mower: 20 minutes, 99 calories
- **Rake and weed by hand:** 45 minutes, 276 calories
- Set your default printer farther away from your desk at work: 2 minutes, 9 calories

health than the less active participants. You can get the beauty and health benefits of more movement simply by taking more steps during your day. Your optimal goal, say health experts, is to take 10,000 steps a day. Use the following tips—combined with the walking programs in "Youth-Booster #3: Get Yourself Going With Cardio," page 191—to help you hit the mark.

- Go down the hall and talk to colleagues instead of e-mailing:
  2 minutes, 9 calories
- Strategizing with a coworker? Suggest that you **walk as you brainstorm**:
  30 minutes, 148 calories
- Use the restroom one flight up or down: 2 minutes, 18 calories
- Spend half your lunch hour taking a walk: 30 minutes, 148 calories
- Carry in groceries one bag at a time instead of making one or two trips:
  8 minutes, 39 calories (**Bonus: Putting away groceries:** 8 minutes,
  24 calories)
- Walk or ride your bike to do your errands whenever you can: 30 minutes,
  135-148 calories
- **Get up and change the channel** instead of using the remote: 2 minutes,
  2 calories
- Make a few circles around the supermarket to get in more steps:
  8 minutes, 39 calories
- Pace (or at least stand) while you talk on the phone: 20 minutes,
  20-99 calories
- Try to make your social life more active: **Meet friends for miniature golf,
  go bowling,** stroll through a museum, walk through a historic neighbor-
  hood or park, rent a paddleboat or rowboat, play pool or Ping-Pong:
  60 minutes, 171-270 calories

Stay on the go all day The difference that incidental activity makes in
your calorie burning and cardiovascular health means it's worth devising
ways to stay active all day. Walk to the mailbox, take the stairs, mow
your lawn, wash your car. These activities alone are not enough to get
you in shape, but you will burn the extra calories responsible for the

tummy rolls and weight creep over the years. Daily activities can be good for your bones, too. A Swedish study found that middle-aged women who gardened, picked berries, shoveled snow, and walked frequently sustained far fewer hip fractures later in life than those who were less active. In fact, these generally active women also fared better (hipwise) than those who engaged in more formal, gym-type exercise.

Stand up for youthfulness When you sit, you don't move much, and thus you don't reap the benefits of physical activity. But there's more to it than that: Research by the American Cancer Society also indicates that parking yourself in a chair has consequences above and beyond missed exercise. In a study that tracked 123,000 people, women who reported sitting more than six hours per day were 37 percent more likely to die prematurely than those who sat fewer than three hours a day—even if they got regular exercise. When participants reported sitting for long hours without engaging in a regular exercise routine, the results were even worse: Women who sat for six hours a day *and* didn't work out were 94 percent more likely to die within the study's 13-year time span than those who sat fewer hours and were very physically active.

According to epidemiologist Alpa V. Patel, Ph.D., lead author of the study, sitting too much may negatively affect cholesterol, triglycerides, blood pressure, leptin (the hormone that governs appetite), and other factors associated with obesity and cardiac disease. If you have a job that requires sitting most of the day (Americans sit nearly eight and a half

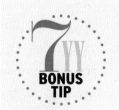

Set an alarm on your computer, smartphone, or PDA to remind you to stand up, stretch, and walk around every half hour.

Top GHRI-Tested Pedometer Picks

If you're a...	Then try...	Because...
Techie	Accusplit Eagle 190 Multi-Function Pedometer	It logs (and lets you track) total steps, distance, calories, and activity time. It also has an extra-large cumulative memory, counting up to 10 million steps.
Minimalist	Yamax CW-300 Digi-Walker	A no-frills pedometer with only two features—timing and step count. Lightweight and easy to use, it includes a filter that prevents arm movements or other quick upper-body motions from mistakenly being counted as steps.
Detail tracker	Omron Pocket Pedometer	Has software so you can view and print your walking stats (steps taken, calories burned, fat burned, and distance covered). The info is updated each time you upload it, so you can log on and analyze your progress for the day, week, month, or year.

hours a day on average), this research should be talking to you. And it doesn't take much to see real improvement: Australian researchers noted that people who got up from their chairs the most had lower C-reactive protein, a marker for age-accelerating inflammation and heart disease, than those who got up the least, regardless of total sitting time. The people who stood up also had trimmer waistlines. "Stand up at least every 30 minutes," suggests lead author Genevieve Healy, Ph.D., of the University of Queensland, Australia. While longer active breaks are probably best, even brief pop-ups help.

Improve Your Balance

Good balance prevents falls. One in three adults 65 and older falls, and loss of balance is the most common reason for emergency-room visits in this age group. You can develop your sense of balance—or improve it—and you don't even need a special workout to do it. Here, easy ways to sneak balance exercises into your day.

- Stand on one foot, then the other, as you brush your teeth.
- Waiting in a slow-moving line? Try walking in place, putting feet down heel-to-toe.
- Balance on one foot as you put on socks or shoes.
- Hike off-road: Stepping around rocks, over tree roots, and through loose gravel improves your balance.
- Walk forward and backward about 10 steps along a straight line (the edge of a sidewalk or an imaginary line).
- Dance—the forward, backward, and side-to-side movements of most forms of dance develop your equilibrium.

Youth Booster #2: Get Strong

Strength training is a proven way to keep your metabolic rate—the number of calories your body burns throughout the day—from dropping with age. Because muscle burns more calories than other types of body tissue, building muscle mass increases your metabolic rate, helping to counteract the 5 percent loss per decade that accompanies age. In fact, most of what we recognize as aging is actually muscle loss.

Strength training works by stressing muscle fibers in ways that prompt them to repair and rebuild themselves. Regular sessions of lifting weights or other forms of resistance training promote a continual remodeling of muscle tissue, increasing your calorie-burning ability while toning and tightening your body. As you sculpt your muscles, you'll be building a firm foundation for skin, reducing and preventing the appearance of wrinkles, droops, and sags.

Strength training can even slow the aging of your cells. It turns out that structures inside cells called mitochondria, which turn nutrients into energy, tend to operate less effectively as the body ages. Scientists believe this slowdown may be involved in muscle loss. To see if resistance training could reverse this effect, Canadian researchers had young adults (average age 26) and older adults (average age 70) train twice a week for an hour each time over a six-month period. When before-and-after muscle samples were compared, the decline in mitochondrial function of the older adults, which had been documented by researchers at the outset of the study, reversed. By the end of the study, the older adults' mitochondrial function was similar to that of the younger adults. The older resistance trainers also became markedly stronger, improving their strength by about 50 percent.

Research is also showing that strength-building may have other longevity-boosting benefits. It can lower blood pressure, build bone (see "What's the Best Exercise to Build Bones?", page 191), help improve cognition, and reduce the risk and symptoms of heart disease, arthritis, and type 2 diabetes. As if that weren't enough, it may help improve balance; falls are the number one cause of broken bones in those over 40.

Your training options The good news about strength training is that there's more than one way to do it, so you don't have to be limited to one type, or even a specific location or kind of equipment—you can strength-train at a gym or at home, and with machines, free weights (like dumbbells), your own body weight (push-ups are a good example), or resistance bands, which we call for in our plan.

We like bands (available in sporting-goods stores and online) because they're more versatile than machines and just as effective. Free weights and machines create tension in only one direction (from either pulling up or pushing down), but bands provide resistance in both directions. One

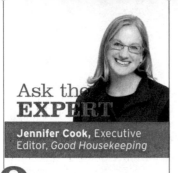

Ask the
EXPERT

Jennifer Cook, Executive Editor, *Good Housekeeping*

Q *I've never lifted weights, but my husband has a set of hand weights at home. What weight should I start with, and can you recommend a good routine?*

Jenny says: Start with light weights (three or five pounds), then move up to eight or 10 pounds as you get stronger. How can you tell when to make the switch? If you can complete two sets of 10 repetitions with good form, you should lift a heavier weight. For an easy but "all-inclusive" circuit that targets trouble spots—abs, butt, upper arms, hips—go to goodhousekeeping.com /weights-women.

type of movement causes muscles to shorten; the other makes them lengthen. When you combine both, you'll sculpt your body double-time. With bands, you can also control the tension to work different muscle groups, adjust the level of difficulty, and add variety to your fitness plan. Bands are portable, too—easy to take with you on a walk (like in our body-toning "Walking Workout #2," on page 196) or slip into a suitcase when you travel.

Start with a medium-tension band. Most bands are color-coded according to resistance level. There's no industry standard, but often yellow corresponds to very light resistance, green to light, blue to medium, red to heavy, and black to heaviest. The thicker the band, the more resistance it provides. Try stretching a band: On a scale of 1 to 10, the exercise difficulty should feel like a 7 or 8. It's a good idea to buy at least two different tensions, since some parts of your body may be stronger than others, and you want to be able to progress. Muscles get stronger when you challenge them—with a heavier weight, greater resistance, or more repetitions. In our plan, you start out with one set of repetitions and then advance to two sets for each exercise. We'll also help you figure out when you should move on to a higher-resistance band.

If you prefer to strength-train with free weights or weight machines, use the weight room at your local gym, or exercise with dumbbells at home. If you've never pumped iron before, sign up for a few sessions with a personal trainer. That way, you'll learn how to get the most out of each move—without risking injury—as well as how to increase the weight or resistance as you get stronger.

Build a routine that works The most important consideration with any workout plan is structuring your routine so it fits into your schedule and you actually do it! The moves below can be done on their own as a dedicated strength workout, or you can incorporate them into an aerobic workout as we suggest in week four of the 7 Years Younger Plan. What's great about these strengtheners is that they simultaneously work your upper and lower body. That will save you time and make your workouts speed by. Do these three moves at least two times a week. After a month, add another set, and make sure that the resistance is challenging enough to fatigue your muscles; you should barely be able to do the last repetition. When you get to a point where you can do all the repetitions fairly easily, switch to a higher-resistance band.

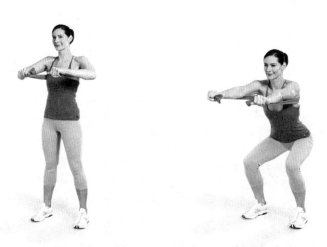

1. **SQUAT WITH CHEST PRESS** Stand with feet shoulder-width apart. Wrap band around shoulder blades and hold an end in each hand, arms at chest level, elbows out. Lower body into a squat, sitting back into heels with knees over ankles, until thighs are nearly parallel to ground. At the same time, press arms straight out in front of you at chest height. Do one set of 8 to 10 reps.

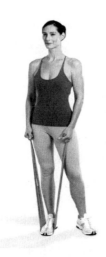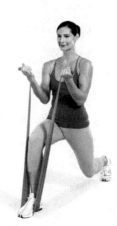

2. **REAR LUNGE WITH BICEPS CURL** Stand with band under right foot. Hold an end in each hand. Step left foot back 3 feet, landing on ball of foot, and lower body until right thigh is parallel with ground. Hold lunge while you curl hands toward shoulders. Do one set of 8 to 10 reps. Switch sides and repeat.

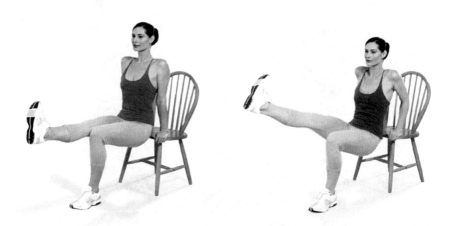

3. **TRICEPS DIP WITH LEG LIFT** Sit at edge of bench (or sturdy chair) with thighs parallel to floor. Lift yourself off bench so you're supported by hands and feet, then raise right leg. Lower body, bending elbows and extending right leg 6 inches to side. Push body back up; bring leg back to center. Do one set of 8 to 10 reps, then repeat with the left leg.

the bottom line

What's the Best Exercise to Build Bones?

Certain forms of exercise are better than others at staving off the bone loss that occurs with aging, reducing your risk of osteoporosis, the brittle bones disease. Here, a rundown of the best bone-builders in each exercise category:

Strength training

As you pull an exercise band, complete a push-up, or heft a weight, your muscles tug on your bones, stimulating the growth of new bone tissue. That's one reason why adding strength training to your exercise schedule is so important. Most aerobic forms of exercise stress the bones in your lower body but not those in your upper body. Strength training lets you work both.

Aerobics

A workout must be weight-bearing in order to build bone. Walking quickly is weight-bearing (strolling, however, doesn't have much impact because your body is used to it); so are jogging and aerobic dance. Jumping rope, stair-climbing, and hiking are other good weight-bearing exercises. Cardio activities that have little bone benefit (but are great for anti-aging results) include swimming, cycling, water aerobics, and using elliptical machines.

Sports

Activities that are great for fracture prevention include racquet sports (which strengthen wrists and, with their pivots and side moves, are great for hips and spine), soccer, volleyball, and basketball. Dancing is good for bones, too.

Youth Booster #3: Get Yourself Going With Cardio

Catch sight of yourself in a mirror after a bout of cardiovascular exercise, the kind that accelerates your breathing and gets your heart rate up, and you'll see the direct effect of your aerobic effort: Your skin glows from increased circulation. Beneath your skin, cardiovascular workouts help

How Hard Should You Be Working?

Listen to your body. The following descriptions correspond to the directions in the three walking workouts. Remember that your stamina will increase as time goes by, so you'll naturally ramp up your efforts.

Warm-up/cooldown
You should be moving along, making a little bit of effort.

Moderate
You can talk comfortably while walking.

Fast
You're a little breathless but can still talk in short sentences.

your circulatory system function better by building new capillaries and making existing ones more efficient at supplying blood and fuel to all your tissues. Improved circulation helps all your organs—from skin to stomach—look and act younger. Research has also shown that aerobic exercise can delay biological aging by 10 years or more, increasing the likelihood you'll stay fit, mobile, and independent as you grow older. And while the likelihood of many diseases—from diabetes to cancer to heart disease—increases with age, cardiovascular exercise counters that risk. If, say, you work out for just a half hour a day—and keep at it over the years—you'll halve your risk of dying from colon cancer. Even if you've never done much physical activity before, you have every reason to get on the fitness bandwagon now.

If you're an exercise newbie, you don't need to do a lot of huffing and puffing to reap benefits—although the more you do, the more years (and pounds) you'll shave off. The three walking workouts that follow are a good place to start. Each takes 20 minutes, and you should do one (or a combination) three times a week. Start off slowly; your ultimate aim in a few weeks' time is to be exercising at least four times a week for 30 to 40 minutes each time and at a pace that makes it slightly hard to have a conversation.

Walking Workout #1: Fat-Blasting Interval Training

Alternating short bursts of all-out effort with bouts of a slower, steady-state speed ramps up your body benefits dramatically. When researchers divided 45 lean and overweight women into a group that cycled steadily and one that switched between sprinting for 8 seconds and light pedaling for 12 seconds over a 20-minute workout, the interval trainers lost *three times* as much fat as the women who exercised at a moderate pace for a full 40 minutes. Without changing their diets, the sprinters also dropped five and a half pounds, on average, while the non-sprinters *gained* a pound. Why does interval training yield better results? "More muscle fibers get worked during those high-intensity intervals," says Martin Gibala, Ph.D., an exercise physiologist at McMaster University. "When you push hard in short bursts, it reactivates nerve fibers, builds new capillaries, and forces your body to repair the muscle. All of that burns a tremendous amount of calories—long after you've completed your session."

Your Fat-Blasting Interval-Training Plan

2 min.	Warm-up
1 min.	Moderate walk
30 sec.	Fast walk
1 min.	Moderate walk
1 min.	Fast walk
30 sec.	Moderate walk
30 sec.	Fast walk
1.5 min.	Moderate walk
30 sec.	Fast walk
3 min.	Moderate walk
1.5 min.	Fast walk
2 min.	Moderate walk
1 min.	Fast walk
2 min.	Moderate walk
2 min.	Cooldown

Laura Goldblum
"Taking care of myself really invigorated my looks"

L aura, 49, thought a lot about how our culture defines beauty and explored her own feelings about growing older while engaged in the 7 Years Younger challenge. "I wanted to figure out what I could do to feel both attractive and comfortable with myself as I got older, but I also thought about what I accept about aging and what I reject," says Laura, a single mother of two. "I reject that I can't have some wrinkles."

Sticking to a workout schedule Laura discovered that it felt good to take care of herself in a healthy way. And working out was a big part of that. Before she began the program, Laura had been going to exercise classes. "I show up, someone yells at me, and I do it," she says. "But when things get in the way, I skip the gym and end up not exercising at all." With its flexibility, the 7 Years Younger program

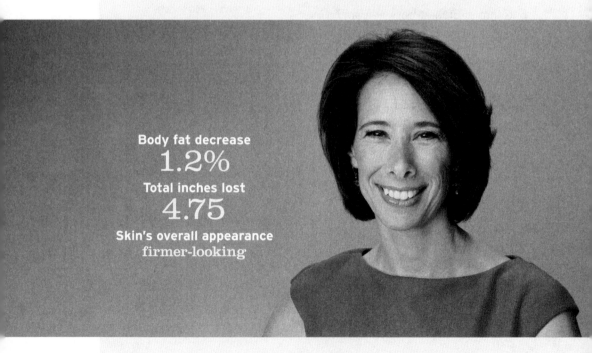

Body fat decrease
1.2%
Total inches lost
4.75
Skin's overall appearance
firmer-looking

allowed her to be less dependent on her gym's class schedule. "It lets you weave exercise into a busy life, which makes a lot of sense," she says. Laura still goes to classes, but the program's walking and strength-training exercises with bands help her fill in the gaps.

Trying out makeup Laura thought she'd skip the makeup portion of the program; she's always preferred her face au naturel. Happily, she decided to test makeup after all. "I actually got into the habit of putting on mascara and lipstick," she says. "It definitely makes a difference."

The five-minute reprieve With family responsibilities swirling around her, Laura appreciated the program's directive to take five minutes a few times a day to breathe and relax. "Before, I tended to do whatever was right in front of me at the time," says Laura. "Taking five minutes here and there has helped me focus on the truly important things I need to do and revealed what I can weed out."

Her life lesson 7 Years Younger reminded Laura how valuable it is to have fun, to pay attention to the present, to get outside, and to be with other people. "Those were the aspects of the program that I really appreciated," she says. "I don't think it's only how many pounds you lose or the wrinkles that you soften that make you look younger; it's the energy you exude. I want to lead an invigorated life, and that comes from taking good care of myself."

For more about Laura Goldblum, see color insert.

Want to be a test panelist for a future 7 Years Younger plan? Sign up today at 7yearsyounger.com/panelist to be considered—and get our free weekly e-newsletter, Your Anti-Aging Tip Sheet!

Even beginners can interval-train; this 20-minute walk (detailed on page 193) is a great introduction. You can do it outdoors or on a treadmill. (See "How Hard Should You Be Working?" on page 192 for a description of what each pace outlined in the workout feels like.)

Walking Workout #2: Walk-and-Tone Circuit Training

Alternating between a cardio activity, such as walking, and strength-training moves compresses two workouts into one session, saving you time. It may also help you work off more weight. In a study from the South Shore YMCA in Quincy, MA, exercisers who used this so-called "circuit training" approach for 25 minutes three times a week for 12 weeks lost a whopping 4 percent of their body fat. And no wonder: You're raising your heart rate and burning calories while building muscle, which can boost your metabolism and help you burn more calories throughout the day. You'll gain firmness and lose mushy inches with this approach.

Your Walk-and-Tone Circuit-Training Plan

2 min.	Warm-up
1 min.	Squat with chest press
2 min.	Moderate walk
1 min.	Rear lunge with biceps curl
2 min.	Moderate walk
1 min.	Triceps dip with leg lift
2 min.	Moderate walk
1 min.	Squat with chest press
2 min.	Moderate walk
1 min.	Rear lunge with biceps curl
2 min.	Moderate walk
1 min.	Triceps dip with leg lift
2 min.	Cooldown

Walking Workout #3: Mood-Boosting, Stress-Busting Cross-Training

Cardiovascular exercise has great mental health benefits, helping to ease depression and counter stress. In the process, it may slow aging as well.

Researchers at the University of California, San Francisco, have been investigating how exercise lessens the negative impact of stress on telomeres, those protective caps on chromosomes that are a measure of cell age. In one of their studies, the researchers looked at people with severe stress—those with post-traumatic stress disorder, victims of childhood abuse, and Alzheimer's caregivers—and found that the participants all had shorter telomeres in their white blood cells, a marker of both poorer immune system health and greater cell aging. But exercise seems to short-circuit telomere shrinkage even for these people: In a study of women who'd been abused as children, those who maintained a regular exercise regimen that included vigorous activity at least three times a week didn't have shortened telomeres.

Your Stress-Busting Cross-Training Plan

3 min.	Warm-up walk: Focus on deep breathing—inhale through nose for two counts, exhale through mouth for five
2 min.	Fast walk
2 min.	Lateral shuffle or rope skip
1 min.	Fast walk
2 min.	Lateral shuffle or rope skip
2 min.	Fast walk
2 min.	Lateral shuffle or rope skip
2 min.	Fast walk
2 min.	Lateral shuffle or rope skip
2 min.	Cooldown

In this workout, we've included a mindful warm-up and inserted some cardio moves that require focus (when your attention is on the present, you're much less likely to worry about the future or what's happened in the past). To cross-train (alternate between two activities), follow the plan above or simply alternate between the shuffle and the rope-skipping. By the walk's end, you'll feel relaxed, refreshed, serene, and strong.

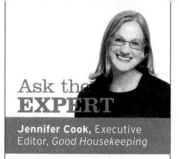

Q *Isn't there some formula for taking my pulse and calculating how hard I'm exercising? Is that the best way to make sure I'm benefiting?*

Jenny says: Tracking your pulse is another way to determine how hard you should be working during a cardio session. Until recently, target heart rate, the pulse rate that promotes heart fitness, has been based on a unisex formula that turns out to be too high for women. To find your female-friendly peak heart rate, calculate 88 percent of your age and subtract that from 206. Then aim to work out at 65 to 85 percent of that number. We've done the math for you at goodhousekeeping.com /target-pulse.

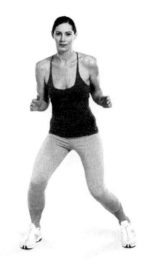

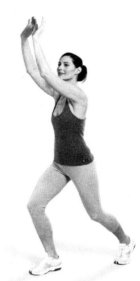

1. LATERAL SHUFFLE Start with feet together, knees bent into a slight squat, and bent arms in front of body. Shuffle as quickly as you can four times to the right. Then do a little hop, jumping both feet off the ground and extending arms overhead as if shooting a basketball. (If you can't jump, pop up onto the balls of your feet as you lift your arms.) Repeat to left, moving as quickly as you can and staying low to the ground. Continue, alternating, for 2 minutes.

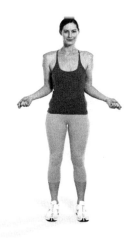
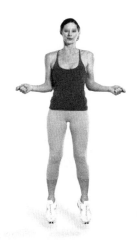

2. ROPE SKIP Stand with feet together, arms at sides. Imagine you're holding a jump rope, and jump in place on balls of feet, making twirling motion with hands. Keep abs contracted as you jump. Continue for 2 minutes.

Youth Booster #4: Find the Core of Your Fitness

Exercises that target the "core" of your body (your abdominal muscles and the muscles in your lower back and mid-back) can flatten your belly, trim your waist, and give you better posture—all of which make you look and move as if you were years younger. When your core is strong, you'll have a lower risk of injury and feel less tired after workouts. "The core stabilizes the body, so if it's weak, you use other muscles to compensate, leading to imbalances that cause fatigue and injury," says Los Angeles–based personal trainer Stephen J. Manak.

Do this trio of core moves three times a week. Aim for 15 reps or as

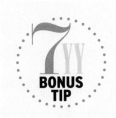

Whether your taste runs to blues or Beyoncé, listening to music while you work out can help you keep at it up to 15 percent longer.

The Cheater's Guide to Exercise

We're not talking about skipping workouts altogether. It's all about finding ways to trick your body into burning more calories without your even feeling it. Try these.

Take 10

If you can't manage 20-minute-or-longer walks, break them up. "The cumulative time you put into short bursts of exercise is equivalent to one long workout," says Martha Gulati, M.D., assistant professor of preventive medicine in the cardiology division of Northwestern University Feinberg School of Medicine in Chicago. "The important thing is to start building an exercise habit." As an ultimate goal, aim to get in two to three 10-minute walks at least four days a week. Even if you have worked out, 10 minutes of walking burns off that much more fat and that many more calories.

Play With Pace

To burn more fat and calories and reap the most cardiovascular benefits, you need to challenge yourself, working out at a level that makes you breathe a little harder and makes your heart beat faster. Speed-walk to the next tree or lamppost; repeat. Or simply choose a route with hills. On the treadmill, try a low incline to kick up your calorie burn-off.

Be Fickle

If you always walk the same route at the same speed and elevation, your muscles adapt and become so efficient that they actually burn fewer calories as you work out. How to tell if your muscles are coasting? If you're not sweating as much at the end of your session, you don't feel that tired after working out, or you're gaining weight even though you aren't eating more or exercising less, you need to shake things up. Try adding intervals (as in our Walking Workout #1), speeding up your pace, adding hill walking or a new activity into the mix—or all of these suggestions.

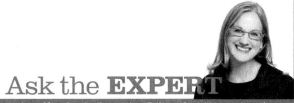

Ask the **EXPERT**

Jennifer Cook, Executive Editor, *Good Housekeeping*

Q *What speed is moderate walking? Three miles per hour?*

Jenny says: Rather than measuring how much ground you're covering, many trainers suggest that you simply use the "talk test": If you find it slightly difficult to talk while you're working out, you're moving at the right pace. No problem chatting with your walking partner? Ramp it up a bit. Getting too breathless to share a funny anecdote? Slow down. The talk test takes into account your state of fitness (as you get more conditioned, you'll need to go faster), the length of your stride, and the terrain (hilly, flat, or some of each) so you don't have to do the math I mentioned in my answer on page 198.

many as you can do while maintaining good form. You'll get to 15 in no time. You'll also see results faster if you put your mind on your middle in your everyday life. Many women let their abdominals get lax when not doing specific core exercises. Simply tightening your core muscles periodically as you walk, carry in the groceries, or sit in front of the computer can make you flat faster.

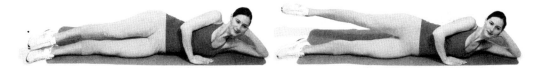

1. **SIDE LIFT** Lie on mat on your left side, lining up shoulders, hips, and knees. Prop up head on left hand, with elbow on mat. Place your right hand in front of you to keep from rolling over. Contract abs. Starting with feet together, lift right leg six inches, then lower. (For a challenge, lift both legs off mat about four inches, then raise top leg.) Do one set of 15 repetitions, working up to two sets. Switch sides and repeat.

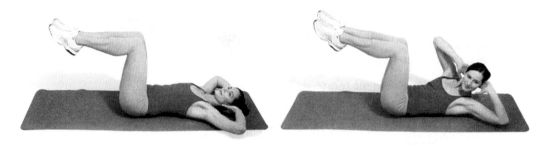

2. **TWISTING CRUNCH** Lie on your back on mat, feet in air with knees bent at a 90-degree angle. Place hands behind head, keeping elbows wide. Lift shoulders off mat, rotating right shoulder toward outside of left knee as you lower knees slightly to the left. Return to center, and repeat on opposite side. Do one set of 15 repetitions, working up to two sets. (If your back arches off the mat, simply place your feet flat on mat, keeping knees bent, and lower as directed from this position.)

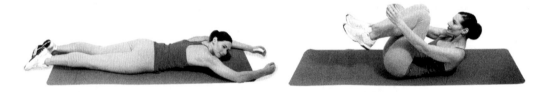

3. **FLIP-FLOP** Lie facedown, arms extended overhead. Inhale and then, exhaling, contract abs and roll over onto your back, arms still overhead. From here, bring knees toward chest and lift shoulders off mat, sweeping arms down to sides. Lower back onto mat, extending arms overhead again, and roll back onto tummy. Do one set of 15 repetitions, alternating the direction you roll each time. Work up to two sets.

Youth Booster #5: Discover How Feeling Flexible Feels Fantastic

Much of what we experience as aging is actually a loss of flexibility. If you don't use your joints, tendons, and ligaments, moving through their whole range of motion, you lose mobility. Not only do you feel stiff, but this loss of flexibility affects how well you function in your daily life. Reaching for things becomes more difficult if your arms and shoulders are tight, while taut hamstrings can lead to lower-back pain. Stretching is like oiling the machinery, says Manak. It helps get blood flowing through your muscles and joints so they have more give, and that can make everything you do—including our walking workouts—a lot easier.

There's another reason it's worth working stretches into your day: They feel good. Stretching is like a moving meditation; it gives you a little time out, and that can help you better handle stress. Your cells, under stress, seem to stop regenerating as quickly, becoming more prone to disease and early cell death. Aging is, in many ways, an accumulation of stress, so anything that relieves the pressure will make you look, think, and act years younger. The five stretches that follow can be done anywhere, anytime. Work them into your day (you don't have to do all of them at the same time) or, if you prefer, do them at the end of your walks.

1. **STANDING HAMSTRING STRETCH** Stand with your legs shoulder-width apart, knees slightly bent. Bend forward from your waist and reach your fingers toward your toes. Don't force the movement; just stretch enough to feel a comfortable tension in the backs of your legs. Hold for 5 to 10 seconds, letting your neck and shoulders relax. Be sure not to bounce. Repeat three times.

2. **STANDING CROSSOVER STRETCH** From a standing position, cross your right foot over your left foot. With your knees slightly bent, bend forward from your waist and reach your fingers toward your toes. Don't force the movement; just stretch enough to feel a comfortable tension in the backs of your legs. Hold for 5 to 10 seconds, then switch sides. Repeat four times.

3. **CHEST STRETCH** Stand in an open doorway, on the side without the door. Open your arms and raise them to shoulder height, placing hands on either side of the doorframe. Lean forward until you feel a stretch through your shoulders and chest. Hold for 5 to 10 seconds. Repeat three times.

Bernadette Pace
"Exercise flipped on my energy switch"

"I can't wait to get home and get on the treadmill and exercise." Bernadette Pace, 53, had had a tough day, and she was telling one of her two grown daughters how eager she was to "burn off" the aggravation. "Mom, say that again," her daughter replied. "You actually *want* to exercise?"

A surprising payoff Eight weeks earlier, Bernadette had been a confirmed exercise-a-phobe. "I've never liked it—I was using my treadmill as a laundry basket," she confesses. But when she began the 7 Years Younger program, something clicked: "Because you 'chunk up' the exercise into intervals, it doesn't get boring." After a few weeks, Bernadette found herself staying on the treadmill even longer than the time she'd allotted for her workout. The payoff: She lost a whopping 10.25 inches from her waist!

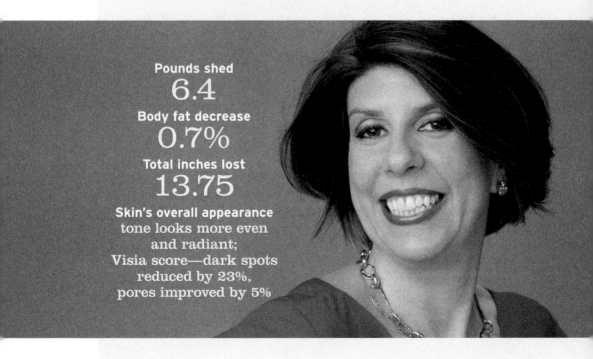

Pounds shed
6.4
Body fat decrease
0.7%
Total inches lost
13.75
Skin's overall appearance
tone looks more even
and radiant;
Visia score—dark spots
reduced by 23%,
pores improved by 5%

Her middle-management strategy Embarking on the program as a non-exerciser (with more weight around her middle than was healthy), Bernadette couldn't do some of the abdominal and strength-training exercises. Instead of giving up, she modified them. "At first, I had to hold on to something to do the squats, and it was too hard for me to start the 'flip-flop' ab exercise from the facedown position, so I started out lying on my side," she says. "Now that I'm stronger, I can do everything the right way."

Frozen assets A long daily commute to her job pretty much guaranteed that Bernadette wouldn't be able to cook for herself every night. So she developed her own time-saving strategy: "I prepared two meals on Sunday, then alternated eating them during the week." (Each one serves four.) She also kept her freezer stocked with the Amy's frozen meals recommended on the weight-loss plan, tossing one in her lunch bag when she didn't have time to pack a homemade meal.

The confidence bonus Bernadette, recently widowed, has been trying to expand her social circle, and her newly glowing skin and replenished energy have helped. "I feel better about myself," she says, "and it's helping me come out of my shell."

Compliment she cherishes When Bernadette posted her "after" photo on Facebook, her brother-in-law commented, "I think you overshot. You were supposed to look seven years younger; you look 10!"

For more about Bernadette Pace, see color insert.

Want to be a test panelist for a future 7 Years Younger plan? Sign up today at 7yearsyounger.com/panelist to be considered—and get our free weekly e-newsletter, Your Anti-Aging Tip Sheet!

4. **CROSSOVER SHOULDER STRETCH** While standing or sitting, extend your right arm in front of you at shoulder height. Grasp your right elbow with your left hand and gently pull your right arm across your body, keeping it at shoulder height, until you feel a comfortable tension. Hold for 5 to 10 seconds, then switch sides. Repeat four times.

5. **TRICEPS STRETCH** While sitting or standing, extend your right arm overhead. Bend your right elbow so your right hand drops behind your back. Grasp your right elbow with your left hand and gently push back until you feel a good stretch in the back of your upper arm. Hold for 5 to 10 seconds, then switch sides. Repeat four times.

Youth Booster #6: Make Your Mind-Body Connection

Adding some type of low-impact mind-body exercise—workouts like yoga and tai chi that have a meditative or mind-focusing component—to your weekly workout schedule can help you lower age-accelerating anxiety, stress, and high blood pressure while also raising your ability to battle damage from free radicals. And if you've found that back pain has crept up on you as you've gotten older, mind-body exercise might just be your ticket to relief. In one study, funded by the National Center for Complementary and Alternative Medicine, 90 people with chronic back pain were assigned to either a yoga group or a standard-medical-care group. Those in the yoga group attended 90-minute yoga classes two times a week for six months. Twelve weeks into the study, again at the six-month mark, and then six months after the study ended, the yoga practitioners all reported less pain. They were also able to function better and suffered from less depression than the standard-medical-care group who did no yoga. Some research suggests Pilates may help with back pain, too.

Although they may be gentler than aerobics, mind-body workouts still strengthen muscles, improve balance, and enhance flexibility.

Most health clubs and recreation centers offer them, but mind-body exercise can also be practiced at home (consider buying or downloading an instructional video). Here are four kinds to try. (Note: You'll see that there may be a range for calories burned. That's because the number of calories you burn depends on your weight and the intensity of your workout.)

Ballet You might not think of ballet as a mind-body exercise, but it has all the hallmarks: This graceful, smooth type of dance is a great way to stretch and strengthen underused muscles and improve flexibility and coordination. The mind-body aspect comes from the focus required for the (mostly) low-impact moves. An added benefit is improved posture; the classic positions help align your body to produce a graceful, taller stance.
Calories burned per half-hour session: 150 to 180

Pilates Named after Joseph Pilates (pronounced puh-*lah*-tees), who developed a series of floor exercises 70 years ago, this workout combines strength, flexibility, balance, and control training with resistance exercises. It's done individually, in groups, or on three specific pieces of specially designed Pilates equipment. Movements look like stretches and emphasize breathing along with muscle flexes. A workout lasts 45 to 90 minutes, and although it's not aerobic at lower levels, advanced students can get cardiovascular benefit. Pilates is usually taught one-on-one, so it can be expensive, but many clubs offer more reasonably priced mat classes (the exercises are done without the large specialized equipment) that are also very effective.
Calories burned per half-hour session: 180 to 220

Tai Chi This ancient Chinese regimen, rooted in the martial arts, improves strength, flexibility, concentration, and balance by combining mental discipline with physical moves. When done correctly, tai chi can raise the heart rate to 60 percent of maximum, qualifying as moderate exercise. Thighs and hips do much of the work, just as in high-impact aerobics—but without the jumping. And it just may keep you young: One study showed that tai chi practitioners slowed their loss of aerobic capacity, a measure of how the heart, lungs, and circulatory system are working.

Calories burned per half-hour session: 125 to 150

Yoga Rooted in ancient Indian philosophy, yoga improves flexibility, muscle strength, and endurance. It consists of deep-breathing exercises and "postures" or "poses" that are held for several seconds to several minutes. Some forms of yoga also involve muscle toning and aerobic movement. The poses can be adapted to any fitness level. As you increase the depth of practice, the benefits increase. Some doctors advise learning yoga in a supervised class because certain positions can cause injury if done incorrectly.

Calories burned per half-hour session: 200

Youth Booster #7: Find the Fun in Fitness

To reap continuous anti-aging benefits from exercise, you have to continue to exercise—that's obvious. But it's sticking to your resolve once the initial excitement passes that makes the difference between those who drop out and those who are in it for the long haul. So, instead of asking yourself

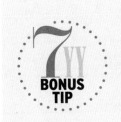

BONUS TIP

Smart scheduling can help you stick to your workouts: An informal survey done at the Mollen Clinic in Phoenix showed that 75 percent of runners and joggers who **worked out early in the day stuck with their programs,** while only a quarter of the nighttime exercisers did.

"Why?" (as in, "Why bother to exercise at my age?") ask "Why not?" (as in, "Why not do something fun that extends my life as a bonus?") Here are some tips for staying inspired and motivated.

Follow the pleasure principle Redefine fitness as fun, and follow your bliss. Inline skating, hula hooping, Zumba, kickboxing, bike riding, spinning, Wii Fit games—they're all fun, and they all burn calories and benefit your health. Research shows that when you're enjoying yourself, you're more likely to stick with an activity, so if walking isn't working for you, try something else that you'll enjoy more.

Exercise family-style You may be more likely to stay active if the rest of your family is on board. "Pick things you can do together, like bicycling, hiking, rock climbing, canoeing, or bowling," says Kelli Calabrese, M.S., exercise physiologist and fitness consultant. "Take a martial-arts class. Everyone's a beginner together; you all start out as white belts and progress from there," she says. Some local parks may offer fitness courses your family could tackle together. Choose a weekend to hike, bike, or canoe in a nearby city or state park. Or check out a local farm and go apple- or berry-picking. Toss around a football, go ice-skating, take a long walk with the dog twice a week—it's not exercise, it's family time.

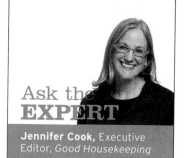

Ask the EXPERT

Jennifer Cook, Executive Editor, *Good Housekeeping*

Q *Is it OK for me to continue my own routine instead of adopting the ones you recommend?*

Jenny says: If your program hits all the key goals outlined in this chapter—firming, calorie-burning, cardio fitness, balance training—you can keep doing it. But why not try some of these moves? If you don't mix it up—you always walk the same route, swim laps at one speed, or have a single strength-training routine—your muscles adapt and become so efficient that they burn fewer calories while you work out. Change it up—and you may also boost your fitness (and weight loss!).

Learn a new skill If you've always wanted to try tennis, ice-skating, golf, cross-country skiing, ballroom dancing, or rowing, taking a course will give you an entrée into a healthy new activity, and the learning process will help keep it interesting. Check local community organizations or the YMCA for affordable classes.

Always exercise on Mondays This sets the psychological pattern for the week and helps you get into the habit of exercise.

Consider the context Do you dislike weight training, or is it just the guys who hang out by the weights that you actually dislike? Maybe it's the grubby showers at your gym that keep you from returning as often as you should. Or perhaps you get bored walking. Examine the external factors that might be discouraging you from exercise, then see what remedies you can come up with (buying a set of dumbbells and ditching your gym membership, downloading books on tape for your walks).

Stay injury-free One common reason people give up on exercise is injury. Suppose you haven't exercised in a while. After a sudden urge to get fit, you might go at it harder than your body is prepared for, twisting an ankle or tearing a muscle along the way. (Even if you avoid hurting yourself, you might feel convinced that exercise is too difficult and quit before you've really started.) No matter how revved up you feel, always start slowly and work at an intensity that feels comfortable. Each workout will help your body adapt so that you can gradually increase the length and/or intensity of your workouts.

Activate Your Anti-Aging Plan Now!

1 **Increase the movement in your daily life** Women who move more throughout the day have greater success at weight loss and maintenance. Set some mini-goals for the week: taking the stairs instead of an elevator or escalator; walking to the store/post office that's farther away. Climbing 10 flights of stairs burns 85 calories in under 10 minutes. Consistent small calorie burn-offs can add up to large weight losses.

2 **Think fun, play, pleasure** When you approach exercise with a positive mindset and use it as an opportunity to enjoy yourself, you're far more likely to develop a regular workout habit. To start, forget about calories and concentrate on enjoyment.

3 **Start strength training** The older you are when you start lifting weights, the faster and more dramatic the results you'll see: Resistance training—especially upper-body moves for women—builds muscle, boosts bone strength, increases flexibility, improves posture, and hikes up your metabolic rate (the number of calories burned every hour of every day).

For more expert anti-aging advice, get our free weekly e-newsletter, Your Anti-Aging Tip Sheet, *at 7yearsyounger.com/newsletter. And join the 7 Years Younger community on Facebook to share your anti-aging story with others at facebook.com/7yearsyounger.*

Age Eraser 6

Chapter Six

Your Brain— Only Better

Feel like some days you're forgetting more than you remember? Surprise: Your brain can actually get better with age. In the 20 or so years that researchers have been intensively studying the brain, the most remarkable discovery has been its plasticity, meaning that the brain itself can change, both producing more cells and increasing the connections between those cells. "We used to think that with age, brain cells shriveled up, died, and that was that," says brain researcher Paul Laurienti, M.D., Ph.D., of the Wake Forest University School of Medicine. "Now we know that even older brains can grow new, stronger connections."

Brain researchers used to believe that everyone lost up to 30 percent of their neurons as they aged, but now it looks as if you not only hold on to most of those neurons, but can make new, "smarter" ones if you try. "Research suggests that it's never too late to start engaging your brain," says Gary Small, M.D., director of the UCLA Center on Aging at the Semel Institute for Neuroscience & Human Behavior and author of *The Alzheimer's Prevention Program*.

In short, your brain keeps developing, at every age, and it reflects what you do with it. Here's your brain-gain plan for now—and the future.

7 TOP MOVES TO TRAIN YOUR BRAIN YOUNGER

Brain Booster #1: Find Your Focus

You've totally forgotten the instructions your boss just gave you. You can't find the phone that was in your hand only two minutes ago. It's easy to think you're losing your memory, but the problem may simply be that you're not focusing on what you're doing/asking/being told.

You're bombarded with information all day; you couldn't possibly remember all of it. But when you focus on something—that is, when you look and listen carefully—it's much more likely the memory will endure. One thing that prevents most people from paying full attention is distraction, anything from your mind wandering (*Did I turn off the oven?*) to the beeping of your smartphone. Many people also engage in what Dr. Small calls "partial continuous attention." Think of someone who is talking to you at a party but looking over her shoulder to see who else is in the room, and you get an idea of what it is. "You seem to be doing one thing, but you're scanning the environment in case something new and more interesting comes through," Dr. Small explains. Trying to juggle these tasks stresses the brain, and that impedes memory storage.

The fix: mindfulness—purposefully paying attention to what's happening in the present moment—so that you are aware of what is going on both inside and around you. Try these four strategies to help get you there.

Notice more to remember more What color hair did the barista who made your latte this morning have? Was your husband wearing a tie or not? Taking time to notice new details keeps your brain sharp. When you walk a familiar route, look up and down both sides of the street. Try to recognize businesses or homes you've never noticed before. Being observant puts you in the present and makes you aware of what requires your attention. "That uncertainty keeps you attentive," says Ellen Langer, Ph.D., a professor of psychology at Harvard University who has written extensively about mindfulness. Even if you'll never need the information, observing and recalling the details of your day gets you off autopilot—and that's going to sharpen your memory.

Say it out loud! Locking the door, taking your calcium, unplugging the iron, transferring the laundry from the washer to the dryer—there's a reason they're called mindless tasks. When you want to get a routine activity lodged into your brain so you don't forget it, say it out loud as you do it ("It's morning; time for my calcium"). And you know that feeling when you walk into a room and stand there wondering why you came in? The same trick—repeating aloud, "I'm getting the scissors," while en route—fends off distraction as you head into the kitchen to get them.

Minimize multitasking If you're not walking the dog to pick up a carton of milk while talking on the phone, you're eating lunch in the car as you shuttle your kids to soccer practice (and listen to the news on the radio). Sometimes there's no choice: To get through your day, you have to do lots of things at once. However, research shows that quickly switching from one thing to another (and back) interferes with so-called "working memory"—your ability to keep in mind something that just happened or absorb something you just learned.

Equally important: minimize interruptions. Think, for instance, of what happens when you're talking to a friend on the phone and your child

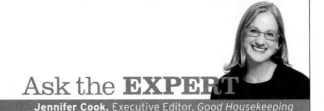

Ask the **EXPERT**

Jennifer Cook, Executive Editor, *Good Housekeeping*

Q *Since I turned 40, I can't seem to remember anything! How do I know I'm not getting something serious, like Alzheimer's?*

Jenny says: Memory problems can feel alarming, but Alzheimer's disease is pretty rare among men and women under age 65. If you find you're forgetting things—like where you put your glasses or what you need to buy at the drugstore—it's far more likely that lack of sleep, distractions, or simply too much multitasking is to blame. Alzheimer's patients have trouble remembering things they just learned and can't recall them even if they're given details to nudge their memory. So if someone reminds you of the name of the woman seated across from you ("Susan"), and you say, "Of course—Susan! We met last year at the soccer playoffs," you've probably got nothing to worry about. However, if it really worries you, bring it up with your doctor at your next checkup.

runs in to ask a question. You answer, then turn back to the conversation. "What was I saying?" you have to ask. The disruption has made your mind come up empty. Some evidence also suggests that juggling more than one mental task gets harder with the years—all the more reason for getting in the habit now of focusing on one thing.

Have a short, intellectually stimulating talk To switch your brainpower to high for a presentation or some mentally challenging work, a quick verbal exchange with a friend beforehand can have the same benefits as mental exercises. Researchers at the University of Michigan divided 76 people into three groups. One group discussed a social issue for 10 minutes. A second group spent 10 minutes doing a crossword puzzle. The third group watched 10 minutes from an episode of *Seinfeld*. Afterward, the volunteers' cognitive performance was assessed with measures of mental processing speed and working memory. The social-

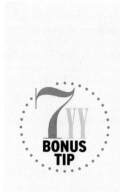

BONUS TIP

Doing activities that boost your mood can sharpen your thinking. In research at the University of Western Ontario, **people who listened to lively music** (Mozart) and watched a happy video (a laughing baby) **performed better than volunteers** who listened to sad soundtrack clips (from *Schindler's List*) or watched neutral videos (*Antiques Roadshow*) or negative ones (earthquake news). The **happy folks bested others on problems** that specifically called for classifying patterns, but you can try it for any project where you need to think innovatively, suggests lead author Ruby T. Nadler.

interaction group did slightly better than the brain-work group, and both groups did better than the TV watchers.

Brain Booster #2: Be Deliberate About Making Memories That Last

Memory-enhancing techniques can make a big difference in how well you remember details, names, and faces. And once you've got the tricks under your belt, continued use of them will reward you with lasting benefits. There's even some suggestion that improving your memory translates into greater intelligence. So you not only remember things, you get smarter, too! These tried-and-true techniques are often used in brain-health programs. Start practicing them today.

Make associations When you give words more meaning by associating them with something you already know, you improve the likelihood that the hippocampus (the brain's control center for learning and memory) will store them as long-term memories. So, say, when you're introduced to someone named Sally, you can make up a rhyme ("Sally in the alley") or connect the name to a song ("Mustang Sally"). Some people swear by devices like mnemonics, memory aids that use patterns or abbreviations. One dog owner never leaves for the morning walk without her three *b*'s (bags, biscuits, ball) and two *t*'s (telephone, tissues). Along the same lines, you might also create an acronym to jog your memory. Where's that store that caught your eye? Remember the familiar abbreviation for Los Angeles—L.A.—and it will trigger the address: "Larch and Ashland."

Divide and conquer If you organize your desk or workspace, you can find things more easily. Similarly, you can organize your brain so you can call forth information more readily. One way to do that is to practice what scientists call "chunking"—in nonscientific terms, breaking things up. This technique is particularly useful in remembering numbers. By repeating a phone extension as "38, 27" instead of "3, 8, 2, 7," you only have to remember two numbers, not four. Another way to chunk info is to categorize. If, for instance, you need to buy salmon, milk, lemons, cereal, and rice, you might group them into "dinner" (salmon, lemons, rice) and "breakfast" (cereal and milk).

Connect names and faces To better remember names and faces, try the following steps:

1. Repeat the person's name as you're introduced ("Hi, Alice").
2. If it's an unusual name, ask the person to spell it or pronounce it again.
3. Connect the name to something—such as someone you know who has the same name (*My sister-in-law is named Alice, too*)—or to an association it conjures up (*I always loved that Alice Cooper song "School's Out"*).
4. Look for a distinctive feature on the person's face and connect it to an image (*Alice has blue eyes, blue like Alice in Wonderland's dress*).
5. Finally, say the person's name again as you finish your conversation ("Nice talking with you, Alice")—but if that feels forced, just repeat the name to yourself as you walk away.

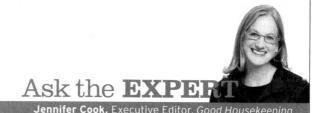

Ask the **EXPERT**

Jennifer Cook, Executive Editor, *Good Housekeeping*

Q *I've tried that trick to remember names, but I wind up recalling the word association and not the name. How can I make this technique work?*

Jenny says: Been there, done that: You recall that the woman's name had something to do with flowers, but was it Rose? Violet? Daisy? When I consulted memory expert Benjamin Levy, author of *Remember Every Name Every Time*, he advised bringing in your right brain—that is, mentally adding a visual image to solidify the verbal association. It can help to find a link that's meaningful to you personally. I love novels, so I'll often think of a book character with the same name as a person I meet. Finally, try practicing the name game when there's no pressure. As you're watching a TV show, for example, make it a point to learn (and recall) the name of every character introduced during the episode.

Create quirky changes Some experts believe that you can build your brainpower by altering the way you habitually do things, thereby activating new circuits and increasing production of neurotrophins, proteins that maintain and protect brain cells. While this is not a specific memory trick, it does boost your overall recall. One change-up that will exercise your brain in a new way is to brush your teeth with your left hand if you're normally right-handed (or vice versa). You might also change your route to work, or take a shower before bed instead of in the morning.

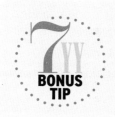

BONUS TIP

Try wearing a watch or favorite bracelet on the other wrist **when you need to remember** something. The oddity of not finding the watch where it should be may serve as a proverbial string tied around your finger.

the bottom line

Are Speed-Dialing, Google, and GPS Ruining Our Memories?

Gadgets now do a sizeable amount of the memory work we once did ourselves, but whether that's making our brains lazy is still an open question. Researchers at Columbia University found that participants who were shown information and then told it would be accessible again on their computers did worse on a memory test than those who thought the information was going to be deleted. In another study, participants were told that statements they typed–answers to a trivia quiz–would be saved into one of five folders on a computer. When their recall was later tested, they were better at remembering where they'd stored the information than the actual trivia itself. The upshot: If you don't have to remember something, you won't–but you will remember where you can find it.

And that's not necessarily a bad thing. The Columbia researchers argue that by emptying your brain of things like phone numbers and facts that you can easily Google, you may free up your gray matter for more profound thinking. They point out, too, that people have always relied on sources outside their own brains to store information, like the memory of a friend, family member, or coworker. That might strike a familiar note. If, for instance, your spouse is the one who always drives to your weekend cottage, you aren't likely to learn how to get there yourself. In the same way, you can now depend on your GPS. "Technology is not necessarily bad for the brain," says UCLA's Gary Small, M.D. "But when we overuse it, it becomes unhealthy." Dr. Small's own research, in fact, has shown that Internet searching may actually make you smarter. In a study published in the *American Journal of Geriatric Psychiatry*, he and his colleagues found that people between the ages of 55 and 76 registered significant activity in areas of the brain responsible for decision-making and comprehension– and more activity than reading elicited–while performing online searches. The benefits were most pronounced in people well versed in Internet use.

Brain Booster #3: Find It Before You Lose It!

It's easy to get the idea that you're just someone who's always losing things. In fact, misplacing items is not a hard-wired trait; you can drastically reduce those misplaced-key moments with better search-and-rescue techniques.

Designate a special place for important everyday items Keys, lipsticks, glasses, phones, money—they all have a way of getting lost. Perhaps because these articles seem so mundane, you don't think about them much, and that's the problem. Inattention is the root of most memory lapses leading to misplaced items. And fatigue or stress can make inattention even worse.

You'll be less likely to misplace items if you habitually put them in one place. Simply having a bowl or other container near the door where you dump your keys, glasses, phone, and other "loseables" can work wonders. Designate certain pockets in your purse for your phone, keys, and wallet. Have an organizer for your bills and mail where you place them right after you've opened them so nothing gets thrown out with the recycling by mistake (making folders for e-mail bill alerts and other important electronic documents can organize you virtually as well). Just the moment it takes to mindfully put things in a designated place will improve your find-it success rate considerably.

Use methodical seeking strategies When, despite your best efforts, you do lose things, Michael Solomon, a self-described "findologist" based in Baltimore, suggests that you "tail thyself"—retrace the steps leading up to the loss. You might even go so far as to put your path into print: Sit down with a piece of paper and pencil and write down everything you did. Take your time and concentrate. Then stand up and repeat your steps.

Also be on alert for the camouflage effect: The item you seek is nearby, just hidden from view. How many times have you scoured the front hall for your keys only to find that they are sitting under the pile of mail you dumped on the kitchen counter? Consider, too, that the lost item might actually be where it's supposed to be. Your lipstick is really in your purse; you're just rummaging through too fast to find it. That bill or memo is still on your desk; finding it just takes a more systematic search through your papers.

"Look once, look well," is how Solomon puts it. It's common to search for something five or six times in the same place, rifling through the same stack of bills for a receipt or upending the contents of a drawer looking for a pill bottle. Instead of ransacking the room, do a thorough search the first time around. Carefully turn over each slip of paper and lift every book in search of the receipt; take the time to pull aside things in a drawer to see if a bottle rolled backward or look under the nightstand where a pill bottle might fall.

Three Find-It Tricks

1. **Find the "safely hidden" but forgotten item** How clever you were to find such a good hiding place; now, don't outsmart yourself. Your husband's birthday gift or your child's graduation present is probably above (or below) eye level and in the dark. Check closets, the top of the fridge, a shelf in the basement.

2. **Check (unintentionally) secret hiding places** Can't find earrings or a favorite moisturizer? Check your suitcase or travel tote bag, both sinkholes for lost items because they might not have been unpacked after a trip.

3. **Have extra keys on hand** Of course you want to find your keys, but you'll have less stress if you know that there's an extra set available. Make a duplicate or two and keep them in a designated place for those times you must leave the house ASAP.

Brain Booster #4: Help Yourself Remember by Staying Calm

It's not unusual to feel frustrated when you can't remember something, especially if you need that information or item in a hurry. But getting upset only exacerbates the problem, in both the long and the short term.

Defuse anxiety The more worried you are about drawing a blank, the harder it is to remember. In fact, when you're frantic, it's possible to look directly at a lost object and not see it. "We become so agitated, we don't perceive what's right in front of us," says Solomon. Before you begin looking for a lost item or trying to recall information, collect your wits and calm down. Refuse to allow your mind to race: Breathe deeply for a few minutes. Make a cup of tea or drink a glass of water. Recite some soothing words. Then tap your mental reserves again; this time you'll be more likely to find what you're looking for.

Short-circuit stress When you get anxious, your body releases a stress hormone called cortisol. A chronically elevated level of cortisol—often the result of living a tension-filled life—has been connected to many health problems as well as memory impairment. When blood levels of cortisol increase, it may damage neurons, interfering with encoding or retrieving information. The anti-anxiety steps outlined above can help you regain your composure—and your memory.

Meditate to remember Just as stress can downgrade recall, relaxation can give it a boost. In the UCLA Laboratory of Neuro Imaging, researchers found that those who meditated regularly had more gray matter (nerve cell–rich tissue in the brain) than people who didn't. Researchers also found that meditators had stronger connections between brain regions and less age-related atrophy. The researchers didn't look at whether the meditators actually did better on memory tests, but their results are intriguing nonetheless—and offer a good reason to take up the practice. Don't procrastinate: It's not clear how long it takes to get the effect, but the people studied had been meditating for a minimum of five years.

Brain Booster #5: Use It or Lose It

Your brain isn't a muscle, but it exists with the same credo: Use it or lose it. And as with a muscle, if you exercise your brain, it's going to get strong and supple. "Brain training is analogous to physical workouts," says brain researcher Sherry L. Willis, Ph.D., a professor in the department of human development and family studies at Pennsylvania State University. "You have to cross-train—work different parts of your brain—and keep adding new challenges."

Like physical exercise, brain training shouldn't be a no-pain-no-gain situation. If it's too hard, it will be frustrating and stressful, which is no good for recall. Nor should it be too easy—that will only lead to boredom and a lack of intellectual enhancement. But choose the right amount of mental stimulation, and it will create fresh connections in your brain. "You can actually generate new cells in the hippocampus," says Peter Snyder, Ph.D., professor of clinical neurosciences at the Warren Alpert School of Medicine at Brown University. Those new cells build cognitive reserves that are important for creating new memories and may protect against memory loss—even dementia—later in life. Here's how to make your brain more fit.

Live a more thought-provoking life Highly educated people tend to have a lower risk of Alzheimer's, most likely because education has gotten them in the habit of being mentally active. Yet you don't need an advanced degree to get your brain moving. For instance, in the Bronx Aging Study, men and women ages 75 to 85 who regularly participated in six activities—reading, writing, playing board or card games, joining in group discussions, doing crossword puzzles, and playing music—were

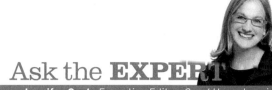

Ask the **EXPERT**

Jennifer Cook, Executive Editor, *Good Housekeeping*

Q *I took a foreign language in high school. Will that help keep my brain fit, even though it was years ago?*

Jenny says: If only! Learning a language does create new brain pathways, which explains why the bilingual among us have stronger memory circuits, a greater ability to pay attention, and better cognitive abilities. But those pathways are like muscles, and can get flabby with disuse. Experts say that having taken Spanish 20 years ago won't do you much good now unless you start putting any knowledge you've retained to use. That doesn't necessarily mean signing up for evening language classes (though if that inspires you, go for it). Take consistent baby steps: When you eat out at an ethnic restaurant, try ordering your meal in that language. Or catch a foreign film: Even watching with the English subtitles will help if you try to match the words to the spoken language. Challenge yourself a little, and you just may see big brain benefits.

less likely to show symptoms of dementia. Taking classes can also be a brain booster, particularly if you learn a second language. Research from the University of Toronto suggests that being bilingual builds brain reserves that may help keep Alzheimer's symptoms at bay for as long as four years. One reason may be that using two languages strengthens the portion of the brain that helps you focus and ignore distractions.

Game your gray matter Crossword puzzles, Sudoku, mazes, computer games, brain teasers, playing the guitar—anything that gets you using your noodle may help keep your brain fit, and it will certainly be fun trying. You will likely get the biggest cognitive boost by using both the left and the right hemispheres of the brain. Right-brain exercises include reading maps, working mazes, playing an instrument, and drawing (the right brain is more involved with spatial tasks). Left-brain exercises heighten your verbal and logic skills and include doing crossword puzzles and playing other types of word games. Puzzles and games that have you working against the clock, like Boggle, Scrabble, or the memory game Simon, may give your brain an extra lift by forcing you to pay attention, work quickly, and think flexibly.

Here are four examples—two left-brain and two right-brain exercises. For answers, see page 234.

Left-Brain Exercise #1

Consider the word SPARKLING. Without rearranging the letters, take away one letter to form a new word. Then take away another letter to form another word. Continue until you have a one-letter word.

Left-Brain Exercise #2

A woman scored 100 points in archery. The target had six rings with the following values: 40, 39, 24, 23, 17, 16. How many arrows did she need to reach the 100 points?

Right-Brain Exercise #1

Move two toothpicks to create four squares, one of which is larger than the others.

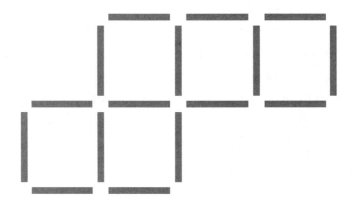

Right-Brain Exercise #2

See how quickly you can do this maze.

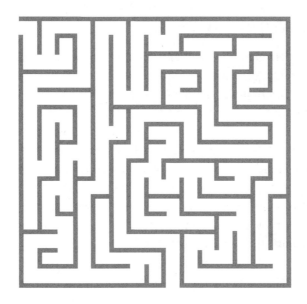

Brain Booster #6: Live a Brain-Healthy Lifestyle

Nothing turns back the clock on brain changes more than the way you eat, exercise, sleep, de-stress, and stay mentally grounded. Keep your brain in the game with these healthy habits.

Hit the sack Anyone who's ever stayed up too late experiences that next-day fuzziness, when it seems like nothing really registers or is available for recall later. That *is* exactly what's happening. Different parts of the brain are responsible for creating different types of memories—a face, a name, or just the recollection that you met someone, explains Gary Richardson, M.D., senior research scientist at the Sleep Disorders Center at Henry Ford Hospital in Detroit. "Sleep is what helps knit all those memories together."

You also need sleep to make long-term memories last. Studies at Harvard

the bottom line

Do Computer Brain-Fitness Programs Work?

Research looking at the effect of these training programs has generated mixed results. For instance, a 2010 study by British researchers that tested two different online brain-training programs on over 11,000 people found that while the testers got better at the tasks they practiced, there was no carryover to other cognitive abilities. (The volunteers had practiced for 10 minutes, three days a week, for six weeks.) Yet in an earlier study, researchers at the Mayo Clinic found that those over the age of 65 who used a brain-training program one hour a day, five days a week, for eight weeks had improvement in both memory and attention. The catch: The study was funded by Posit, the company that markets the brain-training program used by the Mayo researchers.

In fact, the software companies themselves sponsored much of the research that showed just how how well individual computer programs worked. While that doesn't mean the results aren't worth considering, it does suggest that investing in specialized computer training is still a gamble. If you're game to try, there are two key requirements to consider: You must do the exercises consistently and, like any brain challenges, they shouldn't be too easy or too hard.

Medical School have found that when people are given a random list of words to memorize, those who then sleep will recall more words afterward than those who are tested without a chance to sack out. And when it comes to sleep, quality is just as important as quantity. New research suggests that the more fragmented your night's rest, the less likely you are to consolidate memories. (For more on getting a good night's sleep, see page 238.)

Sweat yourself smarter Exercise benefits your brain in numerous ways: Evidence that a fit body translates into a fit mind keeps accumulating.

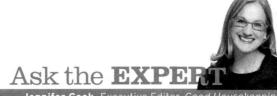

Ask the **EXPERT**

Jennifer Cook, Executive Editor, *Good Housekeeping*

Q *I've been adding more incidental activities every day, per the plan—like walking to do errands and taking the stairs—in order to burn more calories. Will these keep my brain sharp, too?*

Jenny says: It looks that way. Everyday moves like these are gaining new respect among exercise experts. In one Canadian study, researchers who strapped motion detectors to a group of sedentary adults found that those who moved the most during the course of a day had significantly higher cardiorespiratory fitness than those who moved the least; that translates to better brain health. And specifically among older adults, the researchers reported that the most on-the-go participants also had the lowest levels of brain fuzziness, or cognitive impairment.

For instance, when researchers at the University of Illinois looked at the brains of 161 adults, ages 59 to 81, they found that the hippocampus was larger in those who were physically active. "Fitness improvement—even if you've been sedentary most of your life—leads to an increase in volume of this brain region," explains study coauthor Art Kramer, Ph.D., professor of psychology and neuroscience. In another of Kramer's studies, 65 older adults joined a walking group and began walking for 10 minutes three times a week. Each week, they increased the length of their walks by five minutes until, at week seven, they reached 40 minutes per session—the duration they stuck to for the remainder of the study. At the end of one year, high-resolution imaging showed that the walkers had increased brain connectivity and improved scores on cognitive tests. That's proof that you don't have to live at the gym to improve. "Just get out and walk for an hour a few days a week," says Kramer.

Drop the extra weight No one is quite sure why or how excess pounds affect cognition—it may be via reduced blood flow to the brain—but there's some evidence that shows they do count: In a French study, those with a high body mass index (BMI) scored lower on memory tests and had bigger mental declines than people with lower BMIs. Johns Hopkins researchers have also found that obesity, especially fat around your middle, can increase your risk of dementia by 80 percent on average. Losing weight seems to reverse this worrying trend. A Kent State University analysis of people who'd had weight-loss (bariatric) surgery showed that patients had improved memory performance at a 12-week follow-up. Will nonsurgical weight loss produce the same results? A 2011 multicenter review of studies looking at the association found that the biggest brain benefits occurred in those who were obese; it's less clear whether the effect holds true for those who are overweight.

Track your numbers Low levels of HDL (so-called "good" cholesterol) are linked to memory loss and dementia. (Exercise raises HDLs—another reason why it's critical for cognitive health.) But you should watch your total cholesterol level, too: Having high cholesterol in your 40s increases your chances of developing Alzheimer's later in life. Keeping total cholesterol low and HDLs high also reduces your risk of cardiovascular disease, which in itself has brain-health consequences. "Cardiovascular disease seems to be a low-grade inflammatory response in the body that causes wear and tear on brain cells," explains Dr. Small.

Manage your vices Moderate drinking may benefit the brain somewhat, but excessive drinking doesn't only muddle your thinking; it kills off brain cells. Smoking also takes a toll on your mental faculties. Smokers have more memory problems than nonsmokers as well as a greater yearly decline in cognition and a higher risk for Alzheimer's. Just one more reason to quit smoking.

Give yourself a break Regular time-outs—exercise, strolling in a park, scrolling through family photos, closing your eyes to do some mindful breathing—will reduce your stress level and, in so doing, protect your memory. Research shows that chronic stress can shrink one of the key memory centers of the brain.

Floss daily Otherwise you may start forgetting names, dates, and your grocery list. In a study of more than 2,300 men and women age 60 and over, those who scored the lowest on simple arithmetic and memory tasks—making mistakes similar to patients with early Alzheimer's disease–had been exposed to a particular gum disease–causing bacteria the longest. (The researchers could tell from blood tests.) The cognitive connection? The body responds to this pathogen with inflammation, which stiffens blood vessels, raising the risk of heart attack, stroke, and memory problems. "When it comes to preventing dementia and other chronic diseases, it may be just as important to brush, floss, and go to the dentist as it is to take your blood pressure medication," says James M. Noble, M.D., of Harlem Hospital and Columbia University Medical Center.

Move your eyes back and forth It can help jog your memory. In one study, British researcher Andrew Parker had 100-plus students listen to a

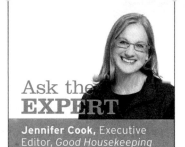

Ask the
EXPERT

Jennifer Cook, Executive Editor, *Good Housekeeping*

Q *High blood pressure runs in my family. Does that affect memory, too?*

Jenny says: Hypertension *has* been linked to memory problems. Since you know you're at risk, you can take steps now to lower your odds or to wrestle down a rising pressure. Some switches that have proven to be helpful: Eat a healthy diet that's rich in fresh fruits and vegetables as well as low-fat sources of dairy and protein; avoid processed foods, which are often high in sodium; reach and maintain a healthy weight; and exercise consistently. To track your progress, see your doctor for blood pressure checks regularly.

voice reading 20 lists of 15 words each. The students then looked over a list of words and were asked to pick out the ones they'd just heard. Those who tried this trick—moving their eyes from side to side for 30 seconds before they were asked to recall the words—performed 10 percent better on the memory test. The eye movements seem mainly to impact a form of recall called episodic memory, says Parker, a senior lecturer at Manchester Metropolitan University in Manchester, U.K. Episodic memory involves recalling specific experiences like what you did yesterday, last week, or last year. Why would moving your eyes enhance recall? One theory is that it helps the two hemispheres of your brain interact more efficiently. The best way to use the technique is on an as-needed basis. Find yourself standing in the grocery store wondering why you came in? Try moving your eyes back and forth.

Brain Booster #7: Eat Smart for Your Brain

What you consume every day can improve daily cognitive function as well as potentially help you prevent Alzheimer's and other forms of memory loss in your later years. The 7-Week Plan, beginning on page 277, covers all your anti-aging bases, but it's helpful to know which foods keep your cranium in top working condition. Here are the top brain bites, and why you should work them into your diet.

Fish People who have higher blood levels of DHA (an omega-3 fatty acid found in cold-water fish like salmon, sardines, and mackerel) have a 47 percent lower risk of dementia than those with the lowest levels, reported a Tufts University study of about 900 older women and men. Eating fish three times a week led to the highest DHA levels.

Legumes Black beans, pinto beans, garbanzo beans, and lentils are all rich in folic acid, a B vitamin that improved memory and information-processing speed in a study of more than 800 women and men conducted by researchers in the Netherlands.

Fruits and veggies A French study of 1,640 healthy women and men reported that participants who ate the most flavonoids—antioxidants found in fruits and vegetables as well as in coffee, tea, chocolate, and wine—had the smallest drops in brain functioning over 10 years.

Blueberries While upping your total intake of produce can help, loading up on blueberries is a particularly good idea. They may have the chemical power to create new pathways for connection in the brain. The number of these connectors tends to drop off with age, but in animal studies, blueberry consumption has been shown to help restore them, says Jim Joseph, Ph.D., director of the neuroscience lab at the USDA Human Nutrition Research Center on Aging, Tufts University.

Cocoa When researchers at the University of Nottingham, England, scanned the brains of 16 women who'd just finished a cup of cocoa, they found that blood flow to some brain regions rose—and stayed high—for two to three hours. This study used a blend of cocoa that's not available commercially, but research suggests that cocoa and other forms of dark chocolate available in markets may have similar powers.

Coffee Prefer coffee to cocoa? Swedish and Finnish researchers found that moderate coffee consumption (three to five cups a day) cut dementia risk 65 percent.

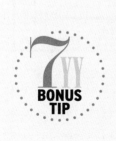

The rates of Alzheimer's are lower in India, and prodigious curry-eating may be one reason why. **Yellow curries are full of the spice turmeric, which is chock-full of curcumin.** This active ingredient has been shown to attack the amyloid plaques that build up on the brain and cause disease. You can use turmeric to color dishes like deviled eggs or vegetable sautés. It's also found in bright yellow mustards.

Answers to exercises on pages 226-227:

Left-Brain Exercise #1:

Sparkling

Sparking

Sparing

Spring

Sprig

Prig

Rig

Pi

I

Left-Brain Exercise #2

Six   (17, 17, 17, 17, 16, 16 = 100)

Right-Brain Exercise #1:

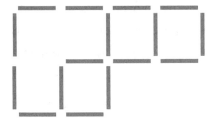

Right-Brain Exercise #2

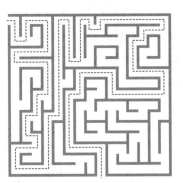

Activate Your Anti-Aging Plan Now!

1 **Minimize multitasking** What passes for efficiency may in fact be distracting you. Simply focusing more on the one thing you're doing—and not on anything else—can sharply improve your brainpower.

2 **Create a "memory place"** Set a bowl or basket in your entryway and use it for frequently used (and frequently lost) items, such as keys, glasses, and cell phone. You'll instantly raise your find-it quotient.

3 **Go out for a brisk walk** You'll boost circulation to the brain and keep your cognitive function high. Exercise also improves cardiac health, keeping arteries clear so the brain gets plenty of blood. Physical activity also helps you de-stress, which can keep you focused and sharpen your memory. Take a new route, and you'll stimulate your brain to make new connections.

For more expert anti-aging advice, get our free weekly e-newsletter, Your Anti-Aging Tip Sheet, *at 7yearsyounger.com/newsletter. And join the 7 Years Younger community on Facebook to share your anti-aging story with others at facebook.com/7yearsyounger.*

Age Eraser 7

Chapter Seven

Say Goodbye
to Stress

Feeling good—calm, content, engaged in the world around you—makes you feel younger. And where the mind leads, the body follows. Anything you do to reduce stress, better your outlook on life, strengthen your relationships, and be generous to others will have physiological payoffs, helping you look younger and more vital. Studies have found that women with lower levels of stress have telomeres (the protective caps on chromosomes that indicate a cell's age) that represent, on average, one less decade of aging compared with those of their more tense counterparts. The stress-busting strategies in this chapter—everything from deep breathing to discovering a volunteer opportunity that you love—can make you less easily ruffled, more resilient, and altogether happier. Just like your younger, more carefree self.

Stress-Buster #1: Get Your Beauty Sleep Every Night

When you catch the proverbial 40 winks each night, *everything* improves. Your skin becomes firmer and better hydrated, so it has a youthful glow. Sleep enhances memory, so your mind stays quick and agile, and it reduces inflammation in the body, helping to fight age-accelerating conditions such as wrinkles, heart disease, diabetes, and arthritis. Most people need anywhere from six to eight hours of sleep. Find out what works for you and then try to consistently hit that mark. To enjoy a nightly age-defying snooze, try to:

Develop better before-bed habits

- **Stick to a schedule** It will be easier for you to fall asleep at night if you turn in and wake up at the same time every day. If you occasionally miss your bedtime during the week, you can use the weekend to catch up, but you'll feel most rested if you keep the same hours nightly.
- **Chill** A cool bedroom lowers your core body temperature, which initiates sleepiness. The ideal temperature is 65°F. Start there and then adjust up or down as necessary.
- **Log off** That little charging light emitted by computers, mobile phones, answering machines, and PDAs is enough to suppress melatonin, the sleepiness hormone, so try to end screen time at least an hour before bedtime. Keep ambient light low, too, and

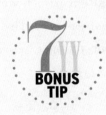

Earplugs, the squishable foam-pellet type, help **block everything from street noise and TV** to snoring. Highest in GHRI tests for their muffling ability and comfort: Hearos Ear Plugs Ultimate Softness Series.

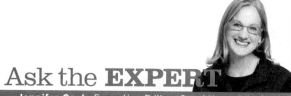
Q *If I have trouble sleeping, can I get the same health and longevity benefits from a sleeping pill?*

Jenny says: You will certainly feel better—and function at a higher level—the next day. But the studies that have looked at the long-term health benefits of getting enough rest usually base the results on people sleeping well at least four nights a week. And while sleeping pills are OK once in a while, taking them frequently, especially for extended periods of time, isn't a good idea. After a while, you may need to up the dosage. Better to address the underlying issues that keep you from sleeping well, through changing your habits or sleep environment to overcome your insomnia.

don't watch TV in bed. Turn off appliance lights (face your alarm clock away from you; charge other devices in another room), and invest in a sleep mask or even blackout curtains if streetlights are visible.

- **Eat earlier** Stop eating one to two hours before bedtime. The digestion process increases blood flow to the digestive tract and makes it difficult to stay asleep. The one exception: If you're having trouble drifting off, a *light* combo of protein and carbs may help. Carbohydrates help your brain use tryptophan, an amino acid that causes sleepiness. And proteins help your body build tryptophan. Snack on peanut butter on toast or low-fat cheese and crackers.

- **Skip the nightcaps** Alcohol is a known sleep disruptor, especially when drunk right before bed. It can increase the amount of time you spend tossing and turning in the wee hours of the night. And according to research at the University of Michigan, it's more of a problem for women than for men.

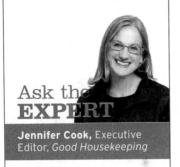

Ask the EXPERT

Jennifer Cook, Executive Editor, *Good Housekeeping*

Q *Before bed, I like to read on an electronic device. Should I be turning that off earlier, too?*

Jenny says: Regular books (or non-backlit e-readers) may be better for your zzz's than a laptop or light-up tablet computer. Light interferes with the production of the drowsiness hormone melatonin, which is why sleep gurus advise that if you have trouble nodding off, you keep your bedroom as dark as possible.

- **Reserve your bed for sleep** (and sex, which some people find can make it easier to fall asleep). But nothing more. That way the power of suggestion (bed = sleep) will be more likely to take hold. You'll walk into your bedroom, see your bed awaiting you, and feel like nodding off.

- **Wind down** The more active your mind, the less shut-eye you'll get. Give yourself time in the evening to relax, even if that means you have to set an e-mail and household-chore cut-off time of 7 or 8 P.M.

- **Keep your bed pet-free** A Mayo Clinic survey found that 53 percent of people who share beds or bedrooms with pets have disrupted rest. It's best to keep pets out of your room, but if you don't have the heart to teach your old dog a new trick, set up a cozy bed on the floor.

- **Count blessings, not sheep** In a British study, survey respondents who scored highest in gratitude slept longer than less appreciative participants. The quality of their sleep was also better. Take a few minutes each day to mentally savor the things, large or small, that you're thankful for.

Keep daytime habits that contribute to a restful night

- **Do some heavy breathing** Regular aerobic exercise—like the kind you'll be doing in our 7 Years Younger 7-Week Plan—improves sleep quality. Work out for 20 to 40 minutes, four

the bottom line

Can the Right Sleeping Position Reduce Wrinkles?

Lying on your back keeps your face youthful: Squishing your face up against a pillow night after night as you snooze on your stomach can contribute to wrinkling. A back-lying position also reduces discomfort from gastric reflux (also known as heartburn), a condition that may occur more frequently as you get older—the little muscle that separates the esophagus from the stomach becomes more stretched out, which allows stomach acid to move back up, causing reflux and interfering with sleep.

Sleeping on your back also makes it easier for your head, neck, and spine to maintain a neutral position so you feel less achy and more rested in the morning, says Christopher R. Rose, M.D., medical director of the Covenant Sleep Center in Lubbock, TX.

If it's hard to break the habit of sleeping on your stomach, try propping a pillow under your knees and using a cervical pillow (a special pillow designed to support the neck) to make sleeping on your back more comfortable.

---

times a week, and you'll be sleeping better. Schedule workouts with an eye toward sleep: Exercise helps regulate your sleep/wake cycle, but the stimulation that comes from a workout in the three hours before bedtime may cancel the benefit.

- **Stay engaged** If you're tired, you may be tempted to just veg out with TV reruns. But boredom can actually cause sleep loss. Stay busy and challenged during your waking hours—socially, emotionally, and physically—and you'll sleep more soundly.

- **Cut off caffeine** You don't have to cut *out* coffee and other caffeinated beverages, but you should taper off by 2 P.M. When you hit your afternoon slump, wake yourself up with a short walk instead of a caffeinated drink.

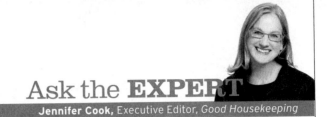

Ask the EXPERT

Jennifer Cook, Executive Editor, *Good Housekeeping*

Q *Night sweats are making it hard for me to get a good night's sleep. How can I cool off my hot flashes?*

Jenny says: As you probably know, flashes are triggered by fluctuating estrogen levels. Hormone therapy does help, but you and your doctor need to review your history and other health issues—such as a family history of breast cancer, heart disease, strokes, or blood clots—to determine whether you're a candidate or not. When I checked with Donna Arand, Ph.D., clinical director of the Kettering Sleep Disorders Center in Dayton, OH, about supplements, she told me that although various kinds have been looked at, their benefits haven't really held up in studies. She suggests keeping your bedroom cool, using layers of light covers (so you can strip down if necessary), and wearing PJ's made from a fabric that draws moisture away from your body. Also, Arand says, try a ceiling fan, which many of her patients find really helpful.

- **Nap the right way** If you're dragging, take a short siesta (10 to 30 minutes), but only if it's early in the afternoon. A late-afternoon nap will likely make it harder to fall asleep that night. Upon awakening, refresh with a spritz of water on your face, or (to save your makeup) pat the back of your neck with cold water.

Stress-Buster #2: Take a Deep Breath

Breathing is connected to your body's stress-response system, so the way you breathe can actually help calm you in times of stress. And stress affects everything: your skin, your heart, your brain, your energy. Learning the most effective breathing method can change the way you think, feel, and react on a daily basis by influencing the information sent to your brain by your nervous system.

The kind of breathing that thwarts the aging effects of stress is diaphragmatic breathing, a method that uses the diaphragm, the muscular sheet just below the lungs, to draw air all the way into the bottom of the lungs. You're doing diaphragmatic breathing if your inhalations raise or inflate your belly. With stress (and age) many people unconsciously ditch diaphragmatic breathing and start breathing more shallowly, contracting the rib cage to draw air into the lungs so that the chest, not the belly, rises. If you breathe that way now—and frequently people who are chronically stressed out or prone to anxiety do—you may just need a little practice to make healthier breathing a habit.

Consciously paying attention to your breathing provides a way to calm yourself, averting a potentially harmful cascade of stress hormones coursing through your body. "Focused breathing," explains Steven Hickman, Psy.D., director of the University of California, San Diego Center for Mindfulness, "brings you into the present." Anxiety is largely about what might happen in the future. But if you can relax and bring your mind to the task at hand, you will feel more serene, a much healthier situation for your body and a much better state of mind to be in when you need to get something done.

Pranayama, a yoga-breathing technique, has been shown to lower depression, improve mental alertness, and reduce both physical and psychological anxiety. Practice this easy exercise for a few minutes each day, and you'll feel better prepared to handle whatever ups and downs come your way:

Lie on your back on a mat on the floor or on your bed. Place your hands on your belly and inhale slowly through your nose, letting the air fill your belly. Count to five as you inhale, then exhale (also through your nose) on the same count, expelling all the air. As you breathe, pay attention to your inhalation and exhalation, focusing on the rise and fall of your belly. You can practice pranayama anywhere, anytime. It's just a matter of slowing down and focusing on your breath.

Diane Durando
"Taking charge of my well-being makes me look years younger"

I t's an understatement to say that the past 10 years of Diane's life have been challenging—she lost her brother, sister, and mother, and one of her two children was born premature (now a toddler, she's doing well). By the time Diane, 41, embarked on the 7 Years Younger program, it had been years since she'd paid any attention to her own well-being. "This program changed my philosophy and my priorities," she says. "From now on, I'm going to be a little more greedy about taking time for myself."

Reaping the benefits of more sleep Before 7 Years Younger, it wasn't unusual for Diane to get into bed with a BlackBerry in one hand and a computer on her lap. "It was working for my life and my career, but not for my body," she says. "I was famous for being an insomniac." But putting all her electronics away and winding down

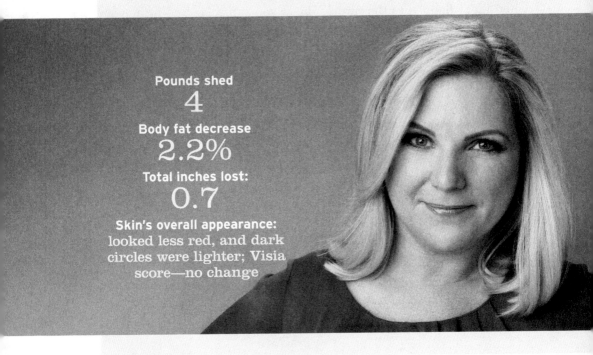

Pounds shed
4
Body fat decrease
2.2%
Total inches lost:
0.7
Skin's overall appearance: looked less red, and dark circles were lighter; Visia score—no change

for an hour before bed helped immeasurably. Her sleep now: "Much more restful," she says, and you can see it in her face. "A lot of people have mentioned that my skin looks younger or healthier or has a glow to it, and I think better sleep is one reason why."

Mindful, not mindless, munching The 7 Years Younger weight-loss plan was a wake-up call for Diane, who hadn't realized how many calories she'd been eating. "When 3 P.M. rolled around, you could find me at my desk snacking mindlessly—not junk food necessarily, but without regard to calories or portion size," she says. "I'd eat almonds, but did I measure them? No. Now I do."

An exercise in efficiency Diane had been wearing her hair the same way for as long as she could remember. When our beauty crew lopped off a good five inches, she flinched a little—then rejoiced. "I love it, and it's so much quicker to style. It's given me an extra 10 minutes in the morning to do some ab moves, squats, and lunges," she says.

Her life motto Diane takes a positive view of what's ahead. "Habits don't change overnight; it's a journey," she says. "I have a road map now, and I feel as though I'm on my way."

For more about Diane Durando, see color insert.

Want to be a test panelist for a future 7 Years Younger plan? Sign up today at 7yearsyounger.com/panelist to be considered—and get our free weekly e-newsletter, Your Anti-Aging Tip Sheet!

Get Grounded

When you find yourself in the middle of a situation that's got you worked up and stressed out, ask yourself this question: *Where are my feet?* "It literally grounds you, and it's just a silly enough question that you'll remember it even when you're really anxious or panicky," says Hickman, who has advised anxious patients in the emergency room to focus on their feet. "It's a reminder to come back to where you are if you're lost in worry."

Stress-Buster #3: Make Time for Meditation

You had a fight with your sister, and the contractor didn't show. Then the dog dug up your tomato plants. Meditating not only calms you down, but can also change your perspective and how you handle stressful situations altogether. And every step you take toward reducing stress will also reduce your risk of heart disease, lessen the chance that you'll turn to food for comfort (and gain extra pounds), and even keep your skin looking younger.

Meditation works much the same way breathing exercises do, but it also allows you to go deeper. If breathing exercises are like taking a walk around the block, meditation is like going to the gym for an hour—both are beneficial (and both are good habits to get into), but the latter is going to have a greater impact on your health and how young and vibrant you feel. For instance, in an Australian study, researchers found that people who practiced meditation regularly for eight weeks had greater improvements in work stress, anxiety, and depression. Meditation may even help you cope better with menopausal symptoms. In a University of Massachusetts Medical School study, women who were experiencing hot flashes and night sweats participated in weekly two-and-a-half-hour mindfulness classes focusing on body awareness, meditation, and stretching. By the end of the eight-week study, they didn't have fewer hot flashes than a control group, but they were less stressed and anxious, slept better, and were less bothered by their hot flashes and night sweats.

If you practice meditation regularly, you're not likely to get as worked up by things like a sister's stubbornness or a contractor's negligence or a bad dog. In stressful situations, we often operate on autopilot, but handling problems in a more deliberate way can be far more effective and less likely to send your stress level soaring. "Meditation helps you do that by cultivating mindfulness," says UCSD's Hickman, "so that you can be less emotionally reactive and have the presence of mind to deal with difficult things."

Test-Drive This Meditation

There are different ways to practice meditation. The following is a meditation in the mindfulness tradition. It may take several weeks for you to get into a daily habit. Start by trying to meditate for 10 minutes, working up to 20—or even longer, if possible.

1. Sit quietly in a comfortable position.
2. Close your eyes.
3. Become aware of your breathing. Breathe slowly and naturally, drawing air into your belly and exhaling.
4. Focus on your breathing, and any time your mind wanders away from your breath, take note of what's on your mind and bring your focus back to your breathing. Acknowledge your thoughts without judging, condemning, or rejecting them. Each time, bring your focus back to your breath and begin again.
5. When you are finished, sit quietly for a minute, then open your eyes and rise slowly.

Mindful meditation is not about breathing; it's about the *awareness* of breathing. If you're finding it hard to focus, you might try repeating a word, a prayer, or a short phrase that's meaningful to you.

There are many community meditation classes available, as well as audio files online that you can download. The Mindful Awareness Research Center at UCLA, for instance, has free downloadable guided meditations of varying lengths (marc.ucla.edu/body.cfm?id=22), and there are several guided meditations on YouTube. Look for those by Jon Kabat-Zinn, Ph.D., professor of medicine emeritus at the University of Massachusetts Medical School and a pioneering researcher in mindfulness.

Stress-Buster #4: Repeat the Words That Mean the Most to You

Affirmations—meaningful phrases that you repeat to yourself—have always seemed to have a place in the pantheon of self-esteem-boosting techniques. But it turns out that reciting something significant to yourself can also be a stress-buster, helping to avert waves of anxiety and tension that can have a cumulative and deleterious effect on your body.

The power of a positive phrase Repeating affirmations counters stress by breaking the train of anxious thought, says Herbert Benson, M.D., director emeritus of the Benson-Henry Institute for Mind Body Medicine in Boston. In studies at the University of California, Santa Barbara, students who practiced self-affirmation had lower levels of stress hormones on exam days than students who didn't. Research also suggests that the technique can rewire some anxiety circuits in the brain. "What we think can change the structure of our brains through what scientists call neuroplasticity," explains Andrea Sullivan, owner of BrainStrength Systems, a consulting, coaching, and public-speaking service. "When we repeat an affirmation, our prefrontal cortex sends signals throughout the brain telling it to come into alignment with our intention. In effect, we are rewiring our brains in accordance with new, empowering thoughts that help us produce the results we want."

The best thing about affirmations is that you can use them anytime, anywhere, both in times of sudden need and long-term, as a vaccination against stress. Choose a positive statement (and positive means "I'm happy" rather than "I'm not upset") that is brief, so you can remember it easily when you need to focus. We asked women across the country what words of wisdom they summon to restore perspective when they're about to spiral out of control. Borrow theirs or, better yet, coin your own.

When life looks like it's falling apart, it may just be falling into place.

"When my husband and I left Houston to restore an 1856 ranch in the Texas Hill Country, it seemed like everything that could possibly go wrong did. I was starting to have doubts about our decision. But then I realized that all of these 'bad things' had to happen—and this affirmation came to me." —*Beverly Solomon, Lampasas, TX, creative director*

Will this matter five years from now? No? Then get over it.

"I use it whenever little disasters stress me out. It helps me keep perspective on what's important: family, friends, staying centered." —*Hali Chambers, Luray, VA, massage therapist*

This isn't as important as you're making it; don't allow it to rent space in your head.

"I used this phrase many times in the throes of child-rearing challenges. During a hard time at work, telling myself the job wasn't as important as I was making it helped me relax." —*Brenda Nixon, Columbus, OH, author and speaker on parenting*

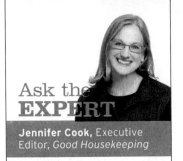
Q *I feel silly saying affirmations out loud. Does it work if you just say them to yourself?*

Jenny says: What's important is what works for you and for the moment. For daily stress prevention, taking a moment to pause and think about your affirmation or writing it down may soothe your tension. However, if you want to disrupt a negative dialogue that's escalating in your mind, speaking your phrase or at least whispering it loudly to yourself may be more effective.

Don't worry about the mule going blind; just keep the wagon loaded.

"I love this little mantra that my father learned from his father, who grew up on a farm in Texas. The basic message is, 'Put one foot in front of the other, and keep moving forward.' The saying always makes me smile even in the worst of times." —*Mary Ann Lowry, Thousand Oaks, CA, life coach*

Support is a phone call away.

"I keep a support-system note card pinned to my office bulletin board and on my refrigerator. On it is contact information for friends, babysitters, housecleaners, doctors, handymen, and counselors. All I have to do is call!" —*Renée Peterson Trudeau, Austin, TX, life-balance coach*

How badly do I want what's on the other side of this brick wall I just hit?

"When I've tried and tried to reach what appears to be an unattainable goal, I ask myself what's preventing me from achieving it. What's my brick wall, and how can I get over, under, or around it? What do I need to do that fits within my moral and ethical framework that can help me achieve the desired outcome?" —*Betsy Hiebert, Winnipeg, Manitoba, small-business owner*

If everything is important, then nothing is.

"The saying keeps me on an even keel and helps me prioritize the plates that are spinning above my head so I know which ones I can drop and pick up again later." —*Kelly Stettner, Springfield, VT, nonprofit director*

The write stuff Besides having a phrase handy, it can also help to write down affirmative values. "One idea that has emerged from our research is that when someone is experiencing stressful times, writing about important values that are not connected to the stress may be helpful," says David Sherman, Ph.D., an associate professor of psychology at the University of California, Santa Barbara, and lead author of the affirmation study. A useful exercise: Write about other key facets of life—values or relationships—and think about why they are important. That can help give you perspective on a stressor or anxiety-provoking event (like an impending job interview) and make it less physiologically taxing.

Stress-Buster #5: Remember to Look on the Bright Side

Optimists tend to handle stress better, have higher levels of self-esteem, and live longer. Optimism helps prevent illness, too: When you're able to look on the bright side of life, you're less likely to experience the adverse feelings that stress your body. "Negative emotions like hostility and bitterness are bad for overall health and specifically for the heart," says Stephen Post, Ph.D., director of the Center for Medical Humanities, Compassionate Care, and Bioethics at Stony Brook University in New York. In fact, women with sunny dispositions enjoy better heart health, experiencing far less arterial narrowing than more dour women.

Optimism and pessimism seem like inborn personality traits, and to some extent they are. But they're changeable, too. Research shows that

the bottom line

Spirituality's Anti-Aging Payoff

One of the reasons, researchers believe, there are so many vital, energetic centenarians on Okinawa is because the culture fosters a deep spirituality. Spirituality can give you a way of dealing with the twists and turns in life, and if you're involved with a spiritual community, you have a ready-made support system—two factors that foster low stress and good health.

Regularly attending a house of worship also seems to confer benefits of its own. Looking at the results of a survey of more than 3,000 adults, sociologists concluded that religious people were more satisfied with their lives—precisely because of the social network they built through their faith. An earlier study from Duke University Medical School found that older people who attended religious services once a week were 46 percent less likely to die over six years than people who went to services less often. Attendance is only part of the picture, though; it's the underlying belief system that provides comfort and improves health, says Duke researcher Harold G. Koenig, M.D.

Even if organized religion isn't for you, private spiritual practices like meditation and prayer can be a healthy addition to your life. Best of all: "The combination of the two is linked to the best outcomes," says Dr. Koenig.

you can actually become a more optimistic person by practicing different mood-enhancing techniques. If, when bad things happen, you tend to give them a lot of weight and, conversely, when good things happen you expect them to be temporary and consider them unimportant, you can benefit from some optimism training. Here are two positivity enhancers to try:

Imagine your best self

Visualizing yourself having the best of all possible lives can make you more optimistic about your future and help ward off symptoms of depression. For years, researchers have been using a type of optimism training called "best possible self." In a Dutch study, psychologists put the following version of "best possible self" to the test and found that it both increased optimism and improved the study participants' mood—immediately as well as over time. Here's how to do it:

- **Part I:** Think about three aspects of your life: your personal state of being, your relationships, and your work life. Now, if you were to be your best possible self, what would your future in those three areas look like? Think of all possible aspects in each area and write down your answers. Start each sentence with, "In the future I will..." Make your goals realistic and attainable, and remember, this is your best possible self.
- **Part II:** Turn those statements into a story and write the story of your best possible future.
- **Part III:** Take five minutes each day for two weeks and visualize the story you've written. As the image takes hold you'll feel not only more hopeful about the future, but more cheerful, too.

Reach out to the world

Join a community group, try a new activity, accept party invitations, strike up a conversation with a stranger—do anything that expands your

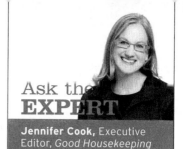

Ask the EXPERT

Jennifer Cook, Executive Editor, *Good Housekeeping*

Q *I've always been a skeptic. Will that affect my longevity?*

Jenny says: Emotions are only a part of your personal long-life equation. As long as you follow a healthy lifestyle and get regular medical checks, you'll be on the right track. Still, you might want to push your needle toward more positivity. A recent Australian study found that adults who took a few minutes to reflect on three positive things that had happened that day were more content and optimistic after just a few weeks. These don't have to be momentous things—just pleasurable or meaningful activities, like enjoying your morning cappuccino or connecting with an old friend on Facebook.

Kathy Coleman
"The less I stress, the younger I look!"

One night during the 7 Years Younger program, Kathy found herself home alone and thought she'd act on one of the recommendations we'd given her: watch a funny movie. "Another time I might have felt guilty about not doing something productive, like working or putting in a load of laundry, but on that night, I just lay back and watched *Crazy, Stupid Love*," says Kathy. "And I felt great!" The 52-year-old married mother of two relished the time for herself and its stress-reducing benefits. Movie night also represented what she liked best about the program. "It's an all-around plan, not just diet and exercise; it allows you to start in one place, then add other components down the line," she says. "This program lets you feel successful in a lot of different areas."

No more skin sins By the end of eight weeks, Kathy had gone from being a skin-care minimalist to having a detailed routine. "Before

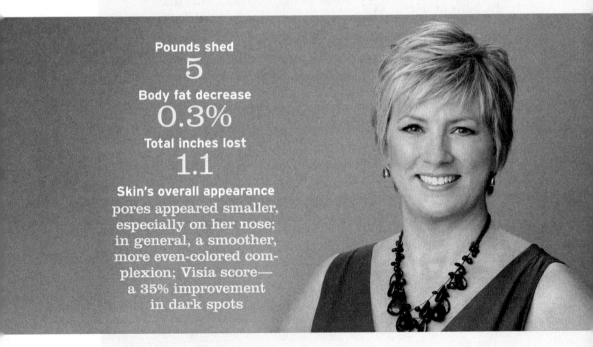

Pounds shed
5
Body fat decrease
0.3%
Total inches lost
1.1
Skin's overall appearance pores appeared smaller, especially on her nose; in general, a smoother, more even-colored complexion; Visia score— a 35% improvement in dark spots

7 Years Younger, I rarely washed my face or used any products at night; my complexion was dry and looked blah. Now I do all the steps at night, including using a serum, and I exfoliate consistently," she says. "I've been very close to 100 percent compliant since starting."

Small changes, big difference Kathy didn't drastically overhaul her makeup or her exercise habits (she already was walking for fitness and doing yoga regularly). However, the little tweaks she made to her routine were notable, to both her and others. She swapped her regular foundation, which was thick and pancake-y, for a tinted moisturizer, and now loves the feel of the lighter product on her skin. She also incorporated the resistance-band exercises into her exercise sessions: "I like the variety they added."

Weighing the weight-loss plan "This plan offers a lot of flexibility and variety," says Kathy—who lost a very respectable five pounds. Like most of our panelists, Kathy loved the breakfast options; her favorite was the Egg Scramble (page 322), made with spinach and feta cheese: "Adding the vegetables and cheese to the egg really bulked up the meal. It seemed like a lot of breakfast for relatively few calories."

For more about Kathy Coleman, see color insert.

Want to be a test panelist for a future 7 Years Younger plan? Sign up today at 7yearsyounger.com/panelist to be considered—and get our free weekly e-newsletter, Your Anti-Aging Tip Sheet!

horizons (see Stress-Buster #6 for more ideas on enlarging your social circle). The reason: Acting gregarious can make you feel more outgoing, which is linked to a more positive mood. If you're in a good mood, you're likely to be more optimistic, too.

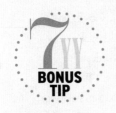

In research at the University of Maryland, scientists found that **laughing can increase blood flow by 22 percent** and may protect against heart problems and reduce stress. Keep a funny picture of your dog on your computer or watch a funny YouTube video to get your grin on.

Stress-Buster #6: Surround Yourself With Friends

Friends can help you live a more fulfilling life, and a longer one to boot. In fact, research shows that friendship can be as beneficial to your well-being as quitting smoking, losing weight, and exercising—and it may help you outlive people who have a less active social life. In an analysis of 148 studies that involved more than 300,000 people from all over the world, researchers at Brigham Young University in Provo, UT, found that people who had relationships were, on average, 50 percent more likely to be alive at the end of the seven-and-a-half-year study period. But the review didn't only find that having friends was beneficial. It also showed that lack of friendships had health risks roughly equivalent to that of smoking up to 15 cigarettes a day and double that of obesity.

Friendship also seems to have benefits above and beyond that of family ties. In one Australian study looking at the link between friendship and longevity, having children and a close family network had no effect on how long participants lived; it was having friends that conferred benefits.

Julie Ann Raab

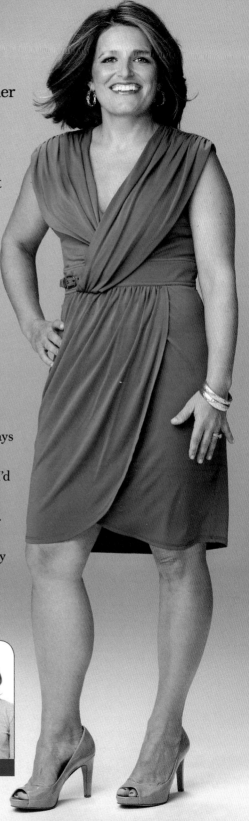

Julie Ann, 40, always felt younger than her age—until recently, when she started to look and feel her years. To reverse the trend, she took steps to eat right, tackled her age spots head-on with products that worked, and tweaked her fitness routine. At the end of eight weeks, her brown spots had paled, her skin was considerably smoother, and she had lost inches around her middle.

JULIE ANN'S PLEDGE

With this pledge, I dedicate myself to the 7 Years Younger program for the next eight weeks.

MY GOALS:

1. To lose weight and keep it off, and find new ways to get in better shape.
2. To focus more time on taking care of my skin. I'd love to get rid of the brown spots that came after being pregnant and being out in the sun too much.
3. To focus on being more easygoing. Life can be chaotic, and I need to figure out how to refocus my energy during a stressful day.

For more on Julie Ann Raab, see page 34.

Pounds shed	Body fat decrease	Total inches lost
1	3%	2.5

Skin's overall appearance
dark circles looked lighter;
Visia score—pores improved by 13%,
skin discolorations reduced by 7%,
and texture improved by 45%

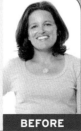

BEFORE

Diane Gurden

With her kids in school full-time, Diane, 43, was ready to start paying attention to herself. She wanted younger skin, a more modern look, and a trimmer body. She was open to change—she tried new foods, exercised more, gave up the lipstick she'd worn for nearly 30 years—and demonstrated resiliency. Even a five-day power outage didn't knock her off course.

DIANE'S PLEDGE

For the next eight weeks I will:

TRY my best to cook new, healthy recipes so my family and I start eating more nutritionally balanced diets.

ADD exercise to my calendar daily to improve strength, mental health, and overall outlook and perspective.

EMBRACE skin-care and makeup techniques more appropriate for a woman in her 40s.

FOCUS on my goals rather than just being a caretaker for everyone else in my life.

For more on Diane Gurden, see page 142.

Pounds shed	Body fat decrease	Total inches lost
12	4.3%	5.5

Skin's overall appearance
more radiant and bright

BEFORE

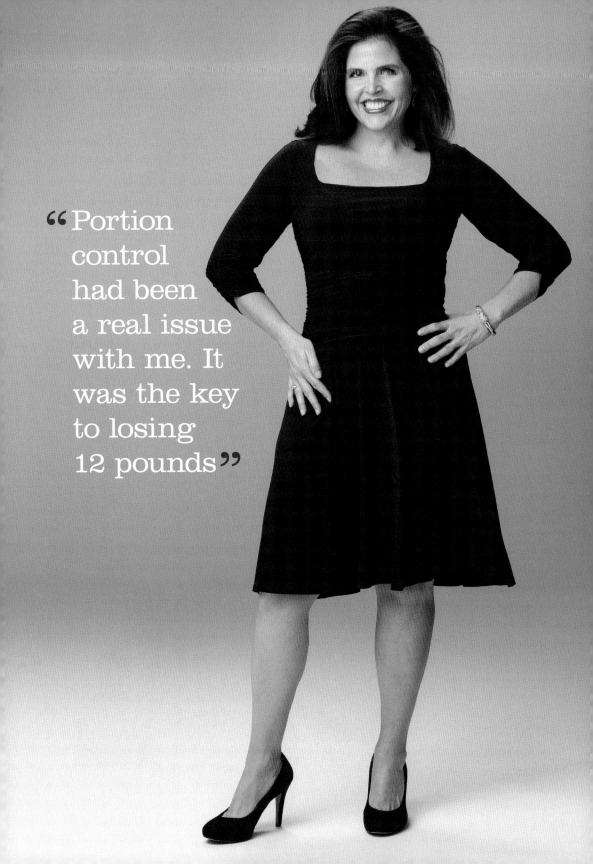

"Portion control had been a real issue with me. It was the key to losing 12 pounds"

Tessa Jean

Tessa's motto is "You're never too young for anti-aging." Focusing on the big 4-0 ahead, Tessa, 34, armed herself with good ideas on how to turn her nutritional know-how into actual meals, an overhaul of her skin-care and makeup routines, and a much-improved sleep schedule. By the end of the program, Tessa was slimmer, glowing, and pleased with the doable road map for future self-care.

TESSA'S PLEDGE

I **PLEDGE** to commit to ME: Tessa Jean will be the priority for the next eight weeks in a holistic manner.

I **PLEDGE** to stretch first thing every morning and give thanks for waking up.

I **PLEDGE** to eat a HEALTHY breakfast that contains protein, whole grains, fruit, and healthy fats.

I **PLEDGE** to drink at least eight glasses of water every day, and I will NOT go to bed until this goal is met.

I **PLEDGE** to live in the moment, to concentrate on the flavors of the food, to concentrate on the task in front of me, and to focus on quality over quantity.

I **PLEDGE** to work out at least four days a week and focus on the endorphins being released as I exercise.

I **PLEDGE** to aim for eight hours of sleep and NOT get less than six.

I **PROMISE** to challenge my mind and keep it active by paying attention to my surroundings.

I **PROMISE** to maintain positive thoughts and a positive outlook on life.

For more on Tessa Jean, see page 48.

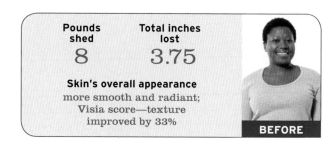

Pounds shed	Total inches lost
8	3.75

Skin's overall appearance
more smooth and radiant;
Visia score—texture
improved by 33%

BEFORE

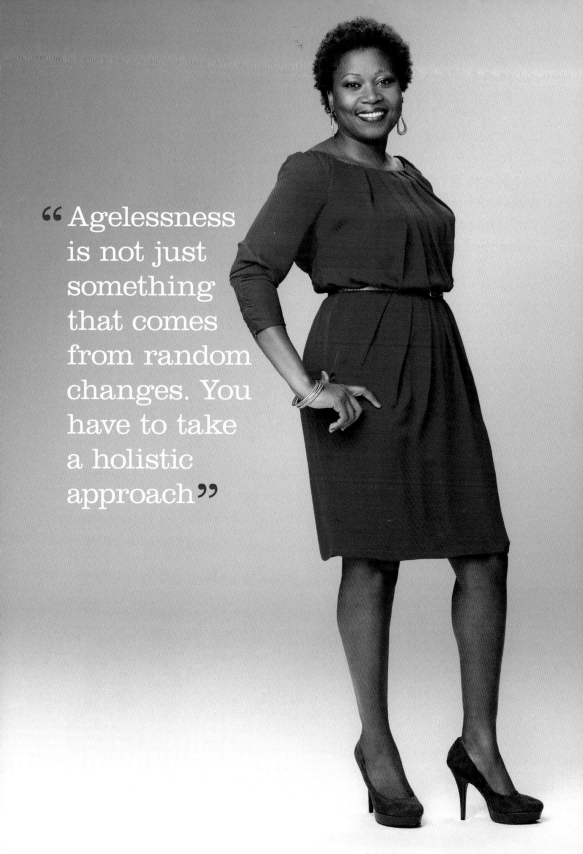

" Agelessness is not just something that comes from random changes. You have to take a holistic approach "

Lauren Mintzer

At the outset of the 7 Years Younger program, Lauren, 44, said if she could change one thing in her life "it would be to have more energy to do all the things that I need to do." Her other goal was to address her wrinkles and brown spots. By adding just a few additional products and a little more time to complexion care, she saw a noticeable difference. And joining a gym gave her the energy boost she craved.

LAUREN'S PLEDGE

I hereby dedicate the next eight weeks to following the 7 Years Younger program to the best of my ability.

I WILL demonstrate just how much I love myself by eating better, taking care of my skin and hair, and exercising daily so that by the end of the program I will be able to look great and be fit!

MY GOAL is to look and feel the very best I possibly can. I want to be able to fit comfortably into the size 6 dresses that I will be trying on for my daughter's bat mitzvah.

I HOPE to bring out the brightness of my skin so that when I look at all the photos taken on her special day, I will feel good about myself.

I KNOW I will have challenging moments during the process. But I hope keeping my goal in mind will help me to stay on course, since I am doing this program for me.

I WILL post this promise so that I can see it every day. I know that doing so will help me through the process.

For more on Lauren Mintzer, see page 112.

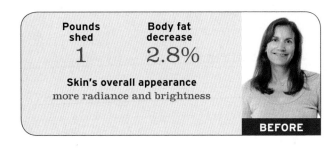

Pounds shed	Body fat decrease
1	2.8%

Skin's overall appearance
more radiance and brightness

BEFORE

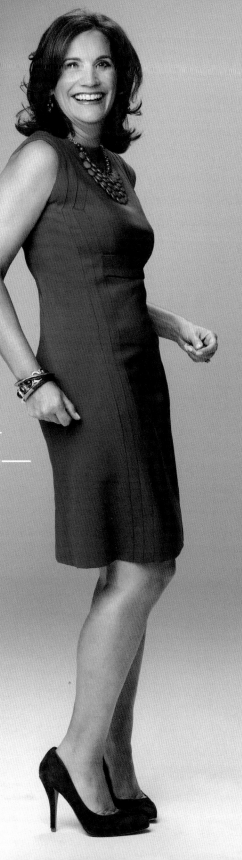

"I went a little crazy with exercise. I joined a gym and I've been spinning and kickboxing and doing lots more— it's fantastic!"

Rachel Dorfman

The last five years had held a lot of heartbreak for Rachel, 37, aging her beyond her years. To reverse the tide, she wanted to shed pounds, feel more grounded, and find the right products for her hair and skin. Our program helped her navigate back to regular exercise and clued her in to simple but effective skin- and hair-care routines. Life stresses, she knows, will come and go; now she's developed better tools to handle them.

RACHEL'S PLEDGE

As part of the 7 Years Younger program, I pledge to spend the next eight weeks adopting healthier habits to get my life back on track.

I'VE LEARNED there are things in life you can control and things you can't. With this program, I pledge to focus on finding new ways to schedule time for myself. This is my opportunity to examine the choices I've been making health-wise and to remember what it feels like to take care of myself—something I've been ignoring for a while. I pledge to make myself a priority, knowing that if I can't take care of myself, I will never be able to take care of anyone else.

I ALSO PLEDGE to move in the direction of getting in better shape, even if that means I have to sacrifice immediate pleasures such as a glass of wine or watching TV at night.

I'D REALLY LIKE to find ways to simplify my life, so that I can find more time to relax. I think the 7 Years Younger plan is my starting point to achieving all this.

For more on Rachel Dorfman,
see page 78.

Pounds shed	Body fat decrease	Total inches lost
7.4	3.8%	10.25

Skin's overall appearance
Visia score—7% improvement
in dark spots

BEFORE

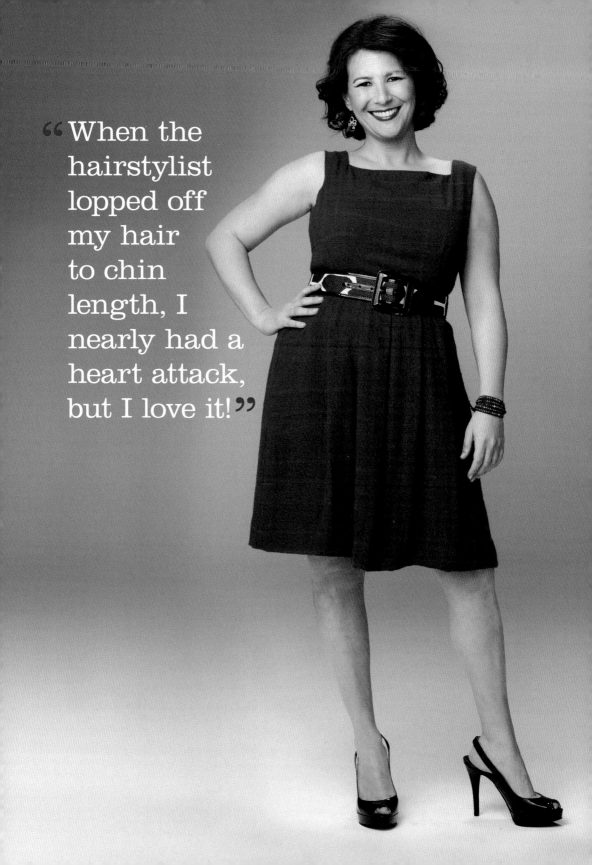

"When the hairstylist lopped off my hair to chin length, I nearly had a heart attack, but I love it!"

Laura Goldblum

Laura, 49, had already incorporated solid age-defying habits into her life when she joined the team of testers, but she knew she could use some tutoring in dealing with her skin, hair, and makeup. Ultimately, she found a way to keep her natural style while applying beauty techniques that took years off her face. Now she's ready for the adventure of the rest of her life.

LAURA'S PLEDGE

I hereby dedicate the next eight weeks to following the 7 Years Younger program.

MY GOAL for this program is to find new strategies that will help me look and feel my best. I'm turning 50 this year, and I want to hit my next decade looking and feeling great!

I'm very active and try to eat healthy, but I don't pay enough attention to my physical appearance in terms of makeup and skin-care products. I care about how I look, but as a single mom on the go, I don't always have the time—or the skills—to make it happen. Therefore:

I PLEDGE to take better care of myself and invest more time in maintaining my skin and hair each day.

In a typical day, I spend a lot of time just taking care of my kids and our lives. When I have a routine, I'm good at staying on track with diet and exercise. When life gets busy, though, it's tough! This program is an opportunity for me to refocus and make a healthier lifestyle a top priority.

For more on Laura Goldblum, see page 194.

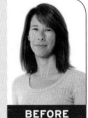

Body fat decrease	Total inches lost
1.2%	4.75

Skin's overall appearance
firmer

BEFORE

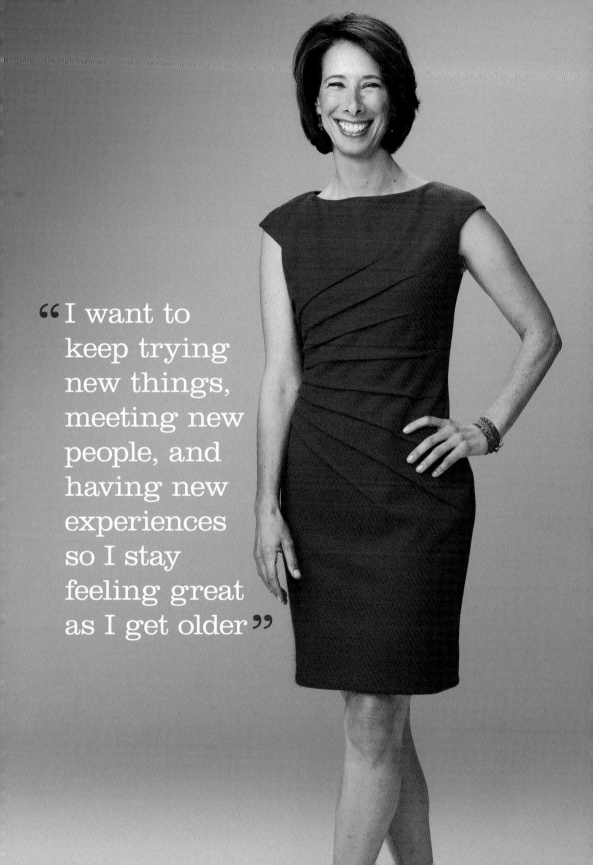

"I want to keep trying new things, meeting new people, and having new experiences so I stay feeling great as I get older"

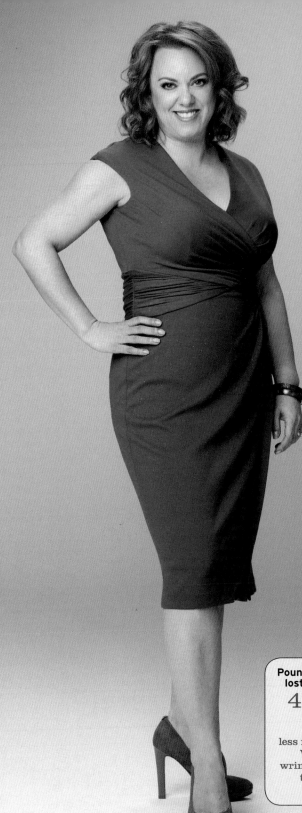

Fern Richter

Chalk it up to weight creep or a few new lines, but "frumpy" was Fern's recent self-assessment. So Fern, 42, got busy exercising, saying OK to a hair makeover, diligently following a skin-care routine, and discovering ways to eat that tamed her appetite. "I was loving food too much," she says. And while we can see the difference, the best part is that Fern feels different deep down.

FERN'S PLEDGE

This program is just for me. It will be hard to stop doing for others and start doing for myself.

I PLEDGE to try to do all I can for my skin—I have been neglectful.

I PLEDGE to exercise as much as possible.

I PLEDGE to make better food choices— eat a big breakfast; a later, bigger lunch; and not so much for dinner.

I PLEDGE to let some things go and do more for myself!

For more on Fern Richter, see page 100.

For more on Fern Richter, see page 100.

Pounds lost	Body fat decrease	Total inches lost
4	0.1%	5.25

Skin's overall appearance
less red-looking and less visible pores; Visia score—18% reduction in wrinkles, especially fine lines around the corners of the mouth; 21% improvement in texture

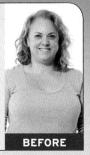

BEFORE

Diane Durando

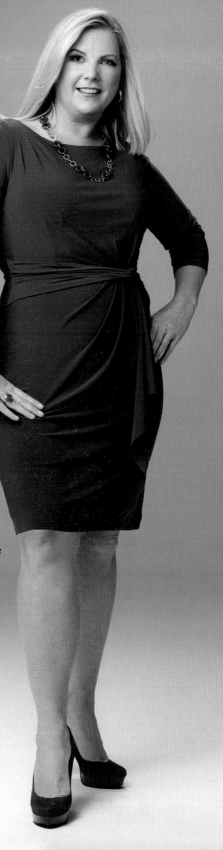

Initially fearful (*Will I have time to do every-thing?* she wondered) yet fiercely deter-mined, Diane, 41, came away with doable strategies to help her age gracefully. She emerged several pounds lighter, looking and feeling refreshed, and most important, she had a heightened understand-ing of how to perpetuate her gains.

"I was coming off a back injury—would I be able to handle the exer-cise? Turns out I could," she says.

DIANE'S PLEDGE

I look on this program as an act of kindness and dedication to myself. By dedicating time and effort to my overall well-being, I am subsequently giving my family a happier and healthier mom/spouse/daughter. WHILE LIFE HAS DEALT many challenging moments along the way, *this* challenge is one in which I have the ability to determine the outcome. I understand that with each new day, I have another chance to continue the transformation.

AT THE END of this program, I hope to have created new habits that will last a lifetime...and it wouldn't hurt to show the world my old sassy self again, inside and out!

For more on Diane Durando, see page 244.

Pounds shed	Body fat decrease	Total inches lost
4	2.2%	0.7

Skin's overall appearance
looked less red, and dark circles were lighter

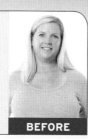

BEFORE

Bernadette Pace

As a widow of two years, Bernadette, 53, was ready for a fresh start. She wanted to downsize her body, revitalize her social life, and look more sophisticated (no more $15 haircuts and tracksuits). In just eight weeks, Bernadette lost over 13 inches, developed smarter eating habits, and began to emerge from her shell.

BERNADETTE'S PLEDGE

I, Bernadette Pace, hereby agree and commit to the following steps to improve accountability to myself and increase my chances for success by dedicating the next eight weeks to following the 7 Years Younger program.

I **DO** hereby commit to living a healthy lifestyle of being active and demonstrating self-control when it comes to eating.

I **WILL** focus on my goal of exercising no less than 30 minutes daily three to five times a week, and take full responsibility for my overall health and well-being.

I **WILL** devote time to and learn how to lead a healthier life, and I will put what I learn in the 7 Years Younger program to use.

I **WILL NOT** let slipups convince me that I am a lost cause. When I slip up, I will remain focused and get back on track.

I **WILL** adhere to the daily beauty routine provided in the 7 Years Younger program and look forward to seeing a transformation.

I **WILL** enlist my daughters to help me stay on track and motivate me.

I **WILL** stick to the program for the long haul. I want to prove to myself I can do it, I want to feel beautiful, and I want my family to be proud of me.

I **WILL** post this pledge on my bedroom mirror where I will see it every day to strengthen my resolve and transform myself into the best person I can be.

For more on Bernadette Pace, see page 204.

Pounds shed	Body fat decrease	Total inches lost
6.4	0.7%	13.75

Skin's overall appearance
tone looks more even and radiant;
Visia score—dark spots reduced by
23%, pores improved by 5%

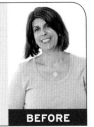

BEFORE

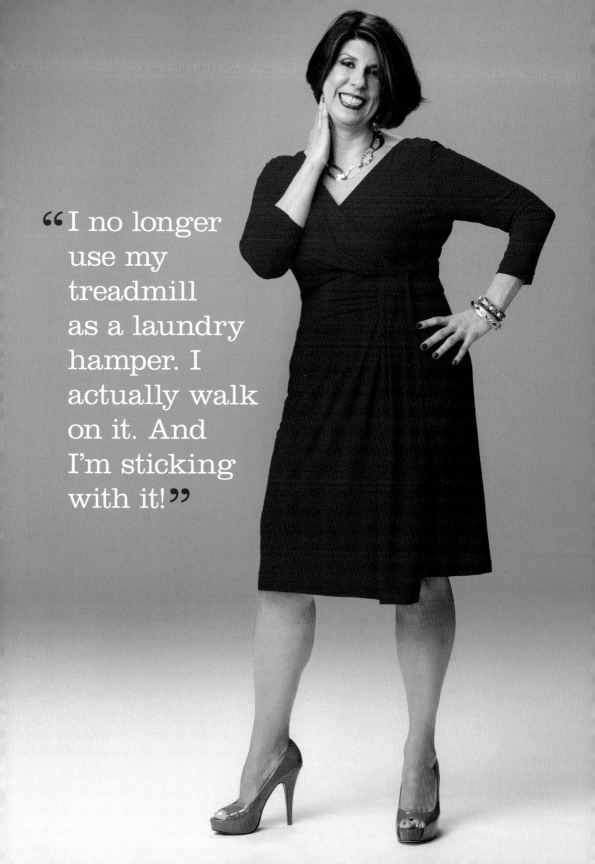

"I no longer use my treadmill as a laundry hamper. I actually walk on it. And I'm sticking with it!"

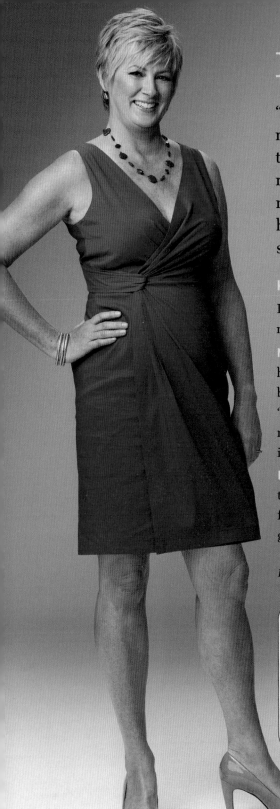

Kathy Coleman

"One day I looked in the mirror and saw my mother," says Kathy, 52. "Not that there's anything wrong with that, but it hit me that I had to start taking better care of myself." A rejuvenating skin-care routine, healthier eating, more laughter, and less stress led to visible improvements.

KATHY'S PLEDGE

I would like to dedicate the next eight weeks to making some permanent changes.

MOST IMPORTANT, I would like to alter my eating habits. I believe I am fully aware of the difference between right and wrong, and I pledge to commit to "right"! My secondary goal is to commit to a healthy nighttime skin-care routine—no more going to sleep in makeup!

I WILL invest the time and energy needed to follow the program, because I'm doing it for me; doing it for me also means doing it for my family. Looking great will be the bonus for being healthy.

For more on Kathy Coleman, see page 254.

Pounds lost	Body fat decrease	Total inches lost
5	0.3%	1.1

Skin's overall appearance
pores appeared smaller, especially on her nose; in general, a smoother, more even-colored complexion; Visia score—35% improvement in dark spots on her face

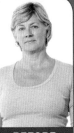

BEFORE

the bottom line

Can Your Glass Be Too Full?

It's healthy to be an optimist, but some evidence suggests that you can take the whole glass-is-half-full thing too far. In the Terman Study, an eight-decades-long study of 1,500 Californians initiated by Stanford University psychologist Lewis Terman, the kids who were cheerful and fun-loving—call them cockeyed optimists—grew up to live shorter lives on average than their diligent and prudent cohorts. It turns out that the happy-go-lucky ones, who figured that everything was always going to be fine, took too many risks with their health, while their conscientious fellows were more likely to check out that funny-looking mole or worry a little more about that odd pain in their side, explains Howard Friedman, Ph.D., distinguished professor of psychology at the University of California at Riverside and coauthor of *The Longevity Project: Surprising Discoveries for Health and Long Life from the Landmark Eight-Decade Study*, which chronicles the Terman Study. What's key is finding the balance between optimism and conscientiousness. But if you're worried that being conscientious is going to turn you into a dull, serious adult, Friedman has good news: The diligent children in the Terman Study grew up to be happy, too. "Their behavior actually produced positive moods," he says. And they weren't boring at all. "They were the people who had the most interesting lives, with many going on to leadership positions. You don't advance to become a CEO, general, or governor by being a screw-up," says Friedman.

Make new friends, look up the old ones It's easy to get in a social rut, even when you're not finding your social life gratifying. Getting out of that rut, though, doesn't take a lot of effort. Here are nine ways to connect.

1 **Follow up** How many times have you met another woman you really liked, only to say a wistful "nice meeting you" as you depart? Next time, take steps to keep the connection: Suggest

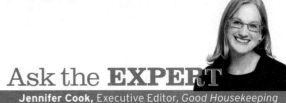
Q *I just don't have time to make new friends. How wide a circle do I really need?*

Jenny says: There's no magic number, but research does suggest that it's a "more is more" situation, in which the greater the number of connections you have, the more you benefit, and the deeper those connections are, the more rewards you'll reap. So if you're too time-strapped to make new friends, focus on deepening your existing ties. Or reconnect with your family: Friendships tend to depend on circumstances like work and geography, while family members are likely already deeply invested in you no matter what.

meeting for coffee or a walk ("I'd love to hear more of your book recommendations") or doing something that you have in common (try her yoga class or ask her to try yours; if you love the same restaurant, make a lunch date).

2 **Write or follow a blog** Many friendships are started up by people who have the same interests and who write about them online.

3 **Volunteer** Besides getting the anti-aging benefits of good works (see page 260), volunteering introduces you to other like-minded people. The best way to turn lending a hand into a new social network is to choose an ongoing "job" (like regularly helping out at a clinic or museum) rather than one-shot stints (like serving Thanksgiving dinner at a shelter or attending an environmental cleanup day). While the short stints are good for meeting people, too, you'll have more time to develop social ties if you choose a volunteer opportunity where you see the same people again and again.

4 **Join a club** There are clubs for virtually every kind of activity: chess, bridge, swimming, walking, cycling, bookstore-sponsored book clubs, plein air (outdoor) painting clubs. If you don't find a ready-made club in your area, start one (a cooking and recipe-sharing club, a book club, a movie club—the possibilities are endless).

5 **Be a habitual exerciser** A certain kind of bonding often takes place among exercisers. If you're a regular in aerobics class or at the gym, chances are you will become friendly with your fellow exercisers.

6 **Take a class** Remember how easy it was to meet people when you were in school? It's still easy. Follow up on an interest you have, anything from history or literature to pottery or dance. Learn to be bilingual, and you'll be doing your brain a favor, too (see page 225).

7 **Seek commonalities** Two things that can drive people apart—politics and religion—can also draw them (tightly) together. This might be the time to become a more active member at a place of worship or center for spirituality. Or to volunteer for a political campaign. Nothing makes for faster friends than a common cause.

8 **Meet up** Where are people congregating? Meetup.com is a website that lets you connect with others. You can type in your location and interest, and the site will let you know about clubs and happenings (everything from snail's-pace runners' groups to crochet and knitting meet-ups) in your area.

9 **Reconnect with old friends** You already communicate through Facebook, but don't leave it at that. Make the effort to get together with people you once hung out with. There's a reason you liked them then; you'll probably still like them now.

Stress-Buster #7: Find Ways to Give Back

Altruism, doing something for somebody else, is selfless—it's not about you. But when you're kind to others, your body responds in a very positive way. In fact, researchers recognize a "biology of compassion" involving the immune system, brain, and hormones that can make you younger. In particular, helping others seems to boost disease-fighting antibodies, one possible reason why people who volunteer at two or more organizations get a boost in longevity comparable to that gained by exercising four times a week. One more reason to volunteer: It just feels good.

Get started Not sure how to begin? Check for opportunities at your church, temple, or mosque. Sign up for Big Brothers Big Sisters or any other group in which you can be a mentor. "People tend to find greater meaning in activities that pass the torch to a younger generation," says Stony Brook's Stephen Post. Maybe because their involvement is so rewarding, 87 percent of mentors engage in at least one other volunteer activity—and reap extra health benefits.

Get inspired Hearing about others' volunteer activities can help you learn about opportunities that you never even knew existed. The website doinggood.com has inspiring stories and videos. After reading/viewing, follow up by going to the page that helps you find volunteer opportunities in your area.

Make it a family affair One thing that can keep you from volunteering is that it takes away from family time. But what if you brought your family with you? The website doinggoodtogether.org can help you find philanthropic activities suitable for kids.

Activate Your Anti-Aging Plan Now!

Want a taste of what it feels like to be cool, calm, karmic? Try these tips:

1 **Notice your breathing** a few times a day; if you happen to be stressed when you check in with yourself, try a breathing exercise to regain serenity.

2 **Reach out and connect** with someone—a friend, a family member, a stranger. Making meaningful connections helps vaccinate you against the aging effects of stress.

3 **Build a positivity habit** When something nice happens to you, no matter how small, take a moment to enjoy the feeling. Let it fill your mind and heart. All too often, we brush off positive events as random or accidental and cling to negative ones. Try to shift the balance toward the positive.

For more expert anti-aging advice, get our free special report, 50 Ways to Stress Less & Live Longer, *at 7yearsyounger.com/stressless.*

Your
Jumpstart Plan

Chapter Eight

7 Days to a Younger You!

We've brought together everything you need into a smart, simple weeklong program that will deliver results—*now*! Your Jumpstart Plan will have you feeling and looking younger after just one week. Think of this as a do-it-yourself spa getaway—eating delicious and nutritious food, indulging in beauty pampering, and making time to be active and exercise. You'll have more energy and stamina from eating better and exercising more consistently, and like our testers, you'll likely drop a pound or two—or even more. Plus, there are plenty of makeup, hair, and de-stressing shortcuts that will help you look and feel younger, pronto. Most important, devoting seven days to caring for your skin, hair, body, brain, and overall health puts you on the fast track to making age-defying practices a habit.

Your Jumpstart week introduces the plan's fundamentals: eating well and exercising consistently. With each new day, you'll add more anti-aging steps so that by week's end you'll have built up your anti-aging

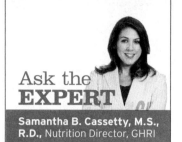
toolkit and will already be turning back the clock. The plan is set up to deliver the best, most immediate results. But pay close attention to your body's reactions so you can adopt the changes more gradually if you feel the need to do so. Go at your own comfortable pace so you don't overdo it and fall off-track. Everyone has a different starting point, especially when it comes to exercise, and your goal is to introduce changes that produce immediate, encouraging results *and* that you can follow long-term.

Exercise

Your goal is to do the ab shapers on page 199 and to walk for 20 minutes each day. You can do the 20 minutes all at once or break it up into two 10-minute walks (or four 5-minute walks). If you're already an exerciser, keep doing your regular routine and just add in a daily walk.

Anti-Aging Eating

This weeklong kickoff is designed to fast-track you to dropping unwanted pounds for good. The plan is packed with food (and loads of anti-aging goodness and wrinkle-fighting antioxidants) but low in calories to help you win at weight loss. There's no counting (fiber, calories, carbs, points) required. We've done the math, so you are eating roughly 300 calories at breakfast, 400 at lunch, and 500 at dinner. Just eat and enjoy. At meals and throughout the day, drink water, seltzer (including flavored varieties, as long as there are no added sugars or caloric flavorings), zero-calorie sodas, and coffee or tea (hot or iced).

Jumpstart Meal Plan

Proof that anti-aging eating can be a pleasure: Each meal on this plan sounds more scrumptious than the last! You'll find all the recipes (which serve four) for the plan in Chapter 10 (see page 321). We even kept tabs on cooking time— everything will be on the table in 30 minutes or less for the entire program.

Day	Breakfast	Lunch	Dinner
1	Breakfast Bowl *(page 322)*	Protein Plate *(page 328)*	Almond-Crusted Chicken with Rainbow Slaw *(page 337)*
2	Cozy Oats *(page 322)*	Pita Pizza *(page 328)*	Flank Steak with Red Wine & Oven Fries *(page 351)*
3	Grab & Go *(page 322)*	Souped-Up Soup *(page 328)*	Pork Chops Marsala *(page 345)*
4	Egg Scramble *(page 322)*	Mediterranean Tuna Salad *(page 328)*	Pasta Primavera *(page 361)*
5	Sweet Stuffed Waffle *(page 323)*	Turkey Wrap *(page 330)*	Shrimp & Asparagus Stir-Fry *(page 358)*
6	Cereal-Yogurt Parfait *(page 322)*	Roast Beef Sammy *(page 328)*	Salmon with Gingery Cabbage *(page 355)*
7	California Breakfast Wrap *(page 324)*	Microwavable Meal *(page 328)*	Turkey Burgers *(page 344)*

JUMPSTART AND 7-WEEK PLAN SUPPLIES CHECKLIST

Now that you've got the 7 Years Younger Plan in your hands, you need just one more thing: your calendar. You'll need to choose a target date to start the plan, so pick a time that's as free as possible from distractions—vacations, work presentations, holidays, etc. And give yourself plenty of preparation time to go on the plan; about two to three weeks should do. During the weeks leading up to your start date, stock up on the tools and supplies you'll need to follow the plan. (Start with the helpful checklists on pages 267-268. Then click on **7yearsyounger.com/shop** to access our online store for all the items and products you'll need.)

Also, spend some time preparing psychologically. According to the "Stages of Change" model, which has been used by psychologists for decades to analyze how people make lasting lifestyle shifts, a "contemplation" phase (which precedes any actual change in habits or behaviors) is crucial to staying the course. During your contemplation period, ask yourself:

- "What are my reasons for starting the 7YY plan?"
- "What changes do I hope to accomplish?"
- "Can I identify any potential pitfalls or obstacles and plan for ways to get back on track?"
- "What are some of the things I can do now to make it easier for me to complete the plan?"
- "Who among my friends and family can I count on for support during the plan?"
- "Who in my social network can I turn to for support?" (Don't forget to check our resources at 7 Years Younger on Facebook at facebook.com/7yearsyounger.)

Congratulate yourself for and acknowledge each positive step you take to prepare for the plan during these countdown weeks, whether it's purchasing skin products, eliminating high-fat and high-sugar treats from your pantry, buying a new workout bra, or easing into exercise by trying to fit in a daily walk. Regular reinforcement revs up your commitment and heightens your belief in your abilities, so you'll be all set to go when your start date comes around.

SHOPPING LIST
Cleansers & Moisturizers

Jumpstart Plan
- [ ] Cleanser such as Cetaphil Gentle Cleanser
- [ ] Exfoliating cleanser such as Olay Pore Minimizing Cleanser & Scrub
- [ ] Facial moisturizer with sunscreen such as Elizabeth Arden Ceramide Lift and Firm Day Cream Broad Spectrum Sunscreen SPF 30 OR Chanel Ultra Correction Lift Lifting Firming Day Cream SPF 15 (see page 59)
- [ ] Anti-aging night cream with retinol or peptides such as Vichy LiftActiv Retinol HA Night (see page 60)
- [ ] Hand cream such as Boots No7 Protect & Perfect Day Hand Cream (see page 60)

7-Week Plan
- [ ] Anti-aging serum such as Boots No7 Protect & Perfect Intense Serum (see page 58)
- [ ] Anti-aging body moisturizer such as Fresh Sugar Açai Age-Delay Body Cream (see page 58)

Makeup*

Jumpstart Plan
- [ ] Concealer (see page 72)
- [ ] Eyelid primer (see page 77)
- [ ] Soft pencil or eyeliner brush with eye shadow (see page 77)
- [ ] Eyelash curler (see page 82)
- [ ] Lengthening mascara (see page 82)
- [ ] Foundation or foundation stick (see page 70)
- [ ] Clear lip liner (see page 83)
- [ ] Lip brush (see page 84)
- [ ] Lipstick (medium hue)

7-Week Plan
- [ ] Foundation (see page 70)
- [ ] Blush (see page 74)
- [ ] Eye makeup remover (see page 81)
- [ ] Bronzer (see page 76)
- [ ] Lip balm (see page 85)
- [ ] Brow pencil (see page 76)

For anti-aging makeup recommendations from the Good Housekeeping Research Institute, get our free special report, Best Anti-Aging Makeup, at 7yearsyounger.com/makeup.

Hair

Jumpstart Plan

- ☐ Hair glaze such as John Frieda Clear Shine Luminous Glaze (see page 106)
- ☐ Shampoo and conditioner such as Biolage Rejuvathérapie Age Rejuvenating Shampoo and Conditioner OR Pureology Nanoworks Shampoo and Conditioner (see page 116)
- ☐ For volume, if needed: such as Nexxus Diametress Luscious Volume Shampoo and Conditioner (see page 116)
- ☐ Deep conditioner such as Biolage Rejuvathérapie Age Rejuvenating Intensive Masque (see page 117)

7-Week Plan

- ☐ For frizz, if needed: a spray, cream, or mousse containing dimethicone such as Living Proof No Frizz Weightless Styling Spray
- ☐ Haircolor such as Revlon ColorSilk with UV Defense OR Couture Colour (see page 117)
- ☐ Shine spray, serum, or color extender such as L'Anza Healing Strength Neem Plant Silk Serum (see page 116)
- ☐ For dry hair/flyaways, if needed: one travel-size bottle of leave-in conditioner (see page 97)

Other

7-Week Plan

- ☐ Teeth whitening kit such as Crest 3D White Advanced Vivid Whitestrips with Advanced Vivid Technology (see page 90)
- ☐ Exercise band, 6 feet, medium tension (see page 187)
- ☐ Pumice (see page 57)
- ☐ At-home peel kit such as Boots No7 Glycolic Peel Kit (see page 58)
- ☐ Self-tanner (optional, see page 50)

Find these top anti-aging products at 7yearsyounger.com/shop.

Day 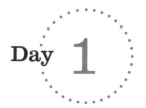 1

Kick off your get-younger week by gently cleansing your complexion. These easy steps will make your skin feel (and look) as if you've just had a facial. Next up: getting a better night's sleep. Sleep works almost across the board to turn back the clock. It's critical for good health, and you'll look much more vibrant when you're well rested. The walks you'll begin now may help you sleep better, too.

Your Jumpstart Checklist

- [ ] **Jumpstart Meal Plan (see page 265)**

- [ ] **Skin care**

  In the morning...

  - ■ **Wash with a cleanser** labeled "gentle," "sensitive," or "calming." Twice a week, use an exfoliating cleanser instead of the gentle one (see page 23 for details on exfoliating).
  - ■ **Moisturize** with a moisturizer-sunscreen, applying it while your skin is still slightly damp. This helps skin retain moisture, allowing for maximum line-erasing and plumping of cells.

  In the evening...

  - ■ **Cleanse** with the same gentle product you used in the morning.
  - ■ **Apply an anti-aging night cream** that contains retinol or peptides (see page 30 for suggestions).

- [ ] **Sleep-well strategy**

  - ■ **Stop drinking caffeine** after 2 P.M.; it can take six to 12 hours for caffeine's stimulating effects to clear your system.
  - ■ **Start keeping a consistent sleep schedule** Try to go to bed at the same time and wake up at the same time. Keep it up all week—a regular schedule will make it easier for you to fall asleep at night.
  - ■ **Eat dinner before 8 P.M.** If you're actively digesting, you may find it difficult to fall and stay asleep.
  - ■ **Turn off all your electronics**—computer, e-reader, smartphone, TV—at least an hour before bed. The light suppresses melatonin, the sleepiness hormone. Lower your room lights and use this time to gently unwind.
  - ■ **Cool your bedroom** This lowers your core body temperature, which initiates sleepiness. Try 65 degrees to start, and adjust up or down as necessary.

JUMPSTART

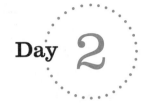

Day 2

Systematically cleansing your skin will make it look fresher and feel smoother—just the palette for these anti-aging makeup tricks. As you'll see in the mirror, a little makeup can go a long way toward making you look younger. In addition, you'll ramp up your calorie-burning by working more activity into your day.

Your Jumpstart Checklist

☐ **Exercise (see page 264)**

☐ **Jumpstart Meal Plan (see page 265)**

☐ **Skin care (see page 269)**

☐ **Sleep-well strategy (see page 269)**

Add

☐ **Look-younger makeup steps**

These two shortcuts focus on your most expressive features–eyes and mouth–and help you look years younger in minutes!

Age-proof your eyes

1. Use concealer to hide dark undereye circles. Pick a creamy formulation in a shade that's close to your skin tone (not too light) and gently dab (or brush) it on from the inner corner of the eye to the midpoint beneath the pupil. Now feather it out, blending away any obvious demarcation lines.

2. Apply a flesh-colored eyelid primer to even out skin tone and create a smooth surface. Glide a thin layer onto your entire top eyelid up to your brow.

3. Line the rims of your eyes using a soft pencil or an eyeliner brush with eye shadow. To line the tops, point your chin up and look down, so your lids are half-closed but you can still see them, and apply the liner. Avoid thick bands of liner, which close up the eye area. Along your bottom lashes, line with a color that's a shade or two lighter than the one you used on top.

4. Choose a powder shadow color that flatters your skin tone: Beige, taupe, and sage are all good options. Neutrals with subtle luminescence will have the most eye-brightening effect. Sweep the color up to the crease. If you want a more dramatic, eye-opening effect,

brush a slightly darker color into the crease.

5. Curl your lashes. Hold gently for 15 seconds.

6. Apply a lengthening mascara to brighten and open up eyes. For smudge-free and clump-proof application, press the wand against the base of your lashes for a few seconds, then jiggle the brush back and forth as you draw it out to the tips.

Age-proof your lips

These steps will brighten your mouth and play down lines:

1. Pretreat the area just above your upper lip with foundation or foundation stick to prevent lipstick from bleeding into any lines near your lips. Use your fingertip to lightly dot it on.

2. Carefully trace the outermost border of your mouth with a clear or nude liner that's the same shade as your lips. Clear liner not only defines lips, but also helps stop lipstick migration into surrounding fine lines.

3. Using a lip brush, apply a medium shade of lipstick. Pick a hue with some brightness to it: roses, natural pinks, berries, and true red can all be flattering. Just opt for sheer shiny or satiny finishes instead of mattes, which are drying and tend to sink into lines. Dip the brush into your lipstick and dab a little on the center of your lips, then spread it to the corners.

☐ Everyday activity

Whenever you have the opportunity to move, take it. To get going, incorporate three incidental exercise moves into your day. (See page 182 for more choices.) Your aim is to burn 100 calories a day with everyday steps. It all adds up: By week's end, you'll have burned an extra 700 calories! (Calorie counts are calculated based on a 150-pound woman.)

- Park at the outer edge of parking lots and walk briskly to your destination; 2 minutes, 11 calories
- Trade elevators for the stairs; for every minute climbing stairs, 9 calories
- Walk up escalators; for every minute walking up an escalator, 9 calories

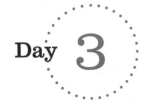

Day 3

Start off your day with a brief meditation. The anti-aging benefit: Taking the time to slow down for a few minutes de-stresses and relaxes your whole body—including tiny facial muscles that clench, forming lines and creases. Next on the quick-change agenda is a speedy trick to make hair shinier, livelier, and more youthful.

Your Jumpstart Checklist

☐ **Exercise (see page 264)**

☐ **Jumpstart Meal Plan (see page 265)**

☐ **Skin care (see page 269)**

☐ **Sleep-well strategy (see page 269)**

☐ **Look-younger makeup steps (see page 270)**

☐ **Everyday activity (see page 271)**

Add

☐ **Five-minute meditation**

1. Sit quietly in a comfortable position.
2. Close your eyes.
3. Become aware of your breathing. Breathe slowly and naturally, drawing air into your belly and exhaling.
4. Focus on your breathing, and any time your mind wanders away from your breath, take note of what's on your mind and gently bring your attention back to your breathing. Acknowledge your thoughts without judging, condemning, or rejecting them.
5. Continue the meditation for five minutes or as long as you can (with practice, you will likely be able to sit longer).
6. When you are finished, sit quietly for a minute, then open your eyes and rise slowly.

☐ **Hair shine enhancer**
You'll love this shine shortcut: After washing your locks, apply a glaze. Before your eyes, you'll see hair regain luster and bounce. Your whole face will look lifted and younger. Basic care can also keep hair looking and acting younger:

■ **Shampoo** Use a dollop of shampoo no bigger than a quarter, and don't allow the lather to sit on your hair for long—shampoo can sap hair's moisture. Work the product in using warm water, then rinse. Wash only every other day (or even less frequently) unless you have oily hair. Lots of flyaways are a sign that you are washing too often.

- **Condition** Make sure your conditioner tackles the same problem your shampoo does (i.e., don't pair a volumizing shampoo with a conditioner that's moisturizing and will weigh hair down). Apply a dab of conditioner (just enough to coat your hair) from mid-shaft to the ends (roots have their own moisturizing sebum). Use a wide-tooth comb to distribute and gently detangle; then rinse.

- **Deep-Condition** Once this week, try a deep conditioner in place of your regular conditioner. The extra conditioning can remedy dryness and dullness, leaving your hair softer, shinier, and stronger.

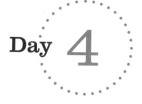

Day 4

Get your brain thinking younger starting today; use memory-enhancing tricks to improve your recall right away. Also, to boost the body-shaping effects of healthier eating, try some bloat-deflating steps to get a flatter belly fast.

Your Jumpstart Checklist

- ☐ **Exercise**
  (see page 264)

- ☐ **Jumpstart Meal Plan**
  (see page 265)

- ☐ **Skin care (see page 269)**

- ☐ **Sleep-well strategy**
  (see page 269)

- ☐ **Look-younger makeup steps**
  (see page 270)

- ☐ **Everyday activity**
  (see page 271)

- ☐ **Meditation (see page 272)**

- ☐ **Hair care**
  (as needed, see page 272)

Add

- ☐ **Instant memory tricks**
  1. **Associating** Link words to something you already know to increase the likelihood that your brain will store them as long-term memories. If, for instance, you're introduced to someone named Ellen, you can

make up a rhyme about her name. Or you can use mnemonics, memory aids that use patterns or abbreviations: "Don't leave home without two l's— lunch and laptop."

2. **Chunking** Your brain can process only so much information at one time, so breaking up incoming facts into chunks can help. By repeating a phone extension as "38, 27" instead of "3, 8, 2, 7," you only have to remember two numbers, not four. You can chunk info by categorizing as well. To remember everything you need for the gym, think head (your earphones and music player), body (workout clothes), and feet (shoes and socks).

☐ **Deflate belly bloat**

■ Practice chewing slowly, and sip instead of gulping liquids. Eating and swallowing quickly means you ingest more air, which can bloat your belly.

■ Pass on using a straw; you'll suck down air with your drink.

■ Refrain from chewing gum. Although it has pluses for weight loss and teeth cleaning, you'll generate and ingest air bubbles as you chew.

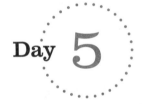

Day 5

Treat yourself to a time-out; put your feet up while you give your hands an anti-aging massage and spend a few minutes focusing on your breath.

Your Jumpstart Checklist

☐ **Exercise** (see page 264)

☐ **Jumpstart Meal Plan** (see page 265)

☐ **Skin care (see page 269)**

☐ **Sleep-well strategy** (see page 269)

☐ **Look-younger makeup steps** (see page 270)

☐ **Everyday activity** (see page 271)

☐ **Meditation (see page 272)**

☐ **Hair care (as needed)** (see page 272)

☐ **Instant memory tricks** (see page 273)

☐ **Belly-bloat deflators** (see page 274)

Add

☐ **Hand-moisturizing massage**

Apply a hand cream with emollient ingredients, such as shea butter or petrolatum, and humectants like glycerin that help draw moisture to the skin. Give yourself a light hand massage, letting the moisturizer plump up the top layers of skin and leaving hands with a younger look.

☐ **Deep breathing**

Lie on your back on a bed. Place your hands on your belly and inhale through your nose, counting to five. Feel the air fill your belly. Exhale through your nose on the same count. Continue, focusing on the rise and fall of your belly.

Days 6 and 7

Today and tomorrow, hold steady. You've just started a lot of healthy new habits, and you need time to incorporate them into your daily routine. But you're well on your way to looking and feeling years younger!

Your Jumpstart Checklist

☐ **Exercise**
(see page 264)

☐ **Jumpstart Meal Plan**
(see page 265)

☐ **Skin care (see page 269)**

☐ **Sleep-well strategy**
(see page 269)

☐ **Look-younger makeup steps**
(see page 270)

☐ **Everyday activity**
(see page 271)

☐ **Meditation**
(see page 272)

☐ **Hair care (as needed)**
(see page 272)

☐ **Instant memory tricks**
(see page 273)

☐ **Belly-bloat deflators**
(see page 275)

☐ **Hand massage**
(above)

☐ **Deep breathing**
(above)

The Road Map
to the Rest
of Your Life

Chapter Nine

The 7-Week Plan

Congratulations on completing your Jumpstart Plan! You're now on your way to achieving your goal of looking and feeling 7 years younger. Your next step is this 7-Week Plan, where you'll spend the first week developing your baseline routine by building on everything you did during the Jumpstart week. During the remaining six weeks, you'll add to that routine by introducing powerful anti-aging safeguards. Think of Week 1 as laying the foundation of youthfulness, Weeks 2 through 7 as a time to refine and enhance your routine so you get even more noticeable and lasting results. As you go, you can customize the plan: Add steps at a pace that suits you, and take time to incorporate everything into your life. As long as you stay consistent, you're going to feel rejuvenated and see a younger you reflected back in the mirror by the time you reach the program's end. Keep going after that, and you'll enjoy even more remarkable improvements.

WEEK 1: COMMIT TO CONSISTENCY

Small changes that you include consistently in your daily routine will deliver big results! That's the key to moving forward on your youth-boosting path. This first week kicks off your foundation plan—your baseline routine that will carry you through the next seven weeks. You should develop your own personal routine to repeat and follow over time. Reminding yourself of your greater goal—to use this plan as a springboard to a new, younger you—will help keep you on track.

Skin Care

You'll constantly thank yourself for cleansing, exfoliating, and moisturizing your skin: It will glow with health when you're bare-faced, and when you wear makeup, it will look even better! Our application tips won't hide your glow; they'll enhance it.

Daily Repeat the Jumpstart skin-care routine (page 269).

To your evening routine, ADD An application of a nighttime serum (see page 30).

Beauty

The feedback you're getting in the mirror—younger-looking skin, brighter eyes, and softer lips—is a major motivator. This week, extend the anti-aging effects of the right makeup.

Daily Repeat the Jumpstart makeup routine for eyes and lips, (see page 270)

At least three times a week, try

Wearing Foundation

- Choose a hydrating or satin-finish liquid foundation in a shade slightly warmer (think: golden) and deeper than your natural skin tone.

- Using a foundation brush or a damp sponge, apply foundation over your entire face, including under the eyes, up to browbones, along your jawline, and onto your neck.

Applying Blush
- Choose a highly pigmented powder—you'll only need a touch and will avoid powdery buildup that ages you.
- Using a blush brush, lightly swirl the blush a little high on the apples of your cheeks.

Hair Care

Regularly Repeat the Jumpstart shampoo, conditioning, and deep-conditioning routine (see page 272).

Weight-Loss Meal Plan

Each day of the week Follow the 7 Years Younger weight-loss plan. It is designed to fit seamlessly into your lifestyle. The menu is full of age-defying nutrients, but the best part is, we've refreshed some classic family favorites—like steak, pasta, and chicken quesadillas—to fit with the program. And no meal takes longer than 30 minutes, tops, to prepare. As you enjoy delicious and filling fare, you'll be peeling off pounds and rewinding time. Just choose one breakfast (300 calories), one lunch (400 calories), and one dinner (500 calories), plus two snacks (125 calories each) every day (calorie counts are approximate). If you aren't filling your plate with several of the dairy-rich options, consider taking a calcium supplement. Women need 1,000 to 1,200 mg every day, but you can reduce your supplement (to, say, 500 mg) if you're doing OK on the dairy front. Here's what's ahead for your first week:

Week 1

Day	Breakfast	Snack	Lunch	Dinner	Snack
1	Trail Oats (*page 323*)	Chips & Cheese (*page 338*)	Supermarket Sushi & Salad Bar (*page 330*)	Linguine with Carrot-Turkey Ragout (*page 360*)	Berries & Chocolate (*page 335*)
2	Peaches & Cream (*page 323*)	On the Run (*page 335*)	Burger Day (*page 327*)	Pomegranate-Glazed Salmon (*page 354*)	Soy Mix (*page 336*)
3	Breakfast Bowl (*page 322*)	Mini Babybel Light (*page 336*)	Mediterranean Tuna Salad (*page 328*)	Vegetable Lasagna Toss (*page 362*)	Roast Beef Rolls (*page 336*)
4	Cereal & More (*page 322*)	Cottage Cheese with Melon (*page 336*)	Spring Salad (*page 328*)	Turkey Burgers (*page 344*)	Trail Mix (*page 335*)
5	Monte Cristo (*page 323*)	Chips & Salsa (*page 336*)	Protein Plate (*page 328*)	Roasted Shrimp Scampi (*page 357*)	Banana Split (*page 335*)
6	Pronto Plate (*page 323*)	Coffee Break (*page 335*)	Spicy Butternut Squash Soup (*page 328*)	Almond-Crusted Chicken with Rainbow Slaw (*page 335*)	Berries & Chocolate (*page 335*)
7	Grab & Go (*page 322*)	Hard-Cooked Egg (*page 336*)	White Pizza (*page 330*)	Flank Steak with Red Wine & Oven Fries (*page 351*)	Watermelon Salad (*page 335*)

Tester's INSIDE TIP

"To help curb my appetite before meals, I drink a cup of hot tea. The flavorful herbal varieties are particularly satisfying. My current favorite is peppermint. It's great to sip as I'm making a meal, so I don't sample too much."

—Tessa Jean

Daily, as needed Deploy a smart swap, one of the many smart strategies designed to help you reach your weight-loss goals. This exclusive fruit-swap list lets you make seasonal adjustments and allows for personal preferences so that you can follow the plan all year long. If, for example, a snack includes half a sliced apple, you'll know you can switch it for half a medium-size banana, a cup of blueberries, or a kiwi instead.

Fruit Swaps

150-calorie fruits

1 mango

1 extra-large banana

2 cups pineapple chunks

½ avocado

100-calorie fruits

1 cup cherries

1 medium apple

1 small pear

1 medium banana

1 cup grapes

50-calorie fruits

1 cup cantaloupe

1 cup honeydew

1 cup watermelon

1 small orange

1 cup blueberries

15 strawberries

½ grapefruit

1 kiwi

1 cup raspberries

Exercise

Two days a week Repeat the 20-minute walk in the Jumpstart Plan (or 20 minutes of walking, broken up into 5- or 10-minute segments).

Continue with the ab shapers introduced in the Jumpstart week. (see page 199).

Two days a week, ADD Walking Workout #1: Fat-Blasting Interval Training (see page 193). Aim for 20 minutes this first week; if you find yourself fading mid-workout, walk for a shorter total time or reduce the number of fast-walk intervals. You'll actually be exercising for a little less time than you did in the Jumpstart week, but you'll be working harder—and speeding up fat loss.

Daily, ADD Two more everyday activities to the three you implemented in the Jumpstart week, for a total of five. (See page 182 for choices.)

 Tester's INSIDE TIP

"I began taking exercise breaks instead of coffee breaks at work. I walk around the parking lot of my office, and I see people looking at me like I am crazy! I roll up my pants, dance to the music on my iPod, and stop to use the resistance band for exercises. Quite a sight, I assure you—but soon I will be that crazy skinny, young lady who walks around the parking lot!" **–Fern Richter**

Brain Fitness

Making memory-enhancing techniques second nature can help stave off future mental freezes.

Daily Keep practicing the two instant memory tricks from the Jumpstart Plan (see page 273).

Daily, ADD A memory challenge: Quiz yourself about details. Start to notice distinct elements in your environment, then task yourself to remember them later. What was your boss wearing yesterday? What color is the house on the corner? What flowers were on the table at the last restaurant you visited? Paying closer attention will take your brain off autopilot and put you in the present so that you absorb more information.

De-stress

Daily

- Repeat the daily sleep-well strategy from the Jumpstart Plan (see page 269).
- Keep practicing the meditation or do the deep-breathing exercise from the Jumpstart Plan (see page 272 and page 275, respectively).

"Getting to bed earlier takes some discipline and organization, but it makes a world of difference. I've been up at 6 A.M. sharp every day now for three weeks! There's also a spillover effect: My energy is much higher, I don't get tired in the afternoons, and my friends keep complimenting me on how radiant my skin looks." **—Tessa Jean**

You're off to a great start! For more advice and support, join our community at facebook.com/7yearsyounger.

WEEK 2: KEEP BUILDING NEW ROUTINES

In Week 1 you established the basic routines and made them part of your daily schedule. Now, take advantage of this foundation to piggyback another, related step. This week, you'll extend your care to other parts of your body.

Tester's INSIDE TIP : *"You think that you'll start taking care of your skin or exercising or eating better when everything calms down, but the truth is, things never calm down. You just have to make those things a priority and get them on your schedule."*
—Diane Gurden

To Week 1 activities, ADD

Skin Care

Daily, several times a day Give your hands a moisturizing massage. Station bottles or tubes of moisturizer near the bathroom and kitchen sinks. Aim to moisturize after washing hands.

Tester's INSIDE TIP : *"I'm outdoors a lot. The best sunscreen is one that stays put and doesn't drip, so I always look for one with zinc oxide. I put it on the backs of my hands to prevent spots."*
—Julie Ann Raab

Beauty

Daily Now that you're wearing makeup more regularly, make sure you're using a gentle eye makeup remover (see page 81). Drying pads and wipes can age the thin, delicate skin around your eyes—just the opposite of what you're working for.

Hair Care

As needed A new layer to add to your shinier, healthier hair: Consider updating your style with the right cut. Make an appointment with your hairstylist to get an updated, anti-aging look (see page 109).

Tester's INSIDE TIP : *"I've spent a little more time concentrating on my hair, makeup, and outfit each day. I hate to say, 'I put on lip gloss and it's had a profound effect on my life,' but taking extra time to make sure I feel good before I walk out the door in the morning has made me feel more confident and added a bit of a spring to my step. It's given me confidence at work, as well."* —Rachel Dorfman

Exercise

By now, you've experienced the anti-aging effects of regular workouts; you're feeling more energetic and stronger. This week, tap into exercise as a spread stopper. Trimming excess weight is not just cosmetic; weight, especially around the midsection of the body, is associated with an increased risk of diabetes, heart disease, and stroke. That's why you're replacing one of the straightforward 20-minute walks with another day of Walking Workout #1: Fat-Blasting Interval Training (see page 193). For each Fat-Blasting workout, lengthen your session by five minutes. Stretching before or after a workout keeps your muscles ready to move. Your exercise schedule will now look like this:

- **One day a week** 20-minute walk (or 20 minutes of walking broken up into 5- or 10- minute segments).
- **Three days a week** Walking Workout #1: Fat-Blasting Interval Training—add an extra five minutes to the workout by increasing the first five *moderate* walking intervals by one minute, i.e.,

2 minutes (warm-up)	1.5 minutes (moderate walk)
2 minutes (moderate walk)	30 seconds (fast walk)
30 seconds (fast walk)	2.5 minutes (moderate walk)
2 minutes (moderate walk)	30 seconds (fast walk)
1 minute (fast walk)	4 minutes (moderate walk)

Continue as the original workout outlines. Your total routine should now take you 25 minutes.

- **Two days a week, ADD** Two sets of 15 repetitions each of the three belly-flatteners (page 199). Your core—the muscles of your abdomen, back, and pelvic floor—should be strong enough to do another set. As your core strengthens, you'll trim your waist and lower belly so your clothes will fit better. Your balance will also improve.
- **One or two days a week, ADD** The stretching moves (page 202). Squeeze in an extra session by doing flexibility moves as you watch television or listen to the news. Classes like yoga, tai chi, and Pilates are also great opportunities to increase your muscles' range of motion.

Brain Fitness

A few times a week, ADD A brain game. Instead of watching TV during downtime, play a few games and do some brain-stimulating activities. Crossword puzzles, Boggle, Scrabble, and memory games work the left side of your brain; drawing, playing an instrument, and doing mazes work the right side (see page 225).

Tester's
INSIDE
TIP

"To combat 'brain fog,' I have been playing Sudoku and Scrabble, as well as shopping without lists. I also try to make some sort of association when meeting someone new. I've actually gotten better at Sudoku and am seeing an improvement as I practice more. I hardly ever take my list with me to the market anymore and, after reviewing what's on it before I leave, I remember everything about 90 to 95 percent of the time!" **–Bernadette Pace**

De-stress

Daily Repeat the daily sleep-well strategy from the Jumpstart Plan (see page 269).

Daily Keep practicing the meditation from the Jumpstart Plan (see page 272) or do a deep-breathing exercise (see page 242).

"I'm a big believer in taking a deep breath during stressful situations and giving myself 5 to 10 minutes to get a grip. I also find that just stepping out of the room puts things in perspective and allows me to look at things in a more positive light." **–Diane Durando**

Weight-Loss Meal Plan

As you prepare and enjoy this week's meals, start to train your eye on proper portions. Pause for a moment and look at your meal and how much space on the plate it takes up. Practice eyeballing serving sizes in order to prevent overeating at parties or restaurants.

Week 2

Day	Breakfast	Snack	Lunch	Dinner	Snack
1	New York Bagel *(page 323)*	Cheese Plate *(page 336)*	Stuffed Sweet Potato *(page 330)*	Chicken Quesadilla with Avocado-Tomato Salsa *(page 341)*	Ice Cream Waffle *(page 335)*
2	Egg Scramble *(page 322)*	Banana Pudding *(page 335)*	Microwavable Meal *(page 328)*	Shrimp & Asparagus Stir-Fry *(page 358)*	Chips & Cheese *(page 336)*
3	PB&A *(page 323)*	Asian App *(page 336)*	Spinach Salad with Tuna and Avocado *(page 331)*	Pork Chops Marsala *(page 345)*	Popcorn *(page 336)*
4	On the Road *(page 323)*	Kind Mini Fruit & Nut Delight Bar *(page 335)*	Asian Bowl *(page 327)*	Turkey & White Bean Chili *(page 343)*	Parm Plate *(page 336)*
5	PB&J B'fast *(page 323)*	Kashi TLC Fruit & Grain Bar *(page 335)*	Hot Roast Beef Hero *(page 328)*	Whole Wheat Penne with Broccoli & Sausage *(page 363)*	Trail Mix *(page 335)*
6	Mixed Fruit Smoothie with Whole-Grain Blueberry Muffin *(page 325)*	Mini Babybel Light *(page 336)*	Fast Fuel *(page 327)*	Stuffed Portobellos *(page 369)*	Vanilla Ice Cream with Strawberries *(page 335)*
7	English Muffin Stack *(page 323)*	Coffee Break *(page 335)*	Veggie Wrap *(page 330)*	Shrimp & Spicy Tomatoes *(page 359)*	Pear with Cheese *(page 336)*

As needed Deploy a smart swap. The plan is completely portable, so if you feel like eating out (or ordering in), you can still stick to the suggested calorie counts. Some popular possibilities:

Applebee's

- Grilled Dijon Chicken and Portabellos, plus a small side of Seasonal Veggies
- California Shrimp Salad (½ order; includes dressing)

Chili's

- GG Salmon with Garlic & Herbs (includes Rice and Seasonal Veggies)
- Chicken Fajita with 1 Flour Tortilla (no condiments) and Mandarin Oranges

Olive Garden

- Venetian Apricot Chicken with 1 cup Minestrone Soup
- Seafood Brodetto

P.F. Chang's

- Chicken Lettuce Wraps (½ appetizer order), 1 cup Hot & Sour Soup, and 1 Banana Spring Roll (¼ order)
- Asian Grilled Salmon on Brown Rice (½ order), Shanghai Cucumbers, and 1 Mini Great Wall of Chocolate

Tester's INSIDE TIP

"Business lunches were a little hard, but I would just look for dishes that were grilled or ask for things steamed and the dressing on the side. Most restaurants were accommodating. Looking at the menu online also helped me plan healthier options."—Bernadette Pace

WEEK 3: BEAT BOREDOM

Progress on all fronts is not always steady, so putting in the effort across the board is the key to steamrolling through any impasses. Be on the lookout for signs of boredom. One of its classic manifestations: dreading, instead of embracing, your routines. A quick fix: Readjust your focus to a new area.

To Week 2 activities, ADD
Skin Care

As needed Troubleshoot. Instead of focusing on adding another step to your daily routine, home in on what's irking you about your complexion. Whether it's acne, age spots, or redness you have to deal with, take the advice on trouble spots in Chapter 1 (page 27) and begin treatment.

Beauty

Daily Makeup is a terrific aid, but this week, fix your sights on brightening your smile. Keep your teeth looking younger and whiter by brushing twice daily and flossing once a day. Rinse your mouth with water after every meal, especially if you've had a glass of wine. As your teeth get whiter, experiment with different lip colors. A sparkling grin can lift your whole face—and your attitude.

Hair Care

As needed Fine-tune your approach to styling: Adjust your products to meet the changing needs of your hair, such as shifts in dryness/oiliness or basic texture. To cut down on frizz and keep hair smooth, use a spray, cream, or mousse containing dimethicone (or one of the other "-cone" ingredients). You may also need to go easy on daily use of hot tools such as blow-dryers, hot rollers, and flat irons. If your hair isn't frizz-prone, let it air-dry till it's slightly damp and then, after you've spritzed on a heat-protection spray, use a blow-dryer and a big, round brush to smooth out your style. Air-drying increases frizz, so if it's a concern, blow-dry straightaway, but avoid washing and styling every day.

Exercise

The tried-and-true advice for keeping boredom at bay is to mix up your routine. If your walking resolve is weakening, try one of our fitness switches (see chart below) to keep you engaged. A little reverse psychology can also keep you motivated: Researchers at the University of British Columbia found that when people thought about exercising, they tended to focus on the first few minutes—and started to dread the session. But *after* a workout, participants rated it positively. Finding a happier way to ease into exercise—like starting your playlist with your favorite songs, or focusing on how good you'll feel afterward—can help get you through those first moves and make you stick with the session.

Instead of walking, why not try 30 minutes of...	You'll burn...*
Watching the sunrise while stretching	90
Canoeing	126
Biking to the store	143
Catching fireflies with your kids	179
Hiking to a picnic spot	215
Skinny-dipping when the kids are asleep	215
Snorkeling	186
Golfing (and carrying the clubs)	205
Walking on the beach	149
Dancing after dinner	205
Snowshoeing	228
Sledding with your kids	260
Horseback riding	149

* Number of calories burned by a 150- to 155-pound woman.

"I hurt my back right before I started the program, so I wasn't able to do all the exercises. To make up for it, I tried to walk more whenever I could. For instance, instead of just going down the hall to the corporate cafeteria, I'd walk several blocks to pick up lunch." **–Diane Durando**

This week, focus on the no-sweat aspect of your fitness routine. Stretching literally takes five minutes, but it can help unkink the muscles you've been taxing during your walking program. Stretching also sends vital nutrients and blood to joints, tendons, and ligaments, keeping them mobile and supple. Do the five stretches (page 202) at least once every other day.

Regularly, ADD Five more minutes of walking to your Fat-Blasting workouts. To mix it up, try relocating your walk to an area with hills. Your exercise schedule will now look like this:

- **One day a week** 20-minute walk (or 20 minutes of walking broken up into 5- or 10-minute segments).
- **Three days a week** Walking Workout #1: Fat-Blasting Interval Training—add five more minutes to the workout (from Week 2) by increasing the first five *moderate* walking intervals by one minute, i.e.,

2 minutes (warm-up)	2.5 minutes (moderate walk)
3 minutes (moderate walk)	30 seconds (fast walk)
30 seconds (fast walk)	3.5 minutes (moderate walk)
3 minutes (moderate walk)	30 seconds (fast walk)
1 minute (fast walk)	5 minutes (moderate walk)

Continue as the original workout outlines. Your total routine should now take you 30 minutes.

- **Two days a week** Add another set—for a total of three—to your belly-flatteners.

De-stress

Daily Giving yourself a regular pep talk can help you deal with daily ups and downs. Develop your own personal positive phrase (see page 248) that you keep in the back of your mind—and/or write down and post on your computer monitor, bathroom mirror, or car dashboard—and repeat to yourself whenever you need to calm and collect yourself or just need some inspiration.

Tester's INSIDE TIP

"I stressed over some parts of the program, like when I didn't lose weight for a couple of weeks. But instead of freaking out, I kept telling myself, This is an adventure, and a journey, and a beautiful gift that I am giving to myself. *I'm trying to focus less on results and more on the day-to-day. Even small changes are important, and success with this program is not necessarily about losing weight; it's about my skin, my hair, my emotional health, and building in time each day that's just for me!"* **—Rachel Dorfman**

Weight-Loss Meal Plan

At this point on the plan, you know what meals work for you, your family, and your schedule. It's fine to make a few swaps, but keep an eye on maximizing variety.

Week 3

Day	Breakfast	Snack	Lunch	Dinner	Snack
1	Sweet Stuffed Waffle *(page 323)*	Roast Beef Rolls *(page 336)*	Souped-Up Soup *(page 328)*	Pork à l'Orange *(page 348)*	Greek Yogurt with Honey *(page 335)*
2	Cereal-Yogurt Parfait *(page 322)*	Soy Mix *(page 336)*	Roast Beef Sammy *(page 328)*	Scallops & Parsnip Puree *(page 356)*	Mezze *(page 336)*
3	California Breakfast Wrap *(page 324)*	On the Run *(page 335)*	Protein Plate *(page 328)*	Chicken Bruschetta *(page 339)*	Kettle Corn *(page 335)*
4	Bagel Spread *(page 322)*	Watermelon Salad *(page 335)*	Pita Pizza *(page 328)*	Roasted Cod & Mushroom Ragout *(page 353)*	Banana Split *(page 335)*
5	Cozy Oats *(page 322)*	Chips & Salsa *(page 336)*	Deli Twist *(page 327)*	Beef & Peppers Stir-Fry *(page 350)*	Whole Grain Fig Newtons *(page 335)*
6	Asparagus Omelet *(page 322)*	Coffee Break *(page 335)*	Turkey Wrap *(page 330)*	Salmon with Gingery Cabbage *(page 355)*	Ice Cream Waffle *(page 335)*
7	Whole-Grain Pancakes *(page 326)*	Parm Plate *(page 336)*	Cheesy Chili *(page 327)*	Pasta Primavera *(page 361)*	Berries & Chocolate *(page 335)*

"I traded lunch for dinner. When I didn't have time to cook— which was most of the time—I'd have one of the lunch suggestions, like the veggie-packed turkey sandwich or Amy's 300-calorie lasagna. That helped keep me on track and losing weight." **–Fern Richter**

Daily, as needed Deploy a smart swap. This week, practice distinguishing between actual physical hunger and emotional hunger, to help you keep boredom from sidetracking your efforts to eat healthier and lose weight. Our at-a-glance chart makes it a snap.

Actual vs. Emotional Hunger: What's the Difference?

Actual	Emotional
Originates in the stomach and is accompanied by physical sensations: rumbling, emptiness	Originates in the mind or mouth
Arises gradually	Arises suddenly
Moderate time frame	Immediate time frame (eat now!)
Characterized by an openness to eating different foods	Characterized by a craving for a specific food
Results from a physical need	Results from an upsetting emotion, event, or situation
End result: satisfaction, satiety	End result: guilt, remorse, anger

WEEK 4: MAXIMIZE YOUR MOTIVATION

Acknowledging your hard work—and rewarding yourself for it—can help you stick with your resolve to look and feel years younger. For starters, you can make your accomplishments more visible. You probably use sticky notes to remind yourself of all kinds of things, so why not a reminder like "I've lost weight!" or "I'm walking four times a week and feeling stronger!" or "I've trimmed an inch from my waist!"? Post positive notes on your computer, on your refrigerator, at your desk, on the bathroom mirror. Or, put a red check or star on your calendar for an at-a-glance sense of accomplishment. If you've lost weight or trimmed off some inches, reward yourself with a massage, a manicure, or even a new workout outfit.

To Week 3 activities, ADD

Skin Care

Once a week Even if you're wearing boots now, sandal weather is never far away: Remove calluses from your feet (see page 57). You'll feel pampered, but even more important, your balance may improve as calluses are removed.

Beauty

As needed Looking younger should give you plenty to smile about; now make that smile shine. Start using a whitening toothpaste, a whitening kit, or a professionally administered treatment (see page 88).

Hair Care

As needed Make an appointment to have your hair colored. All the basic care you've been giving it sets the foundation for hair that shines with a youthful vibrancy. If you're a color newbie, see page 99 for advice on anti-aging coloring. If you already color your hair, try a new shade (as a rule, lighter, warmer hues take away years; darker, severe shades add them). If you have gray hair and don't color it, keep your shade bright by switching to a shampoo labeled "anti-yellow." Keep the texture smooth and soft by using conditioner formulated for curly or coarse hair (see page 98).

Tester's INSIDE TIP

"After years of buying any old shampoo and conditioner, I started using ones formulated for blondes. Now my hair has the luster it used to have when I was in my 20s and 30s. Taking the time to find the right products really pays off."
—Diane Durando

Exercise

Keep doing your stretches (page 202) four or even five times a week. When your muscles are flexible, you move more easily and effortlessly throughout your days.

Regularly, ADD Replace two of your Fat-Blasting workouts with Walking Workout #2: Walk-and-Tone Circuit Training (see page 196). Strength-training with resistance bands gives your body more tone, more strength, and more skin-smoothing muscle. Since you don't want to lose the gains in stamina that you've made in the past weeks, add 10 minutes of walking to those workouts before the cooldown. You should also add on another day of belly-flatteners.

Tester's INSIDE TIP

"The scale doesn't tell the whole story. Even when it didn't seem like I'd lost weight, I'd put on a pair of pants I hadn't worn for a while and think, These were pretty uncomfortable last time; now they feel pretty good. *That kept me doing the workouts regularly!"* —Laura Goldblum

Your exercise schedule will now look like this:

- **One day a week** 20-minute walk (or 20 minutes of walking broken up into 5- or 10-minute segments).
- **One day a week** Walking Workout #1: Fat-Blasting Interval Training—30 minutes of intervals as per Week 3.
- **Two days a week** Walking Workout #2: Walk-and-Tone Circuit Training—add 10 minutes of regular walking before the cooldown. Your total routine should now take you 30 minutes.
- **Three days a week** Three sets of 15 repetitions each of the three belly-flatteners (page 199).
- **Four to five days a week** Do the stretching moves (page 202).

Tester's INSIDE TIP

"As the weeks go on, it is a challenge to slot in the time every day to exercise. I actually put it on my to-do list, along with everything else, so it doesn't fall through the cracks. I definitely have better days. For instance, when I knew I had a couple of less busy days, I signed up for spinning classes. The other days I just tried to get my blood pumping somehow! I have a weighted hula hoop, which is a last-ditch workout; if I don't manage to get anything else in during the day, I do that at home, even in front of the TV."
—Diane Gurden

Brain Fitness

Daily Learning keeps your brain in the game. Search online for opportunities in your community: evening classes at local colleges, adult/continuing education at community centers or clubs. Some major universities offer video classes; others have alumni groups with virtual book clubs. Scan the offerings and look for something that helps you learn about a subject you're unfamiliar with—say, a photo-editing computer program, piano basics, French literature, or film theory. Consider enrolling in a foreign-language class (see page 225).

De-stress

As needed Watch a funny movie. It will relieve stress, and laughing can protect against heart problems (see page 251).

Testers' favorite escape movies:

The 40-Year-Old Virgin	*Little Miss Sunshine*
Airplane	*Moonstruck*
Arthur	*My Cousin Vinny*
Blazing Saddles	Any *Naked Gun* movie
Bridget Jones's Diary	*Shrek*
City Island	*Talladega Nights*
Four Weddings and	*This Is Spinal Tap*
a Funeral	*Vacation*
The Hangover (Part 1)	*Wedding Crashers*
Any Jackie Chan movie	*What About Bob?*

Tester's INSIDE TIP : *"Squeezing in a funny movie during a busy week really helped. This week, I saw* Bridesmaids. *It perked me up and made me laugh every time I told a friend about it!"*
—Bernadette Pace

Weight-Loss Meal Plan

To keep your motivation high, use the pleasure principle. That piece of eating advice comes straight from our panelists. "I love the Cereal-Yogurt

Parfait!" says Bernadette Pace. "It feels like I'm eating dessert for break-fast." Kathy Coleman's favorite is the Pita Pizza: "It's easy and satisfying. I have it more than once a week, and I just add different vegetable top-pings for variety." Enjoy the foods you love. By focusing on the pleasures of eating—the tastes, textures, and aromas of food—you'll feel much more satisfied and even boost your metabolism. When Yale researchers gave 46 volunteers a 380-calorie beverage labeled "Indulgence Shake," the participants' levels of the hunger-and metabolism-regulating hormone ghrelin fell sharply, showing they felt full and had an amped-up calo-rie burn. But a week earlier, when the group sipped the same drink, this time marked "Sensi-Shake," ghrelin stayed flat. Perception is everything!

But balance indulgence with common sense: Research shows that those on a moderate-fat-and-calorie diet (like our plan) lose more weight and are more likely to keep it off than those on a stricter low-fat-low-calorie regimen. Drizzle, don't dollop, sauces. Have salad dressing on the side and dip the tines of your fork in it with each bite. When you're at a party, enjoy a spritzer instead of a glass of wine.

As needed Deploy a smart swap. Replace one of your dinners with a store-bought chicken meal—fast and easy. (See pages 302-303).

"Cutting sugar out of my coffee was an easy move to make, and I helped myself over initial cravings by using Splenda. Now it's automatic that I take my coffee black. As a result, I've been feeling a lot more energetic and a lot less tired and moody in the afternoons. I think it might be a product of no sugar-triggered ups and downs." **–Rachel Dorfman**

Week 4

Day	Breakfast	Snack	Lunch	Dinner	Snack
1	PB&A *(page 323)*	Roast Beef Rolls *(page 336)*	Asian Bowl *(page 327)*	Chicken in Lettuce Cups *(page 340)*	Watermelon Salad *(page 335)*
2	Peaches & Cream *(page 323)*	Chips & Cheese *(page 336)*	Mediterra-nean Tuna Salad *(page 328)*	Herb-Grilled Turkey *(page 342)*	Popcorn *(page 336)*
3	Breakfast Bowl *(page 322)*	Endive Boats *(page 336)*	Supermarket Sushi & Salad Bar *(page 330)*	Balsamic Roasted Pork with Berry Salad *(page 346)*	Banana Pudding *(page 335)*
4	Monte Cristo *(page 323)*	Coffee Break *(page 335)*	Roast Beef Sammy *(page 328)*	Grilled Veggie Pizza *(page 366)*	Kashi TLC Fruit & Grain Bar *(page 335)*
5	Trail Oats *(page 323)*	On the Run *(page 335)*	Burger Day *(page 327)*	Red Lentil & Vegetable Soup *(page 367)*	Mezze *(page 336)*
6	On the Road *(page 323)*	Asian App *(page 336)*	Greek Feast *(page 327)*	Turkey Burgers *(page 344)*	Cottage Cheese with Melon *(page 336)*
7	Mixed Fruit Smoothie with Whole-Grain Blueberry Muffin *(page 325)*	Cheese Plate *(page 336)*	Spring Salad *(page 328)*	Roasted Shrimp Scampi *(page 357)*	Pear with Cheese *(page 336)*

7 Quick and Easy Dinners From a Rotisserie Chicken

When just the *thought* of cooking dinner puts you in overwhelm mode, pick up a precooked rotisserie chicken. They're available from most markets or your local chicken takeout. Each satisfying serving of these recipes is 515 calories or less, provided you toss the skin (but high in sodium because of the canned and packaged foods they contain). And with only five ingredients (not including oil, salt, and pepper) and a minimum of chopping, you can have these meals ready in 25 minutes or less—and keep your can-do spirit high.

Arugula & Cranberry Salad

In large bowl, toss 1 package (5 oz.) baby arugula, 1/4 c. dried cranberries, 3 Tbsp. light balsamic vinaigrette, and 1/4 tsp. freshly ground black pepper. Divide among 4 plates. Top with sliced meat from 1 rotisserie chicken. With vegetable peeler, shave 1 oz. Parmesan cheese over all. Serve with whole-grain dinner rolls. Serves 4.

BBQ Chicken Slaw

In large bowl, toss 1 bag (14 oz.) coleslaw mix; shredded meat from 1 rotisserie chicken; 1 can (15.25 oz.) no-salt-added corn kernels, rinsed and drained; 1/3 c. barbecue sauce; and 1 Tbsp. cider vinegar. Serve with or on whole wheat hamburger buns. Serves 4.

Black Bean Burritos

In large bowl, toss half 10-oz. bag chopped romaine lettuce; shredded meat from 1 rotisserie chicken; 1 can (14.5 oz.) no-salt-added black beans, rinsed and drained; and 1 c. fresh salsa. Warm 4 lg. whole wheat tortillas as label directs. Divide chicken mixture among tortillas, and wrap. Serves 4.

Chicken Parm Casserole

Preheat oven to 425°F. In 8" by 8" baking dish, stir together 1 pound frozen cut green beans, thawed; 1/2 c. marinara sauce; and 2 Tbsp. sliced pimentos, drained, until combined. Top with shredded meat from 1 rotisserie chicken and 1/2 c. marinara sauce. Sprinkle with 1 c. shredded part-skim mozzarella cheese. Bake 15 minutes or until cheese melts. Serve with multi-grain dinner rolls. Serves 4.

Soba Salad

Heat 4-quart saucepan of water to boiling on high. Cook 12 oz. soba noodles as label directs. Drain; rinse with cold water. Drain well. Transfer to large bowl, along with 3 c. mixed greens, 3 oz. shredded skinless chicken breast, 2 c. shredded carrots, 4 Tbsp. dry roasted peanuts, $1/3$ c. light ginger salad dressing, and $1/8$ tsp. freshly ground black pepper. Toss until well coated. Serves 4.

Spinach & Beet Salad

In large bowl, toss 1 package (5 oz.) baby spinach; 1 package (8 oz.) pre-cooked, peeled baby beets, cut into quarters; 3 Tbsp. light poppy seed dressing; and $1/8$ tsp. freshly ground black pepper. Divide among 4 plates. Top with sliced meat from 1 rotisserie chicken; 8 Tbsp. dry-roasted, salted soy nuts; and 1 Tbsp. dressing. Serve with whole-grain rolls. Serves 4.

Stuffed Pitas

In large bowl, whisk together $1/2$ c. roasted red pepper hummus, 2 Tbsp. lemon juice, 1 Tbsp. water, and $1/8$ tsp. freshly ground black pepper. Add 2 c. shredded meat from 1 rotisserie chicken and 5 c. Italian-blend mixed greens; toss until combined. Divide mixture among 4 whole wheat pita pockets, toasted. Serves 4.

WEEK 5: ENGINEER YOUR ENVIRONMENT FOR SUCCESS

In order to transform new behaviors into default habits, there are some important questions to ask yourself: Are there any obstacles preventing you from changing? What could help you make positive changes? Of course, friends and family can supply the emotional support you need to be successful. But often, it's your surroundings that can make or break your efforts. For instance, you feel you'd be fitter if only the gym were closer to your home. Instead of resigning yourself to a fate of being overweight, check to see if there's a gym near your office. Or create routines that can be done outdoors, using benches, stairs, hills, even playground equipment. Reorganizing your medicine chest so that your cosmetics, skin-care, and hair-care products are all within reach seems obvious...but have you done it? Keeping the pantry stocked with the ingredients for the eating plan is important and can be outsourced to your spouse or an older child. Retooling the family calendar (whether it's posted on the fridge or online) to include your exercise sessions or "me-time" breaks for meditation can help you stick to your goals and help your family respect your needs.

To Week 4 activities, ADD:

Skin Care

Once a week, if desired Your skin is already smoother and more radiant; now take it to the next level. Give yourself an at-home peel to brighten and smooth your skin (see page 27).

Beauty

Daily Add bronzer to your makeup roster. Dust it along your cheekbones to brighten, lift, and add subtle shimmer to your whole face.

Hair Care

As needed If your hair is dry and brittle despite once-a-week deep-conditioning, step up deep-conditioning to twice a week. Make sure you're not over-shampooing and that you're using a regular after-shampoo conditioner.

As needed Try an at-home hair glaze if you want to give your hair a shine boost (see page 106).

Exercise

You've built a solid five-week fitness foundation; now challenge yourself. Swap the straightforward 20-minute walk for a longer interval-training walk. Consistent stretching will help ease the physical transition to this new activity level. Your exercise schedule will now look like this:

- **Two days a week** Walking Workout #1: Fat-Blasting Interval Training—30 minutes of intervals as per Week 4.
- **Two days a week** Walking Workout #2: Walk-and-Tone Circuit Training—30 minutes as per Week 4.
- **Three days a week** Three sets of 15 repetitions each of the three belly-flatteners.
- **Four to five days a week** Do the stretching moves.

"My daughters swim seven days a week, so I am at the pool all the time, just sitting on my duff watching them have this amazing workout. I came up with the idea of doing strength-training exercises like push-ups, triceps dips, and lunges on the bleachers while I'm there." –Diane Gurden

De-stress

Daily Give yourself a time-out with a cup of green tea. You'll be treating your skin to a cupful of antioxidants and allowing yourself time to calm down. If you don't have time for both tea and meditation (or a breathing exercise), alternate between the two each day.

"On days when I don't bring my lunch to work, I get takeout lentil soup with a side of cooked spinach. I then add the spinach to the soup for a filling meal." –**Fern Richter**

As needed Deploy a smart swap. Sometimes you can't engineer your own environment, but that doesn't mean you have to relinquish control. If you're facing a buffet table, clench your fist—it turns out firming your muscles literally shores up your willpower and helps you overcome temptation. University of Chicago researchers had students hold a pen tightly or loosely while ordering from a snack bar. Those who stiffened their finger muscles felt more in control of their decisions and were more likely to choose healthy options.

Weight-Loss Meal Plan

By planning your shopping and your menus, you're less likely to make a meal of or snack on something that's high in sugar, fat, or calories. In short, you're rearranging your kitchen/pantry/dining room to be a launch-pad for diet success, not distress.

Week 5

Day	Breakfast	Snack (1)	Lunch	Dinner	Snack (2)
1	New York Bagel *(page 323)*	Mini Babybel Light *(page 336)*	Asian Bowl *(page 327)*	Pomegranate-Glazed Salmon *(page 354)*	Kind Mini Fruit & Nut Delight Bar *(page 335)*
2	PB&A *(page 323)*	Parm Plate *(page 336)*	Spicy Butternut Squash Soup *(page 328)*	Flank Steak with Red Wine & Oven Fries *(page 351)*	Berries & Chocolate *(page 335)*
3	Egg Scramble *(page 322)*	Greek Yogurt with Honey *(page 335)*	Stuffed Sweet Potato *(page 330)*	Turkey & White Bean Chili *(page 343)*	Banana Split *(page 335)*
4	Cereal & More *(page 322)*	Hard-Cooked Egg *(page 336)*	Spinach Salad with Tuna & Avocado *(page 331)*	Grilled Portobello Burger *(page 368)*	Ice Cream Waffle *(page 335)*
5	Grab & Go *(page 322)*	Popcorn *(page 336)*	Microwavable Meal *(page 328)*	Vegetable Lasagna Toss *(page 362)*	Trail Mix *(page 335)*
6	Pronto Plate *(page 323)*	Mezze *(page 336)*	Cheesy Chili *(page 327)*	Almond-Crusted Chicken with Rainbow Slaw *(page 337)*	Whole Grain Fig Newtons *(page 335)*
7	PB&J B'fast *(page 323)*	Soy Mix *(page 336)*	Veggie Wrap *(page 330)*	Balsamic Roasted Pork with Berry Salad *(page 346)*	Banana Pudding *(page 335)*

WEEK 6: FOIL SETBACKS

Life will always throw you a curveball or two. You can stress out and scramble to react, or you can be proactive and anticipate that you may encounter obstacles down the road. Create an emergency-response kit so you can rise to the occasion: Have to work through lunch? Keep a pouch of tuna and some crackers or a container of bean-based soup stashed in your desk. Need to skip exercise? Make up that lost session by going longer on other workouts. Or, take a break and walk some stairs. Climbing stairs for 10 minutes burns 90 calories! Look at these challenges as opportunities to stick with your goals and stay flexible. Another key aspect to long-term success is not to let these setbacks undermine your self-confidence. If you fall back to an old behavior, take a hard look at why it happened. What triggered the relapse? What can you do to avoid these triggers in the future?

To Week 5 activities, ADD:

Skin

Daily If you're losing weight, you may want to wear more revealing clothes. Is the skin on your body measuring up to the renewed skin on your face? Switch to an anti-aging body moisturizer (see page 58); apply after showering on slightly damp skin to lock in moisture and fully plump skin. And don't forget to apply sunscreen—to body *and* face.

Beauty

Daily Once you remove your lipstick, how do your lips look? If they're dry, give them a before-bed softening treatment. Gently rub with a damp washcloth to slough off dead skin, then apply a rich lip balm.

"Before, I was using a cream foundation and then blush, and it just seemed like it was a lot of makeup. I switched to a tinted moisturizer and am surprised at how light it feels on my face. I also use a powder bronzer as a blush. I love the results." **–Kathy Coleman**

Hair

As needed Keep your new color vibrant by using either a shine spray or a color extender (see page 106). If you have gray hair, add a finishing mist with shine-enhancing power (see page 105).

Exercise

A little bit more effort can yield big-time body benefits. This week, increase your walk duration by five minutes. Consider adding another session of the belly-flatteners to your schedule. A strong core not only whittles your middle, but reduces the risk of back pain. Your exercise schedule will now look like this:

- **Two days a week** Walking Workout #1: Fat-Blasting Interval Training—add an extra five minutes to the workout (from Week 5, see page 305) by increasing the first five *moderate* walking intervals by one minute, i.e.,

2 minutes (warm-up)	3.5 minutes (moderate walk)
4 minutes (moderate walk)	30 seconds (fast walk)
30 seconds (fast walk)	4.5 minutes (moderate walk)
4 minutes (moderate walk)	30 seconds (fast walk)
1 minute (fast walk)	6 minutes (moderate walk)

Continue as the original workout outlines. Your total routine should now take you 35 minutes.

- **Two days a week** Walking Workout #2: Walk-and-Tone Circuit Training—add five more minutes of regular walking before the cooldown. Your total routine should now take you 35 minutes.
- **Three to four days a week** Three sets of 15 repetitions each of the three belly-flatteners.
- **Four to five days a week** Do the stretching moves.

 Tester's INSIDE TIP : *"Some days, it's difficult for me to fit in the Fat-Blasting walk. When it isn't possible, I'll do sit-ups and leg lifts on the floor while I'm watching TV."* –**Kathy Coleman**

Brain Fitness

Daily Do one thing. It's a mad, mad multitasking world, but if you can try to limit the number of things you do at once, your brain will be the better for it. You'll start remembering more and in greater depth when you're not distracted. Make a conscious effort this week to keep your attention on one thing at a time. Focus only on the person who's speaking to you; turn off the TV while you're on the computer; don't surf the Net when you're talking on the phone.

Weight-Loss Meal Plan

This plan provides plenty of variety, age-erasing antioxidants in the form of fruits and vegetables, and lots of fiber. If you eat foods not on the plan—at breakfast, for instance—don't get down on yourself. Stay positive and get back on track with the next meal (or snack).

Week 6

Day	Breakfast	Snack	Lunch	Dinner	Snack
1	Asparagus Omelet *(page 322)*	Mini Babybel Light *(page 336)*	Pita Pizza *(page 328)*	Linguine with Carrot-Turkey Ragout *(page 360)*	Banana Split *(page 335)*
2	English Muffin Stack *(page 323)*	Coffee Break *(page 335)*	Fast Fuel *(page 327)*	Cod Livornese with Couscous *(page 352)*	Endive Boats *(page 336)*
3	Cereal-Yogurt Parfait *(page 322)*	Roast Beef Rolls *(page 336)*	White Pizza *(page 330)*	Pork Chops Marsala *(page 345)*	Kashi TLC Fruit & Grain Bar *(page 335)*
4	Sweet Stuffed Waffle *(page 323)*	On the Run *(page 335)*	Deli Twist *(page 327)*	Stuffed Portobellos *(page 369)*	Trail Mix *(page 335)*
5	Cozy Oats *(page 322)*	Asian App *(page 336)*	Souped-Up Soup *(page 328)*	Chicken in Lettuce Cups *(page 340)*	Kettle Corn *(page 335)*
6	California Breakfast Wrap *(page 324)*	Whole Grain Fig Newtons *(page 335)*	Protein Plate *(page 328)*	Beef & Peppers Stir-Fry *(page 350)*	Watermelon Salad *(page 335)*
7	Bagel Spread *(page 322)*	Chips & Cheese *(page 336)*	Turkey Wrap *(page 330)*	Pasta Primavera *(page 361)*	Vanilla Ice Cream with Strawberries *(page 335)*

As needed Deploy a smart swap. Foil the all-too-common setback of no time to cook with a fast-food meal that won't sidetrack weight loss. There are plenty of convenience options that fit into the plan. Be forewarned: These meals are high in sodium.

Subway

- 6" Oven Roasted Chicken Sandwich on 9-Grain Wheat Bread with provolone cheese, lettuce, tomatoes, onions, green peppers, and cucumbers (370 calories, 3.5 g saturated fat)
- Veggie Delite Salad with oil and vinegar from the squirt bottles (instead of Fat-Free Italian Dressing; 85 calories, 0.5 g saturated fat)

   Total: **455 calories, 4 g saturated fat**

McDonald's

- Premium Grilled Chicken Classic Sandwich (350 calories, 2 g saturated fat)
- Premium Caesar Salad (90 calories, 2.5 g saturated fat)
- Newman's Own Low-Fat Balsamic Vinaigrette (35 calories, 0 g saturated fat)

   Total: **475 calories, 4.5 g saturated fat**

Domino's

- One slice from a Large Hand-Tossed Veggie Pizza (270 calories, 3 g saturated fat)
- Grilled Chicken Caesar Salad with Light Italian Salad Dressing (170 calories, 3.5 g saturated fat)

   Total: **440 calories, 6.5 g saturated fat**

Pizza Hut

- Two slices from a Large Thin 'n' Crispy Veggie Lover's Pizza (480 calories, 8 g saturated fat)

   Total: **480 calories, 8 g saturated fat**

Panera Bread

- Smoked Turkey Breast Café Sandwich (420 calories, 0.5 g saturated fat)
- Apple (80 calories, 0 g saturated fat)
  Total: **500 calories, 0.5 g saturated fat**

Chipotle Mexican Grill

- Burrito Bowl with Cilantro Lime Rice (130 calories, 0.5 g saturated fat), black beans (120 calories, 0 g saturated fat), chicken (190 calories, 2 g saturated fat), Fajita Vegetables (20 calories, 0 g fat), and Fresh Tomato Salsa (20 calories, 0 g saturated fat)
  Total: **480 calories, 2.5 g saturated fat**

Wendy's

- Small Chili (210 calories, 2.5 g saturated fat)
- Plain Baked Potato (270 calories, 0 g saturated fat)
  Total: **480 calories, 2.5 g saturated fat**

Panda Express

- Kung Pao Chicken (280 calories, 3.5 g saturated fat)
- Side of Mixed Vegetables (70 calories, 0 g saturated fat)
- Hot and Sour Soup (100 calories, 0.5 g saturated fat)
  Total: **450 calories, 4 g saturated fat**

 Tester's INSIDE TIP

"For the nights when I have evening events after work, I'm trying to make small changes. It's either no alcohol or no dessert—I'm finding that every little bit helps."
—Kathy Coleman

WEEK 7: STAY THE COURSE

To stay motivated on the 7 Years Younger plan and beyond, remind yourself of all the benefits you're getting and focus on the *how* of exercising, eating right, and performing your hair, skin, and beauty routines. Research shows that working on your personal stick-to-it strategy—marking it on your calendar, tracking your progress, and rewarding yourself when you succeed—provides the best incentive for continuing a program.

To Week 6 activities, ADD:

Skin Care

As needed Enhance the glow you've nurtured these past six weeks with the kiss of a sunless tan. Depending on the season, you may want to add just a bit of a glow with a gradual self-tanner (see page 58) or get a more bronzed look with a regular self-tanning product (see page 50). Either way, your skin will look brighter.

Beauty

As needed Groom your brows (see page 75). Fill in sparse spots with a brow pencil. Defined, shapely brows lift your whole face.

 Tester's INSIDE TIP : *"My current go-to makeup product is eyebrow gel. Just a little accents my brows and really perks up my whole look."* –Tessa Jean

Hair Care

As needed Your hair should be in great condition now, but just in case you have a bad-hair day, carry a dry/flyaway hair-repair kit: one travel-size spray bottle of leave-in conditioner. Spritz as necessary.

Exercise

Monotony can kill your exercise enthusiasm. To keep it interesting, mix things up: replace one of your Fat-Blasting Interval Training workouts with Walking Workout #3: Mood-Boosting, Stress-Busting Cross–Training (see page 196). Challenge yourself further by increasing your sessions five minutes. Training for a charity walk, or meeting friends at a weekly class, can also keep fitness in your future. Your workout schedule will now look like this:

- **1 day a week** Walking Workout #3: Mood-Boosting, Stress-Busting Cross-Training—40 minutes or whatever is comfortable
- **1 day a week** Walking Workout #1: Fat-Blasting Interval Training—add an extra five minutes to the workout (from Week 6) by increasing the first 10 *moderate* and *fast* walking intervals by 30 seconds, i.e.,

2 minutes (warm-up)

4.5 minutes (moderate walk)

1 minute (fast walk)

4.5 minutes (moderate walk)

1.5 minutes (fast walk)

4 minutes (moderate walk)

1 minute (fast walk)

5 minutes (moderate walk)

1 minute (fast walk)

6.5 minutes (moderate walk)

2 minutes (fast walk)

Continue as the original workout outlined. Your total routine should now take you 40 minutes.

- **Two days a week** Walking Workout #2: Walk-and-Tone Circuit Training—40 minutes (add 20 extra minutes of straight or interval walking before cooldown).

- **Three to four days a week** Three sets of 15 repetitions each of the three belly-flatteners.
- **Four to five days a week** Do the stretching moves.

Brain Fitness

Daily Get organized so that you don't lose things as easily. Position a catchall container near your front door where you can put your keys; designate pockets in your purse for your phone, wallet, and lipstick. Use them! See page 221 for other ideas.

De-stress

Weekly Social interaction, including helping others, is one of your tickets to feeling connected, less stressed, and more youthful. Focus on making your social connections more varied. Join a club, volunteer, reconnect, and meet up with friends. Resolve to be a more active member of society so that, as these seven weeks end, you'll be launched into a more fulfilling (and fun!) life.

Weight-Loss Meal Plan

After this week, you can remain on the plan or transition off it—your choice. If you do go off the plan, try to keep the same meal/calorie structure: a breakfast of 300 calories, lunch of 400 calories, dinner of 500 calories, and two 125-calorie snacks. Eating smaller meals throughout the day keeps your blood sugar steady and your energy levels (and metabolism) high and prevents your weight from creeping up.

Week 7

Day	Breakfast	Snack	Lunch	Dinner	Snack
1	On the Road *(page 323)*	Coffee Break *(page 335)*	Spinach Salad with Tuna and Avocado *(page 331)*	Chicken Bruschetta *(page 339)*	Ice Cream Waffle *(page 335)*
2	Cereal & More *(page 322)*	Pear with Cheese *(page 335)*	Mediterra-nean Tuna Salad *(page 328)*	Chicken Quesadilla with Avocado-Tomato Salsa *(page 341)*	Kettle Corn *(page 335)*
3	Breakfast Bowl *(page 322)*	Hard-Cooked Egg *(page 336)*	Burger Day *(page 327)*	Scallops & Parsnip Puree *(page 356)*	Soy Mix *(page 336)*
4	New York Bagel *(page 323)*	Endive Boats *(page 336)*	Spring Salad *(page 328)*	Herb-Grilled Turkey *(page 342)*	Cheese Plate *(page 336)*
5	Peaches & Cream *(page 323)*	Kind Mini Fruit & Nut Delight Bar *(page 335)*	Hot Roast Beef Hero *(page 328)*	Red Lentil & Vegetable Soup *(page 367)*	Berries & Chocolate *(page 335)*
6	Cereal-Yogurt Parfait *(page 322)*	Mezze *(page 336)*	Microwav-able Meal *(page 328)*	Salmon with Gingery Cabbage *(page 355)*	Watermelon Salad *(page 335)*
7	Whole-Grain Pancakes *(page 326)*	Trail Mix *(page 335)*	Greek Feast *(page 327)*	Whole Wheat Penne with Broccoli & Sausage *(page 363)*	Greek Yogurt with Honey *(page 335)*

As needed Deploy a smart swap. Now that you're looking younger and feeling better than ever, it's natural to worry you'll start to gain back the weight. Relax. While you may have finished with the meal plan, we've designed the program so that you can continue enjoying fabulous foods and all of the benefits that come along with eating this way. Here are five tips to help ease the transition:

- Stick with the meals and recipes you enjoyed on the plan. Preparing and eating them can be a subtle reinforcement of the structure of being on the plan.
- Base new meals on our blueprint: plenty of fresh produce, ample amounts of lean protein, and measured portions of whole grains.
- Discover your stay-young weight and step on the scale once a week to keep tabs on it. If you find the needle is moving in the wrong direction, reboot with the tips on page 372 or simply get back on the meal plan for a few weeks. There will be slip-ups along the way (a whopping piece of red velvet cake or a frantic week at work that squeezes out your time for the gym), but weekly weigh-ins ensure that you'll have to make only a minor correction to lose that pound or so, not undergo a major eating overhaul.
- When you're serving yourself a meal, fill half your plate with fruits and vegetables first; it's practically a guarantee that you'll be getting the bounty of anti-aging, pound-paring produce called for on the 7 Years Younger plan. (At a restaurant? Ask for an extra serving of steamed or raw vegetables.)
- Experiment with new prep methods, herbs, and spices. Taking pleasure in healthy foods is a recipe for lifelong well-being.

Eat to Lose Pounds and Turn Back the Clock

Chapter Ten

Light and Delicious Recipes

Y um—you're going to love these recipes! GHRI Nutrition Director Samantha Cassetty, M.S., R.D., has made the foods you want to eat (pasta, pizza, even desserts) better for you without skimping on flavor or satisfaction. And she's made the foods you know you should eat more of appetizing and simple to prepare, with ingredients that are easy to find. The recipes incorporate all the 7 Years Younger nutrition guidelines and superfoods, complete with their anti-aging active ingredients and wrinkle-fighting antioxidants. You can substitute any recipe for another within each meal category (breakfast: 300 calories; lunch: 400; dinner: 500). Making these meals and snacks staples of your diet in the months and years to come will ensure that you maintain weight loss, brighter skin, and a more youthful body.

BETTER-FOR-YOU
Breakfast Recipes

These recipes will make a breakfast-eater out of you and put more youth-promoting antioxidants in your day! Plus, breakfast-eaters tend to take in fewer calories overall during the day, promoting weight loss.

Asparagus Omelet

In a bowl, whisk 1 large egg and 2 egg whites. In a separate microwavable bowl, microwave 4 washed and trimmed asparagus spears plus 1 Tbsp. water for 2 minutes on High. In a nonstick 8-inch skillet, heat 1 tsp. olive oil over medium-high heat. Pour in egg mixture. Cook, gently lifting edge of eggs with heat-safe rubber spatula and tilting pan to allow uncooked eggs to run underneath, until eggs are set, about 1 minute. Cut 1 slice reduced-fat Swiss cheese into pieces and place the cheese and asparagus over half the omelet. Fold unfilled half of omelet over filling. Serve with ½ sandwich thin, toasted and spread with 1 tsp. light buttery spread.

Bagel Spread

On each half of a toasted 100% Whole Wheat Thomas' Bagel Thin, spread 2 tsp. reduced-fat cream cheese. Serve with 1 hard-boiled egg and 1 c. cubed honeydew melon.

Breakfast Bowl   JUMP START!

1 c. unsweetened Spoon Size Shredded Wheat with 1 c. fat-free milk; stir in ½ c. strawberries, sliced, and 2 tsp. sunflower seeds.

Cereal & More

¾ c. Kashi GoLean topped with 1 small apple, diced; 1 tsp. sunflower seeds; 1 c. fat-free milk; and a dash of cinnamon.

Cereal-Yogurt Parfait   JUMP START!

In a tall glass, layer 1 c. fresh or frozen (unsweetened) blueberries, ¾ c. nonfat Greek yogurt, ½ c. Fiber One cereal, and 1 Tbsp. chopped walnuts.

Cozy Oats   JUMP START!

Mix 1 packet of plain instant oatmeal with ¾ c. fat-free milk and a dash of cinnamon, and microwave on High until hot. Stir in 3 strawberries, sliced; ½ tsp. maple syrup; and 2 Tbsp. chopped walnuts.

Egg Scramble   JUMP START!

Scramble 1 egg and 2 egg whites with ¼ c. baby spinach, cooked, and 1 Tbsp. feta. Serve with 1 whole wheat English muffin and 2 tsp. light spread.

Grab & Go   JUMP START!

1 Kind Peanut Butter & Strawberry bar with a 12-oz. nonfat latte.

English Muffin Stack

Split a toasted 100% whole wheat English muffin and divide ¼ avocado evenly between both sides. Top each side with 1 tomato slice and 2 Tbsp. shredded low-fat Cheddar cheese. Broil in toaster oven until cheese melts. Serve with ½ medium grapefruit.

Monte Cristo

Toast 1 multigrain Belgian waffle (such as Van's) and top with 2 slices lean deli ham and 1 slice reduced-fat Swiss cheese. Broil until cheese melts. Serve with 1½ c. cubed cantaloupe spritzed with fresh lime juice.

New York Bagel

Toast one 100% Whole Wheat Thomas' Bagel Thin; top with 2 oz. reduced-fat cream cheese, 1 oz. lox, 4 tomato slices.

On the Road

1 Subway Egg & Cheese Muffin Melt with 1 Dannon Light & Fit yogurt mixed with 8 almonds (brought from home).

PB&A

Spread 1 Tbsp. peanut butter on 1 slice whole wheat toast. Top with ½ green apple, sliced. Serve with other ½ apple.

PB&J B'fast

In blender, combine 1 small, ripe banana, cut into chunks; 4 strawberries (fresh or frozen); ½ c. fat-free milk; ¼ c. nonfat Greek yogurt; ¼ tsp. vanilla extract; and 3 ice cubes. Serve with 1 slice whole wheat toast spread with 1 tsp. peanut butter and 1 tsp. low-sugar raspberry preserves.

Peaches & Cream

Mix ½ c. part-skim ricotta cheese with 1 tsp. sugar-free pancake syrup and top with 1½ tsp. sliced almonds, toasted. Serve with 1 large peach, sliced.

Pronto Plate

1 Smart Ones Egg, Sausage and Cheese Smart Morning Wrap with ¾ c. honey-dew melon.

Sweet Stuffed Waffle

Toast two Van's 8 Whole Grain Waffles. On one waffle, spread 1 Tbsp. reduced-sugar apricot preserves and ¼ c. part-skim ricotta. Top with remaining waffle.

Trail Oats

½ c. oatmeal made with water, topped with ⅛ c. dried cherries, 2 Tbsp. slivered almonds, and 1 tsp honey.

For even more great recipes, download our free special report, Eat to Look *& Feel Younger, at 7yearsyounger.com/eattolookyoung.*

California Breakfast Wrap

Active/Total Time 15 minutes · **Makes** 4 main-dish servings

4	large eggs plus 2 large egg whites
	Salt and pepper
4	(8-inch) whole wheat tortillas
3½	Tbsp. goat cheese
3½	oz. baby spinach (about 7 c.)

1   tsp. canola oil

1   medium tomato, seeded and finely chopped (about 1 c.)

1   Hass avocado, finely chopped

1   Tbsp. chopped fresh dill leaves

1. In medium bowl, beat eggs, egg whites, and ⅛ tsp. each salt and freshly ground black pepper.

2. On microwave-safe plate, cover tortillas with damp paper towel. Microwave on High 30 seconds or until just warm and pliable.

3. Spread an equal amount of goat cheese on each tortilla; top with spinach.

4. In 12-inch nonstick skillet, heat oil on medium 1 minute. Add egg mixture. Cook 2 minutes or until almost set, stirring gently. Remove from heat; fold in tomato, avocado, and ¼ tsp. salt.

5. Divide hot egg mixture among tortillas. Top with dill; fold in half.

Mixed Fruit Smoothie

Active/Total Time 5 minutes · **Makes** 2 servings

1	c. frozen strawberries	2	tsp. chopped peeled fresh ginger
½	c. fresh blueberries	¼	c. plain low-fat (1%) yogurt
½	c. fresh orange juice	2	ice cubes

1. In blender, combine strawberries, blueberries, orange juice, ginger, yogurt, and ice cubes.

2. Blend until smooth, scraping down side of container occasionally. Serve with 6 almonds.

Whole-Grain Blueberry Muffins

Active Time 15 minutes · **Total Time** 40 minutes · **Makes** 12 muffins

1	c. old-fashioned oats, uncooked	1	c. low-fat buttermilk
1	c. whole wheat flour	¼	c. fresh orange juice
½	c. all-purpose flour	2	Tbsp. canola oil
2	tsp. baking powder	1	large egg
½	tsp. baking soda	1	tsp. vanilla extract
½	tsp. salt	2	c. blueberries
¼	c. plus 1 Tbsp. brown sugar	¼	c. natural almonds, chopped

1. Preheat oven to 400°F. Line 12-cup muffin pan with paper liners.

2. Grind oats in blender. In bowl, whisk oats, flours, baking powder and soda, salt, and ¼ c. sugar. In small bowl, whisk buttermilk, juice, oil, egg, and vanilla. Stir into flour mixture; fold in blueberries.

3. Combine nuts and remaining sugar. Spoon batter into pan; sprinkle with almond sugar. Bake 22 minutes or until toothpick comes out clean. Cool in pan on wire rack 5 minutes. Remove from pan; serve warm or cool completely.

Whole-Grain Pancakes

Total Time 25 minutes · **Makes** 12 pancakes · **Serves** 4

2	ripe peaches, pitted and chopped	2	tsp. baking powder
½	pint (1½ c.) raspberries	½	tsp. salt
1	Tbsp. sugar	1¼	c. fat-free (skim) milk
½	c. all-purpose flour	1	large egg, lightly beaten
½	c. whole wheat flour	1	Tbsp. vegetable oil
½	c. quick-cooking oats, uncooked		

1. In medium bowl, combine peaches, raspberries, and sugar. Stir to coat; set fruit mixture aside.

2. Meanwhile, in large bowl, combine flours, oats, baking powder, and salt. Add milk, egg, and oil; stir just until flour mixture is moistened (batter will be lumpy).

3. Spray 12-inch nonstick skillet with cooking spray; heat on medium 1 minute. Pour batter by scant ¼ cups into skillet, making about 4 pancakes at a time. Cook about 2 minutes until tops are bubbly, some bubbles burst, and edges look dry. With wide spatula, turn pancakes and cook until undersides are golden. Transfer pancakes to platter. Cover; keep warm.

4. Repeat with remaining batter, using more nonstick cooking spray if necessary. To serve, top with 2 Tbsp. fruit mixture.

MAKE-YOU-LEANER
Lunch Recipes

Take a break for lunch, to refresh and recharge until evening. You can also increase your sense of lasting satisfaction from the meal by practicing mindfulness as you eat. Take a moment to notice the colors, textures, and aromas of the meal before you. As you eat mindfully (not automatically), you'll eat more slowly and purposefully, which gives your brain time to register satiety.

Asian Bowl

To one container cooked Minute Ready to Serve Brown Rice, add ½ c. shelled edamame (cooked) and ½ red pepper, diced. Toss with ½ tsp. sesame oil, ½ tsp. rice vinegar, and 1 tsp. reduced-sodium soy sauce. Top with ½ tsp. sesame seeds.

Burger Day

Cook one veggie burger (about 100 calories). Spread 1 whole wheat hamburger bun with 1 tsp. ketchup and 1 tsp. mustard; layer on burger one 1-oz. slice reduced-fat Cheddar, 2 red onion slices, 1 tomato slice, and 1 romaine lettuce leaf.
Dessert ½ mango, chunked.

Cheesy Chili

Cook 1 pouch Tabatchnick Vegetarian Chili according to package directions. Sprinkle with 3 Tbsp. reduced-fat Cheddar. Serve with 1 oz. baked tortilla chips and 2 Tbsp. guacamole.

Deli Twist

Spread 1 Tbsp. red pepper hummus in 1 large (6½-in.-diameter) whole wheat pita and stuff with 2 oz. lean deli turkey breast, 1 red onion slice, and ¼ c. each chopped pepper and cucumber.
Dessert 1 c. strawberries topped with ¼ c. nonfat Greek yogurt, 1 tsp. sunflower seeds, and 1 tsp. honey.

Fast Fuel

One 6-inch Subway Oven Roasted Chicken Sandwich (made with 9-grain wheat bread, veggies, and choice of cheese) with Honey Mustard Sauce.

Greek Feast

Mix ½ c. chickpeas with 5 grape tomatoes, chopped; ¼ cucumber, peeled and chopped; 1 tsp. fresh dill, chopped; 2 Tbsp. reduced-fat feta; and 2 Tbsp. nonfat Greek yogurt. Stuff in a large whole wheat pita.

Hot Roast Beef Hero

Heat ½ tsp. olive oil over medium heat and add ¼ onion, sliced. Sauté until soft and add 2 ounces of deli roast beef, sliced into strips. Cook until browned. Serve roast beef mixture in a warmed whole wheat hot-dog bun and top sandwich with 4 pickled jalapeño peppers. Serve with ½ red pepper, cut into strips, and 1 tsp. light ranch dressing for dipping.

Dessert 1 pear with yogurt dipping sauce made from ⅛ c. nonfat Greek yogurt and ¼ tsp. honey.

Mediterranean Tuna Salad JUMP START!

2 c. romaine topped with ¼ c. garbanzo beans, rinsed; 2 oz. water-packed tuna; ½ cucumber, chopped; 6 grape tomatoes; 1 Tbsp. crumbled feta; and 2 Tbsp. reduced-fat vinaigrette. Serve with 1 mini whole wheat pita.

Dessert 1 c. blueberries with 2 Tbsp. fat-free whipped topping.

Microwavable Meal JUMP START!

1 Amy's Light & Lean Spinach Lasagna, served with salad of 2 c. mixed greens; 4 grape tomatoes; ¼ avocado, sliced; 1 Tbsp. Parmesan; and 2 Tbsp. reduced-fat vinaigrette.

Pita Pizza JUMP START!

Split one large whole wheat pita. On each half, spread 2 Tbsp. pasta sauce. Top with ½ c. frozen chopped broccoli, cooked; 2 black olives, chopped; and ½ c. part-skim mozzarella. Broil until cheese melts.

Protein Plate JUMP START!

1 hard-boiled egg served with ¼ c. hummus, 5 grape tomatoes, 15 sugar snap peas, and 3 reduced-fat Triscuits. Have with one apple cut into slices and served with 1 Cabot 50% Reduced Fat Sharp Cheddar Cheese snack bar.

Roast Beef Sammy JUMP START!

On each half of a toasted whole wheat sandwich thin, spread 1 tsp. spicy mustard. On one half, stack 3 ounces roast beef, 1 slice reduced-fat Cheddar cheese, 2 tomato slices, and 1 romaine lettuce leaf, and top with remaining half. Have with 1 large banana.

Souped-Up Soup JUMP START!

Toss 2 c. baby spinach into a bowl with 1 can lentil soup. Mix, along with ¼ tsp. curry powder and a dash of garlic powder. Microwave on High until hot. Serve with 3 reduced-fat Triscuits.

Spicy Butternut Squash Soup

To 2 c. prepared butternut squash soup (such as Organic Pacific Foods, 90 calories per cup), add ½ ripe pear, chopped, and 1 Tbsp. pumpkin seeds. Have with 11 whole wheat pita chips (such as Athenos).

Spring Salad

Toss 3 c. greens, ¼ c. sliced strawberries, 1½ Tbsp. chopped walnuts, 3 oz. chicken breast, 2 Tbsp. reduced-fat feta, and 2 Tbsp. low-fat balsamic dressing.

Dessert ½ c. nonfat Greek yogurt with 3 Tbsp. pomegranate seeds.

Quick Cook

37 Time-Saving Ingredients

"Convenience food" might bring to mind highly processed meals that aren't particularly good for you but that can be ready in minutes. Meet the new convenience foods: healthy, fresh whole foods that have been partially prepared, saving you considerable time as you pull together a meal. All the recipes in our plan already include these ingredient shortcuts, but here's an at-a-glance guide for speedier prep when you're using your own recipes.

From the Refrigerated-Produce Section

Prewashed Baby Spinach

Prewashed Chopped Romaine Lettuce

Prewashed Baby Kale

Prewashed and Cut Collard Greens

Prewashed Arugula

Prewashed Mixed Greens

Coleslaw/Shredded-Cabbage Mix

Shredded Carrots

Stringless Snap Peas

Microwave-in-a-Bag Green Beans

Precut Broccoli and/or Cauliflower Florets

Precut Peppers

Sliced Mushrooms

Precut Stir-Fry Mix

Diced Carrot, Onion, Celery Mix

Sliced Carrot and Onion Mix

Pre-Peeled and Cut Butternut Squash

Scrubbed Sweet Potatoes

Cooked Beets

Cooked Lentils and/or Black-Eyed Peas

Fresh Tomato Salsa

Peeled Garlic Cloves

From the Dairy Section

Shredded Cheese

Crumbled Feta

From the Frozen Section

Peeled and Cut Sweet Potatoes

Chopped Onions

Carrot, Corn, Pea Medley

Stir-Fry Medley

Cut Green Beans

Sliced Peppers

Broccoli/Cauliflower Mix

Chopped Spinach

Peas

From the Grocery Section

Microwavable Precooked Rice Packets

Canned Corn

Marinara Sauce

Jarred Sliced Pimentos

Stuffed Sweet Potato

Split 1 large baked sweet potato and mash 1½ Tbsp. peanut butter, ⅛ tsp. cumin, ⅛ tsp. cinnamon, and a dash red pepper into pulp. Top with ¼ c. chickpeas and 15 peanuts.

Supermarket Sushi & Salad Bar

1 brown-rice California roll plus 2 c. mixed salad greens; 4 mandarin orange segments; ¼ c. shredded carrots; ¼ c. edamame; and 5 cashews, chopped. Top with 2 Tbsp. reduced-fat Asian-style dressing.

Turkey Wrap   JUMP START!

Spread one La Tortilla Factory 80-calorie Whole Wheat Tortilla with 1 tsp. light mayonnaise; top with 3 oz. deli turkey, two tomato slices, 1 romaine lettuce leaf, ¼ avocado, and 1 slice reduced-fat Swiss cheese. Serve with 1 plum.

Veggie Wrap

Spread 2 tsp. pesto and 2 Tbsp. soft goat cheese on one La Tortilla Factory 80-calorie Whole Wheat Tortilla. Layer ¼ avocado, ½ jarred pepper, ½ c. field greens, and 3 tomato slices on top. Fold to eat. Have with 25 grapes.

White Pizza

Divide evenly between halves of a 100-calorie sandwich thin: 1 tsp. pesto; ¼ c. part-skim ricotta; ½ jarred red pepper, sliced; and 2 tsp. Parmesan cheese. Toast in toaster oven until bottom is crispy and cheese melts. Serve with salad made with 2 c. salad greens, 4 grape tomatoes, and 1 Tbsp. reduced-fat balsamic vinaigrette. **Dessert** 1 c. blueberries topped with 1 Tbsp. fat-free whipped topping and 3 walnut halves, crushed.

For even more great recipes, download our free special report, Eat to Look & Feel Younger, *at 7yearsyounger.com/eattolookyoung.*

Spinach Salad with Tuna & Avocado

Total Time 15 minutes · **Makes** 4 servings

3	Tbsp. fresh lemon juice		2	Tbsp. fresh flat-leaf parsley
1	Tbsp. extra virgin olive oil			leaves, finely chopped
1	Tbsp. water		2	Tbsp. snipped fresh chives
1	tsp. Dijon mustard		1	pkg. (5 oz.) baby spinach
1	ripe Hass avocado, cut in half,		2	stalks celery, thinly sliced
	pitted, peeled		1	medium red pepper, thinly sliced
	Pinch cayenne		1	can (15 oz.) white kidney
	Pinch freshly ground black			(cannellini) beans, rinsed and
	pepper			drained
	Salt		2	cans tuna packed in water
				(5 oz. each), drained well

1. In blender, combine lemon juice, oil, water, mustard, half of avocado, cayenne pepper, and ¼ tsp. salt. Puree until smooth, scraping container occasionally. Stir in parsley and chives.

2. In large bowl, toss spinach, celery, pepper, beans, and tuna with dressing. Divide among serving plates.

3. Thinly slice remaining avocado half and arrange on top of salads.

Side for one 1 mini whole wheat pita

Dessert for one 1 c. blueberries topped with 2 Tbsp. fat-free whipped cream

Anti-Aging BOOSTER

FROZEN-ENTRÉE OPTIONS

There's no need to settle for a soggy deli salad when you want a fast, slimming lunch or dinner. We screened 294 frozen entrées, selecting only those that came in under 400 calories, had no trans fat, and met nutritionist-approved limits for sodium and saturated fat. We ended up with 21 newly launched single-serve meals. Then, over the course of three weeks, we handed out nearly 400 boxes and steam bags and had our crew of lunchtime volunteers microwave and nibble, score, and write detailed reviews. They proclaimed these 13 dishes the best and tastiest.

For flavor variety, try any of these low-cal add-ins:

- Sprinkle 1½ Tbsp. grated Parmesan on your pasta entrée (32 calories).
- Top Southwestern meals with ⅓ cucumber, chopped, mixed with ¼ c. salsa (31 calories).
- Toss 1 Tbsp. sliced almonds on Asian dishes (33 calories).

1 Amy's Light & Lean Soft Taco Fiesta

Just-right spice earned this entrée first place. "Tastes like real Mexican takeout," noted one reviewer, reflecting the enthusiasm of the group. The meal, with its beans, corn, and other veggies, also scores nutritionally, delivering a healthy hit of fiber and vitamins A and C. **220 calories**

2 Amy's Light & Lean Spinach Lasagna

A close second ("pasta had a good taste and texture"), with volunteers noting the "nice portion size," too. A few would have welcomed "more cheese." **250 calories**

3 Amy's Light & Lean Pasta & Veggies

While a couple of participants were disappointed by "too-soft noodles," the "crisp veggies" and "restaurant-quality taste" earned high praise. **210 calories**

4 Lean Cuisine Market Collection Chicken Poblano

Tasters loved the chili-Cheddar sauce, though a number wished there had been more chicken. **330 calories**

5 Healthy Choice 100% Natural Tortellini Primavera Parmesan

The "fresh" veggies won kudos from tasters, as did the sauce. A few felt that "the portion size was small." **230 calories**

6 Amy's Light & Lean Sweet & Sour Asian Noodle Bowl

Ginger and garlic give this Asian meal a kick. "Tasty" appeared in many reviews, as did surprise at how well the veggies held up to microwaving. Some may find it "a little too salty." **250 calories**

7 Healthy Choice 100% Natural Teriyaki Stir-Fry

Tasters enjoyed the extras: "Pineapple and mushrooms were great additions," noted one. Some found the sauce a little too sweet. **250 calories**

8 Amy's Light & Lean 3 Cheese Penne Marinara

A few volunteers thought the portion size was small, but many "loved" the cheese and found this entrée "full of flavor." **270 calories**

9 Helen's Kitchen Veggie Fajita Bowl

"Could use more seasoning," some participants noted. But they enjoyed the ease of cooking (no stirring, which some other entrées required). **250 calories**

10 Amy's Light and Lean Spaghetti Italiano

The lentil-quinoa-tofu meatballs were a nice surprise for some non-vegetarians ("Delish!" said one); others found them "grainy." **240 calories**

11 Amy's Light & Lean Bean & Cheese Burrito

Bean lovers appreciated the abundance, though cheese fans were a bit disappointed. Some felt this entrée would be better as a snack. **280 calories**

12 Helen's Kitchen Fiesta Black Bean Bowl

"Tastes as good as some real meals I've had!" enthused one volunteer. Some testers, however, found the entrée "bland." **290 calories**

13 Organic Bistro Sesame Ginger Wild Salmon Bowl

Tasters wished there had been more sauce, some remarking on the "slightly dry salmon." Still, this got points for "delicious" veggies and quinoa. **300 calories**

SLIMMING, SATISFYING
Snacks

SWEET TREATS

1 Kashi TLC Fruit & Grain Bar
in Dark Chocolate Coconut

1 Kind Mini Fruit & Nut Delight Bar
with 5 grapes

2 100% Whole Grain Fig Newtons

Banana Pudding
Mix ½ small banana, sliced, with 1 container sugar-free vanilla pudding. Crush one vanilla wafer and pour crumbs over the mixture.

Banana Split
Cut 1 small banana in half lengthwise. Spread ½ tsp. peanut butter on one half, ½ tsp. Nutella on the other. Sandwich the two halves.

Berries & Chocolate
Mix 5 raspberries into one 4-oz. container of Oikos Nonfat Chocolate Yogurt

Coffee Break
1 nonfat latte (12 oz.) with 1 Dark Chocolate Hershey's Kiss

Greek Yogurt with Honey
6 oz. nonfat plain Greek yogurt mixed with 1 tsp. honey and a dash of cinnamon

Ice Cream Waffle
Toast one Van's Chocolate Waffle Stick (80 calories) and top with ¼ c. slow-churned vanilla ice cream (100 calories per ½ c.)

Kettle Corn
2½ c. Angie's Light Kettle Corn (120 calories)

On the Run
1 Luna Mini Bar with iced chai-tea latte made with ⅓ c. fat-free milk

Trail Mix
One 100 Calorie Pack Emerald Cocoa Roast Almonds mixed with 1 Tbsp. Craisins

Vanilla Ice Cream with Strawberries
½ c. light vanilla ice cream (about 100 calories per ½ c.) topped with 4 strawberries, sliced

Watermelon Salad
Toss 1½ c. cubed watermelon with 3 Tbsp. crumbled reduced-fat feta cheese

SAVORY SELECTIONS

1 Hard-Cooked Egg

served with 6 oz. low-sodium
vegetable juice

1 Mini Babybel Light

with 4 Triscuits

Asian App

½ c. shelled edamame mixed with 1 tsp.
toasted sesame seeds

Cheese Plate

1 Mini Babybel Original with 15 red
grapes

Chips & Cheese

5 Food Should Taste Good Multigrain
Chips with 1 mozzarella stick

Chips & Salsa

7 Food Should Taste Good White
Cheddar Chips served with 2 Tbsp.
jarred salsa

Cottage Cheese with Melon

½ c. low-fat cottage cheese with ⅓ c.
cantaloupe chunks, plus 1 Ak-Mak
cracker

Endive Boats

Spread 2 Tbsp. Alouette Light Garlic &
Herbs Cheese among 4 endive leaves;
top with 1 Tbsp. pine nuts.

Mezze

One 100% whole wheat mini pita
spread with 2 Tbsp. hummus and
topped with 10 grape tomatoes, halved

One 100-Calorie Bag Popcorn

sprinkled with 2 tsp. Parmesan

Parm Plate

2 cubes Parmesan cheese (about 1 inch
each) served with 5 dried apricot halves

Pear with Cheese

1 small pear, halved, spread with 1 wedge
The Laughing Cow Light Blue Cheese

Roast Beef Rolls

Divide 1 wedge The Laughing Cow Light
Blue Cheese between two 1-oz. slices deli
roast beef. Spread cheese and place
2 slices green pepper on top. Roll,
and serve.

Soy Mix

Combine 2 Tbsp. dry-roasted edamame;
3 walnut halves, broken into pieces; and
1 Tbsp. dried cranberries.

DELICIOUS, AGE-DELAYING
Dinner Recipes

Choice—that's the distinguishing feature of this collection of recipes. You can eat as a family or dine solo, and still savor a meal that meets your anti-aging goals.

Almond-Crusted Chicken with Rainbow Slaw

Active time 20 minutes · **Total time** 30 minutes · **Makes** 4 main-dish servings JUMP START

2	medium oranges	4	tsp. canola oil
4	c. thinly sliced red cabbage (12 oz.)		Salt and pepper
		1	Tbsp. all-purpose flour
2	large carrots, cut into thin matchsticks	½	c. almonds, very finely chopped
		1	large egg white
1	large yellow pepper, very thinly sliced	¼	tsp. ground cumin
		¼	tsp. no-salt-added chili powder
2	Tbsp. snipped chives	4	skinless, boneless chicken-breast
3	Tbsp. white wine vinegar		cutlets (4 oz. each)

1. Arrange 1 oven rack in lowest position; place 15" by 10" jelly-roll pan on rack. Preheat oven to 450°F.

2. Cut peel and white pith from oranges; discard. Cut oranges into segments; transfer to large bowl with their juices. Add cabbage, carrots, yellow pepper, chives, vinegar, 1 tsp. oil, and ¼ tsp. each salt and freshly ground black pepper. Toss well; let slaw stand.

3. Spread flour on medium plate; spread almonds on another plate. In pie plate, beat egg white until foamy.

4. Sprinkle cumin, chili powder, and ¼ tsp. each salt and pepper over chicken. Press one side of 1 piece chicken in flour; shake off excess. Dip same side in egg white; press into nuts. Repeat with remaining chicken.

5. Remove hot pan from oven; brush with remaining oil. Add chicken, nut side down; roast on lowest rack 10 to 12 minutes or until it just loses its pink color. Serve with slaw.

Spicy corn-on-the-cob side Mix ¼ c. light buttery tub spread with ½ tsp. smoked paprika, ½ tsp. red pepper flakes, and a pinch of salt. Cook corn (1 ear per person) and coat with mixture (serves 4).

Side for one Mix 1 Tbsp. light buttery tub spread with ⅛ tsp. smoked paprika, ⅛ tsp. red pepper flakes, and a pinch of salt. Cook corn (1 ear) and coat with mixture.

Alcohol: Is It OK to Have a Drink on the Plan?

If you like to have a glass of wine with dinner or relax with a beer once in a while, we have good news: **There's a place for alcohol in a healthful weight-loss diet,** this one included—as long as you drop one of your daily snacks to make up for a drink's added calories. A "drink" is equal to 5 ounces of red or white wine, 12 ounces of light beer, or 1½ ounces of 80-proof liquor with a low-calorie mixer. Bear in mind that the benefits of alcohol (see page 150) top out at about one drink per day, so keep your intake moderate.

Chicken Bruschetta

Active time 20 minutes · **Total time** 25 minutes · **Makes** 4 main-dish servings

3	cloves garlic	1	small shallot, finely chopped
3	tsp. extra virgin olive oil	1/4	c. packed fresh basil leaves, finely
	Salt and pepper		chopped
4	skinless, boneless chicken-breast	2	Tbsp. red wine vinegar
	halves (6 oz. each)	1	round loaf crusty whole wheat
1³/₄	lbs. tomatoes, chopped		bread (8 oz.), sliced

1. Preheat outdoor grill on medium.

2. Meanwhile, in 9-inch pie plate, mix 2 cloves garlic, crushed with press; 1 tsp. oil; and 1/4 tsp. each salt and pepper, then rub all over chicken.

3. In large bowl, combine tomatoes, shallot, basil, vinegar, 1 tsp. oil, and 1/8 tsp. each salt and pepper. Let stand.

4. Grill chicken, covered, 10 to 13 minutes or until juices run clear when thickest part of chicken is pierced, turning once. Transfer to cutting board. Let rest 10 minutes; slice.

5. Cut remaining clove garlic in half. Rub cut sides all over bread, then brush bread with remaining 1 tsp. oil. Grill 1 minute, turning once. Divide bread and chicken among serving plates; top with tomato mixture.

Roasted cauliflower side Preheat oven to 450°F. In bowl, toss 4 c. cauliflower florets (approximately 1 medium head) and 2 1/2 Tbsp. olive oil. Spread mixture on a jelly-roll pan or cookie pan. Roast for 20 minutes or until browned, stirring occasionally. Serves 4.

Anti-Aging BOOSTER

Side for one Preheat oven to 450°F. In bowl, toss 1 c. cauliflower florets and 2 tsp. olive oil. Spread mixture on a jelly-roll pan or cookie pan. Roast about 15 minutes, or until browned, stirring occasionally.

Apricot dessert 6 dried apricot halves per person.

Chicken in Lettuce Cups

Total time 30 minutes · **Makes** 4 main-dish servings

3	Tbsp. reduced-sodium soy sauce	1	c. frozen shelled edamame (soybeans)
2	tsp. grated peeled fresh ginger		
1	tsp. honey	2	medium stalks celery, chopped
2	tsp. Asian sesame oil	12	large Boston lettuce leaves
1¼	lbs. chicken tenders, cut into ¼-inch chunks		

1. In cup, combine soy sauce, ginger, and honey. Set aside.

2. In 12-inch nonstick skillet, heat sesame oil on medium 1 minute. Add chicken chunks and cook 3 minutes, stirring occasionally.

3. Add edamame to chicken in skillet; cook 2 minutes, stirring occasionally. Stir in celery; cook 2 minutes longer. Add soy sauce mixture; cook 1 to 2 minutes or until chicken is cooked through, stirring occasionally to coat chicken with sauce. Makes about 3½ cups.

4. Arrange lettuce leaves on 4 dinner plates. Divide chicken mixture among lettuce leaves, using a generous ¼ cup per leaf. Fold leaves over chicken mixture and eat out of hand.

Roasted carrot sticks side Preheat oven to 450°F. In bowl, toss a 1 lb. bag of baby carrots with 2 Tbsp. olive oil. Spread mixture on a jelly-roll pan or cookie pan. Roast about 20-25 minutes, or until browned, stirring occasionally. Serves 4.

Side for one Preheat oven to 450°F. In bowl, toss 4 oz. baby carrots (¼ of a 1-lb. bag) with 1½ tsp. olive oil. Spread mixture on a jelly-roll pan or cookie pan. Roast about 20-25 minutes, or until browned, stirring occasionally.

Apples-with-dipping-sauce dessert In a bowl, mix 2½ Tbsp. peanut butter with 2½ Tbsp. unsweetened applesauce. Slice 2 apples and serve with dipping mixture. Serves 4.

Dessert for one In a bowl, mix 2 tsp. peanut butter with 2 tsp. unsweetened applesauce. Serve with ½ apple, sliced, for dipping.

Chicken Quesadillas with Avocado-Tomato Salsa

Total time 30 minutes · **Makes** 4 main-dish servings

2	tsp. canola oil	4	burrito-size low-fat flour tortillas
1	green onion, thinly sliced	1	c. reduced-fat (2%) shredded
1	lime		Mexican cheese blend
	Salt and pepper	¼	avocado, peeled, seeded, and cut
1	lb. skinless, boneless thin-sliced		into ½-inch pieces
	chicken breasts, cut into	¾	c. salsa
	1-inch-wide strips		

1. In 12-inch nonstick skillet, heat oil on medium 1 minute. Add green onion and cook about 6 minutes or until tender, stirring occasionally.

2. Meanwhile, from lime, grate 1 tsp. peel and squeeze 2 Tbsp. juice. Evenly season chicken on both sides with lime peel, ¼ tsp. salt, and ⅛ tsp. ground black pepper.

3. Add chicken to green onion in skillet; cook 10 minutes or until chicken is no longer pink inside. Transfer to bowl; stir in lime juice.

4. Evenly divide chicken mixture and cheese on half of each tortilla; fold over to make 4 quesadillas.

5. In same skillet, cook quesadillas on medium, in 2 batches, 8 minutes per batch or until browned on both sides and heated through. Cut each quesadilla into thirds. Stir avocado into salsa; serve with quesadillas.

Chopped side salad Mix 8 c. chopped romaine lettuce; 1 red pepper, diced; ½ c. canned corn; and ½ c. black beans with ¼ c. low-fat balsamic vinaigrette. Serves 4.

Side for one Mix 2 c. chopped romaine lettuce; ¼ red pepper, diced; 2 Tbsp. canned corn; and 2 Tbsp. black beans with 1 Tbsp. store-bought low-fat balsamic vinaigrette.

Herb-Grilled Turkey

Total time 30 minutes · **Makes** 4 main-dish servings

1	lemon	1	Tbsp. chopped fresh oregano
1	large tomato, chopped		leaves
1	c. bulgur	1	Tbsp. chopped fresh mint leaves
¼	c. loosely packed fresh parsley	2	tsp. olive oil
	leaves, chopped	1	pound turkey-breast cutlets
	Salt and pepper		

1. Prepare outdoor grill for direct grilling on medium. From lemon, grate ¼ tsp. peel and squeeze 2 Tbsp. juice. In small bowl, stir together 1 Tbsp. juice and tomato; set aside.

2. Prepare bulgur: In 3-quart saucepan, heat 2 c. water to boiling on high. Stir in bulgur and reduce heat to low; cover and simmer about 15 minutes or until all liquid has been absorbed. Stir in parsley, ⅛ tsp. salt, ⅛ tsp. freshly ground black pepper, lemon peel, and remaining lemon juice.

3. Meanwhile, in small bowl, combine oregano, mint, and oil. Pat cutlets dry; rub with herb mixture on both sides. Sprinkle with ¼ tsp. salt and ¼ tsp. freshly ground black pepper to season both sides. Grill turkey 3 to 4 minutes or until no longer pink throughout, turning over once. Top turkey with tomato; serve with bulgur.

Grilled zucchini side Cut 4 zucchinis in half and slice lengthwise to make strips. Toss zucchini strips in 1 Tbsp. plus 1 tsp. olive oil and a dash of salt and pepper. On medium-high in an indoor/outdoor grill pan, grill zucchini for 3 minutes per side. Top with 1 Tbsp. plus 1 tsp. pine nuts. Serves 4.

Side for one Cut a zucchini in half and slice lengthwise to make strips. Toss zucchini strips in 1 tsp. olive oil and a dash of salt and pepper. On a medium-high indoor/outdoor grill pan, grill zucchini for 3 minutes per side. Top with 1 tsp. pine nuts.

Nectarine parfait dessert Cut 4 nectarines in half, pit, and top each half with 1½ tsp. nonfat Greek yogurt, 1½ tsp. fat-free whipped topping, and 1 tsp. low-fat granola. Serves 4.

Dessert for one Cut one nectarine in half, pit, and top as above.

Turkey & White Bean Chili

Total time 25 minutes · **Makes** 4 main-dish servings

1	Tbsp. olive oil	1	can (28 oz.) whole tomatoes in juice, chopped
1	pound ground turkey (93% lean)		
	Salt	1	can (15 to 19 oz.) white kidney beans (cannellini), rinsed and drained
1	medium onion, chopped		
4	tsp. chili powder		
1	Tbsp. ground cumin	¼	c. plain nonfat yogurt

1. In 12-inch skillet, heat oil on medium-high until hot. Add turkey and ½ tsp. salt, and cook 6 to 8 minutes or until turkey loses its pink color throughout, stirring to break it up with side of spoon. Add onion and cook 4 minutes. Stir in chili powder and cumin; cook 1 minute.

2. Add tomatoes with their juice, beans, and ½ c. water; heat to boiling on high. Reduce heat to medium and cook, uncovered, 10 minutes, stirring occasionally. Ladle chili into serving bowls and top with a dollop of yogurt. Makes about 6 cups.

Anti-Aging BOOSTER

Salad Mix 8 c. chopped romaine lettuce; 1 red pepper, diced; and ½ c. canned corn with ¼ c. low-fat balsamic vinaigrette. Serves 4.

Side of chips 20 Food Should Taste Good Multigrain Chips (5 per person).

Salad and side for one Mix 2 c. chopped romaine lettuce; ¼ red pepper, diced; and 2 Tbsp. canned corn with 1 Tbsp. low-fat balsamic vinaigrette. Have with 5 Food Should Taste Good Multigrain Chips.

Turkey Burgers

Total time 25 minutes · **Makes** 4 main-dish servings

JUMP START!

½ c. plus 2 Tbsp. plain fat-free yogurt	1 lb. lean ground turkey
2 green onions, green and white parts separated and thinly sliced	1½ oz. feta cheese, finely crumbled
	1½ tsp. ground coriander
	Salt and pepper
½ c. packed fresh mint leaves, finely chopped	2 whole wheat pitas, cut in half
	2 tomatoes, thinly sliced

1. Prepare outdoor grill for covered direct grilling on medium.

2. In small bowl, combine ½ c. yogurt, white parts of green onions, and half of the chopped mint.

3. In large bowl, with hands, combine turkey, feta, coriander, ⅛ tsp. salt, ½ tsp. freshly ground black pepper, green parts of green onions, remaining mint, and remaining yogurt. Mix well, then form into three ½-inch-round patties (each ¾ inch thick).

4. Place turkey patties on hot grill grate; cover and cook 12 to 13 minutes or just until meat loses its pink color throughout, turning once. (Burgers should reach an internal temperature of 165°F.) During last 2 minutes of cooking, add pitas to grill. Cook 2 minutes or until warmed, turning once.

5. Open pitas. Divide burgers, tomato slices, and yogurt sauce among pitas.

Anti-Aging BOOSTER

Romaine salad Toss 1 (12-oz.) bag romaine hearts, torn into pieces; 1 red pepper, sliced; and 16 grape tomatoes with ¼ c. low-fat balsamic vinaigrette. Serves 4.

Salad for one Toss 3 c. romaine lettuce; ¼ red pepper, sliced; and 4 grape tomatoes with 1 Tbsp. low-fat balsamic vinegar.

Crunchy chips side 32 Food Should Taste Good Multigrain Tortilla Chips (8 per person).

Side for one 8 Food Should Taste Good Multigrain Tortilla Chips.

Pork Chops Marsala

Total time 25 minutes · **Makes** 4 main-dish servings

4	boneless pork loin chops, ½ inch thick (4 oz. each), trimmed of fat	1	large shallot, chopped (¼ c.)
	Salt and pepper	½	tsp. dried thyme or 1½ tsp. fresh thyme leaves, chopped
3	tsp. olive oil	1	lb. asparagus, ends trimmed
1	pkg. (10 oz.) sliced cremini or white mushrooms	½	c. reduced-sodium chicken broth
		⅓	c. Marsala wine

1. Evenly season pork chops, on both sides, with ½ tsp. salt and ¼ tsp. freshly ground black pepper.

2. In 12-inch nonstick skillet, heat 2 tsp. oil on medium 1 minute. Add chops and cook 6 minutes or until browned on the outside and still slightly pink in the center, turning over once. Transfer chops to platter; keep warm.

3. In same skillet, heat remaining oil 1 minute. Add mushrooms, shallot, and thyme; cook 5 minutes or until mushrooms are browned and shallot is softened.

4. Meanwhile, place asparagus in glass pie plate with 2 Tbsp. water; cover and cook in microwave on high 3 to 3½ minutes or until fork-tender. Set aside.

5. Add broth and wine to mushroom mixture; cook 2 minutes. Place chops on 4 dinner plates; top with wine sauce. Serve with asparagus.

Soup starter 6 c. prepared butternut squash soup (1½ c. per person).

Rice side 2 c. brown rice (½ c. per person).

Soup and rice for one 1½ c. prepared butternut squash soup, ½ c. brown rice.

Anti-Aging BOOSTER

Balsamic Roasted Pork with Berry Salad

Active time 25 minutes · **Total time** 35 minutes · **Makes** 4 main-dish servings

4 Tbsp. balsamic vinegar	1 pork tenderloin (1 lb.)
2 Tbsp. extra virgin olive oil	Salt and pepper
3 tsp. Dijon mustard	1 lb. strawberries
2 tsp. packed fresh oregano leaves, finely chopped	¼ c. packed fresh basil leaves
	5 oz. baby spinach
2 medium fennel bulbs, cut into ¼-inch-thick slices	½ pint blackberries
1 small red onion (4 to 6 oz.), thinly sliced	

1. Preheat oven to 450°F.

2. In large bowl, with wire whisk, stir together 3 Tbsp. balsamic vinegar, 1 Tbsp. oil, 2 tsp. mustard, and oregano. Add fennel, tossing until well coated. Arrange on outer edges of 18" by 12" jelly-roll pan. To same bowl, add onion, tossing until well coated. Arrange onions in center of pan. Add pork to same bowl and toss until coated; place on top of onion.

3. Sprinkle pork and vegetables with ¼ tsp. salt and ⅛ tsp. freshly ground black pepper. Roast 18 to 22 minutes or until meat thermometer inserted in thickest part of pork registers 140°F. Let pork stand 5 minutes.

4. While pork roasts, hull and slice strawberries. Finely chop basil; place in large bowl.

5. In bowl with basil, whisk together remaining 1 Tbsp. balsamic vinegar, 1 Tbsp. oil, 1 tsp. mustard, and ⅛ tsp. salt until well combined. Thinly slice pork. Add fennel, onion, spinach, and strawberries to bowl with dressing, tossing until well mixed. Divide among 4 serving plates. Top with blackberries and pork.

Side of sweet potato wedges Heat oven to 450°F. Cut 4 small sweet potatoes into ½-inch wedges and coat with 2 Tbsp. canola oil, 1 tsp. cinnamon, and ½ tsp. salt. Roast for 20 minutes, turning once. Serves 4.

Side for one Heat oven to 450°F. Cut 1 small sweet potato into ½-inch wedges and coat with 1½ tsp. canola oil, ¼ tsp. cinnamon, and ⅛ tsp. salt. Roast for 15 minutes, turning once.

Anti-Aging BOOSTER

Protein At Your Fingertips, No Cooking Required

You may have noticed that many of our recipes call for protein sources that require no cooking. These convenient foods can also help you keep up your protein intake once you're no longer following our plan. Here's a list of the handiest, most nutritious, best-tasting protein sources you can buy.

Canned Beans: Chickpeas, White (Cannellini), Black, Pink, Pinto

Canned Tuna in Water

Canned Salmon in Water

Boxed Tofu (Low-Fat)

Frozen Edamame

Frozen Shrimp

Frozen Veggie Burgers or Crumbles

Refrigerated Precooked (Grilled) Chicken Breasts

Refrigerated Deli Meats: Low-Sodium Turkey, Roast Beef, and Ham

Refrigerated Precooked Cocktail Shrimp

Refrigerated Precooked Chicken Sausage

Rotisserie Chicken

Pork à l'Orange

Total time 25 minutes · **Makes** 4 main-dish servings

4	large carrots, cut into 1-inch chunks	1	tsp. extra virgin olive oil
1	whole pork tenderloin (1¼ lbs.)	1	small red onion (4 to 6 oz.), sliced
	Salt and pepper	1	Tbsp. Dijon mustard with seeds
1	large navel orange	1	pkg. (7.4 oz.) heat-and-serve precooked brown rice

1. In 9-inch glass pie plate, combine carrots and ⅓ c. water. Cover with vented plastic wrap and microwave on High 6 to 7 minutes or until tender, stirring once.

2. Meanwhile, cut pork crosswise into 1¼-inch-thick slices. Press each slice with palm of hand to flatten slightly; season both sides with ¼ tsp. salt and ¼ tsp. freshly ground black pepper. From orange, grate ½ tsp. peel and squeeze ½ c. juice.

3. Heat 12-inch skillet on medium-high until hot. Add oil, then pork in single layer. Sprinkle onion in pan around pork; cook 4 minutes or until pork browns. Turn pork over and stir onion; cook 4 to 5 minutes longer or until pork is barely pink in center. Transfer pork to plate, leaving onion in skillet.

4. Add mustard and orange peel and juice to skillet; cook 1 minute, stirring occasionally. Meanwhile, microwave rice as label directs.

5. Divide pork, carrots, and rice among 4 serving plates and spoon sauce over all.

Roasted Brussels sprouts side Preheat oven to 450°F. In bowl, toss 4 c. whole Brussels sprouts, cut into quarters, and 2 Tbsp. plus 2 tsp. olive oil. Spread mixture on a jelly-roll pan or cookie pan. Roast about 15-20 minutes or until browned, stirring occasionally. Meanwhile, in a glass ramekin microwave 1 Tbsp. plus 1 tsp. sliced almonds on High for about 1½ minutes, shaking every 30 seconds. Toss Brussels sprouts with "toasted" nuts. Serves 4.

Side for one Preheat oven to 450°F. In bowl, toss 1 c. Brussels sprouts, cut into quarters, and 2 tsp. olive oil. Spread mixture on a jelly-roll pan or cookie pan. Roast about 15-20 minutes or until browned, stirring occasionally. Meanwhile, in a glass ramekin microwave 1 tsp. sliced almonds on High for about 45 seconds, shaking after 20 seconds. Toss Brussels sprouts with "toasted" nuts.

Anti-Aging BOOSTER

Beef & Peppers Stir-Fry

Total time 30 minutes · **Makes** 4 main-dish servings

1	lb. flank steak, cut lengthwise in half and very thinly sliced	1	c. instant brown rice
		3	tsp. canola oil
4	Tbsp. lower-sodium teriyaki sauce	1	clove garlic, finely chopped
		¼	tsp. crushed red pepper
4	green onions	2	red peppers, thinly sliced

1. In small bowl, toss beef with 1 Tbsp. teriyaki sauce.

2. Thinly slice dark green tops from green onions and reserve for garnish; cut remaining white and light green parts into 1-inch pieces. Cook rice as label directs.

3. In 12-inch skillet, heat 2 tsp. oil on medium-high until hot. Add garlic and crushed red pepper; cook 1 minute. Add green onion pieces, red pepper slices, and 2 Tbsp. water; cook 4 to 5 minutes or until peppers are tender, stirring frequently. Transfer to medium bowl. Keep warm.

4. In same skillet, heat remaining 1 tsp. oil until hot. Add half of beef; cook 1 minute or until beef just loses its pink color throughout, stirring. Transfer to bowl with peppers; keep warm. Repeat with remaining beef.

5. Add remaining 3 Tbsp. teriyaki sauce to skillet; cook 30 seconds, stirring. Add to beef and vegetable mixture; stir to combine. Serve stir-fry over rice. Garnish with reserved green onions.

Anti-Aging BOOSTER

Veggie stir-fry side In a skillet coated with 2 Tbsp. sesame oil, cook 4 c. broccoli florets (approximately 1 large head) and 1 c. baby carrots, sliced lengthwise, for approximately 5 to 7 minutes on medium-high. Mix vegetables with 1 Tbsp. reduced-sodium soy sauce and top with 1 Tbsp. plus 1 tsp. sesame seeds. Serves 4.

Side for one In a skillet coated with 1½ tsp. sesame oil, cook 1 c. broccoli florets and 4 baby carrots, sliced lengthwise, for approximately 5 to 7 minutes on medium-high. Mix vegetables with ¾ tsp. reduced-sodium soy sauce. Top with 1 tsp. sesame seeds.

Flank Steak with Red Wine & Oven Fries

Total time 30 minutes · **Makes** 4 main-dish servings

JUMP START

3	medium russet (baking) potatoes (8 oz. each)	½	tsp. dried tarragon
3	tsp. olive oil	1	medium shallot, minced
	Salt and pepper	¾	c. dry red wine
1¼	pounds beef flank steak, trimmed of fat	1	bag (9 oz.) microwave-in-the-bag baby spinach

1. Preheat oven to 450°F. Cut each unpeeled potato crosswise in half, then cut each half lengthwise into 8 wedges.

2. Spray 15½" by 10½" jelly-roll pan with nonstick cooking spray. Place potatoes in pan and toss with 2 tsp. oil, ¼ tsp. salt, and ¼ tsp. coarsely ground black pepper. Roast potatoes in oven 25 minutes or until fork-tender and beginning to brown, stirring once halfway through roasting.

3. Meanwhile, rub steak with tarragon and ¼ tsp. salt to season both sides. Heat 12-inch cast-iron or other heavy skillet on medium-high. Add 1 tsp. oil and steak; cook 12 minutes for medium, or until desired doneness, turning over once. Transfer steak to cutting board. To same skillet, add shallot and cook 1 minute, stirring. Add wine and heat to boiling; boil 2 minutes or until reduced to ⅓ cup.

4. Cook spinach in microwave as label directs. Thinly slice steak and serve with wine sauce, potatoes, and spinach.

Dessert 4 c. cherries (1 c. per person) or 3 c. grapes (¾ c. per person).

Dessert for one 1 c. cherries or ¾ c. grapes.

Anti-Aging BOOSTER

Cod Livornese with Couscous

Total time 25 minutes · **Makes** 4 main-dish servings

1 Tbsp. extra virgin olive oil	1 Tbsp. capers, rinsed and drained
1 medium red onion (6 to 8 oz.), finely chopped	Salt and pepper
2 cloves garlic, finely chopped	4 skinless cod fillets (6 oz. each)
⅛ tsp. crushed red pepper	¼ tsp. dried oregano
1 can (14 to 14.5 oz.) no-salt-added diced tomatoes	1 c. whole wheat couscous
3 Tbsp. pitted Kalamata olives, chopped	¼ c. packed fresh parsley leaves, finely chopped
	¼ c. packed fresh basil leaves, finely chopped

1. Preheat oven to 400°F.

2. In 12-inch ovenproof skillet, heat oil on medium-high. Add onion and garlic and cook 4 minutes or until browned, stirring occasionally. Add red pepper and cook 30 seconds. Add tomatoes, olives, capers, and ¼ tsp. freshly ground black pepper. Reduce heat to medium and simmer 5 minutes.

3. Season cod with oregano and ¼ tsp. salt. Slide into skillet and arrange in single layer, spooning tomato mixture over it. Roast 10 minutes or until fish just turns opaque in center.

4. Meanwhile, prepare couscous as label directs. Divide among serving plates.

5. Place cod on top of couscous. Stir parsley and basil into tomato mixture. Spoon over cod and couscous.

Anti-Aging BOOSTER

Asparagus side 1¼ lbs. steamed asparagus spears (about 10 spears per person) topped with 1 Tbsp. plus 1 tsp. toasted almonds, ½ c. Parmesan, and 1 Tbsp. plus 1 tsp. lemon zest. Serves 4.

Side for one 10 asparagus spears topped with 1 tsp. toasted almonds, 2 Tbsp. Parmesan, and 1 tsp. lemon zest.

Roasted Cod & Mushroom Ragout

Total time 30 minutes · **Makes** 4 main-dish servings

1   large sweet potato (1 lb.), peeled and cut into ½-inch chunks
2   Tbsp. extra virgin olive oil
2   large shallots, thinly sliced
    Salt and pepper
2   pkg. (10 oz. each) sliced mushrooms

4   skinless cod fillets (6 oz. each)
¼   c. packed fresh flat-leaf parsley leaves, finely chopped
½   c. dry white wine

1. Preheat oven to 450°F.

2. On 18" by 12" jelly-roll pan, combine sweet potatoes, 1 Tbsp. oil, half the shallots, and ⅛ tsp. each salt and pepper. Arrange in single layer on one side of pan. Roast 15 minutes.

3. Meanwhile, in 12-inch skillet, heat remaining Tbsp. oil on medium-high. Add remaining shallots and cook 2 to 3 minutes or until tender and golden brown, stirring occasionally. Add mushrooms and 2 Tbsp. water; cook 8 minutes or until liquid evaporates, stirring occasionally.

4. Arrange cod on other side of roasting pan. Sprinkle with ⅛ tsp. each salt and pepper. Roast alongside potato 8 to 10 minutes or until fish is just opaque throughout.

5. Stir parsley, wine, and ¼ tsp. each salt and pepper into mushroom mixture. Cook 1 minute or until wine is reduced by half.

6. Divide potato and cod among serving plates. Spoon mushroom ragout over cod.

Sautéed spinach side Sauté a 6-oz. bag of baby spinach and 2 tsp. minced garlic in 1½ Tbsp. olive oil. Fold in ¼ c. golden raisins and ¼ c. sliced almonds. Serves 4.

Side for one Sauté 3 c. baby spinach and ½ tsp. minced garlic in 1½ tsp. olive oil. Fold in 1 Tbsp. golden raisins and 1 Tbsp. sliced almonds.

Dessert ½ grapefruit per person.

Anti-Aging
BOOSTER

Pomegranate-Glazed Salmon

Total time 30 minutes · **Makes** 4 main-dish servings

³/₄ c. 100% pomegranate juice
(without added sugar)

¼ c. orange juice

1 c. bulgur

2 c. water

4 pieces skinless center-cut
salmon fillet (5 oz. each)

Salt and pepper

5 oz. radishes

5 dried apricot halves

3 green onions

1. Preheat oven to 450°F. Line 18" by 12" jelly-roll pan with foil.

2. In 1-quart saucepan, heat pomegranate juice and orange juice to boiling on high. Reduce heat to medium-low; simmer 15 minutes or until reduced to ⅓ cup.

3. In large microwave-safe bowl, combine bulgur and water. Microwave on High 10 to 12 minutes or until bulgur is tender and water is absorbed.

4. Arrange salmon in prepared pan; sprinkle with ⅛ tsp. each salt and freshly ground black pepper. Roast 8 to 10 minutes or until fish just turns opaque.

5. Meanwhile, finely chop radishes, apricots, and green onions. Reserve 1 Tbsp. green onion.

6. Add remaining green onion to bulgur along with radishes, apricots, and ⅛ tsp. each salt and freshly ground black pepper; stir to combine. Divide among serving plates. Top with salmon, then glaze. Garnish with reserved green onion.

Snap-pea side Serve with 4 c. sugar snap peas, steamed. Serves 4.

Side for one 1 c. sugar snap peas, steamed.

Anti-Aging
BOOSTER

Salmon with Gingery Cabbage

Total time 30 minutes · **Makes** 4 main-dish servings

1 **Tbsp. olive oil**	2 **tsp. grated peeled fresh ginger**
1 **small onion, thinly sliced**	½ **tsp. ground cumin**
4 **pieces salmon fillet (6 oz. each), skin removed**	1 **bag (16 oz.) shredded cabbage for coleslaw**
½ **tsp. curry powder**	**Salt**
2 **Tbsp. Dijon mustard with seeds**	

1. Preheat oven to 400°F. In 12-inch nonstick skillet, heat olive oil on medium 1 minute. Add onion; cover and cook 8 to 10 minutes or until onion is tender and golden brown, stirring occasionally.

2. Meanwhile, grease 13" by 9" glass baking dish. With tweezers, remove any bones from salmon pieces. Place salmon, rounded sides up, in baking dish. In cup, stir together curry powder, Dijon mustard, and 2 tsp. water; brush evenly over salmon.

3. Roast salmon, without turning over, 15 minutes or just until opaque throughout.

4. While salmon roasts, add ginger and cumin to onion in skillet and cook 1 minute, stirring. Add cabbage and ¼ tsp. salt; cover and cook 11 to 13 minutes or until cabbage is just tender and starts to brown, stirring occasionally.

5. To serve, spoon cabbage mixture onto 4 dinner plates; top with salmon.

Couscous side salad To 1 c. dry whole wheat couscous, add 1¼ c. boiling water. Cover with plastic wrap and let sit 5 minutes. Fluff with fork. Combine with couscous ½ c. garbanzo beans; 2 green onions, thinly sliced; 1 Tbsp. plus 1 tsp. olive oil; 1 tsp. ground cumin; and a pinch of salt. Top with 1 Tbsp. plus 1 tsp. toasted almonds. Serves 4.

Anti-Aging BOOSTER

Couscous for one To ¼ c. dry whole wheat couscous, add ¼ c. boiling water. Cover with plastic wrap and let sit 5 minutes. Combine with couscous ⅛ c. garbanzo beans; ½ green onion, thinly sliced; 1 tsp. olive oil; ¼ tsp. ground cumin; and a pinch of salt. Top with 1 tsp. toasted almonds.

Scallops & Parsnip Puree

Total time 30 minutes · **Makes** 4 main-dish servings

1³/₄ pounds parsnips	1 Tbsp. extra virgin olive oil
1 head Savoy cabbage (1½ lbs.), cored and cut into ½-inch slices	1 lb. sea scallops (8 to 12 large)
	¼ c. reduced-fat sour cream
2 cloves garlic, crushed with press	1 lemon, cut into wedges
Salt and pepper	1 Tbsp. finely chopped fresh chives

1. Fill 4-quart covered saucepan with water; heat to boiling on high. Meanwhile, peel parsnips and remove center core if woody; cut into ½-inch pieces. Add parsnips to boiling water; return water to boiling. Reduce heat to medium; cover and simmer 15 minutes or until tender. Remove and reserve ¼ c. water from pot; drain parsnips.

2. Meanwhile, in microwave-safe large bowl, combine cabbage, garlic, and ¼ c. water. Cover with vented plastic wrap and microwave on High 7 to 8 minutes or until tender. Drain; sprinkle with ⅛ tsp. salt and ⅛ tsp. freshly ground black pepper.

3. While cabbage cooks, in 12-inch skillet, heat oil on medium-high until very hot. Sprinkle ⅛ tsp. salt on scallops. Add scallops to pan in single layer. Cook 4 to 6 minutes or until browned on both sides, turning once.

4. In food processor with knife blade attached, puree parsnips, sour cream, ¼ tsp. salt, ¼ tsp. freshly ground black pepper, and reserved water. Divide among serving plates; top with scallops. Serve with cabbage and lemon. Sprinkle with chives.

Chocolatey banana dessert Slice 4 bananas lengthwise to make 8 halves. Spread 1½ tsp. Nutella over half of each banana (4 halves). Sandwich with the other banana half. Serves 4.

Dessert for one Slice 1 banana lengthwise. Spread 1½ tsp. Nutella over each half and sandwich together.

Anti-Aging BOOSTER

Roasted Shrimp Scampi

Active time 25 minutes · **Total time** 30 minutes · **Makes** 4 main-dish servings

	Salt	¼	c. fresh basil leaves
1	large lemon	12	oz. shelled and deveined shrimp
1	lb. asparagus, trimmed and cut		(26 to 30 ct.)
	into 1-inch pieces	⅛	tsp. crushed red pepper
4	tsp. extra virgin olive oil	1	box (13.25 oz.) whole-grain-blend
2	cloves garlic		spaghetti
¼	c. packed fresh mint leaves		

1. Preheat oven to 450°F. Heat large covered pot of water to boiling; add 1 tsp. salt. From lemon, grate 1 tsp. peel and squeeze ¼ c. juice.

2. In bowl, toss asparagus, 2 tsp. oil, and ¼ tsp. salt. Place in 18" by 12" jelly-roll pan. Roast 5 minutes.

3. Meanwhile, mince garlic, mint, and basil. To same bowl, add shrimp, garlic, lemon peel, pepper, and half of mint, and stir to coat. Push asparagus to one side of pan; arrange shrimp on other side. Roast 5 minutes or until shrimp just turn opaque.

4. Cook pasta as label directs. Reserve ½ c. cooking water. Drain pasta; return to pot with asparagus, shrimp, lemon juice, basil, reserved cooking water, 2 tsp. oil, ⅛ tsp. salt, and remaining mint; toss to coat.

Side of broccoli 2 c. steamed broccoli. Serves 4.

Broccoli for one ½ c. steamed broccoli.

Anti-Aging BOOSTER

Shrimp & Asparagus Stir-Fry

Total time 30 minutes · **Makes** 4 main-dish servings

1 c. quick-cooking (10-minute) brown rice

3 tsp. Asian sesame oil

1½ lbs. asparagus, trimmed and cut into 1-inch pieces

1 lb. peeled and deveined shrimp

1 Tbsp. grated peeled fresh ginger

2 Tbsp. reduced-sodium soy sauce

2 Tbsp. fresh lime juice

¼ c. loosely packed fresh basil leaves, thinly sliced

1. Cook rice as label directs.

2. Meanwhile, in 12-inch nonstick skillet, heat 2 tsp. sesame oil on medium 1 minute. Add asparagus and cook 7 to 8 minutes or until asparagus is tender-crisp, stirring occasionally. Add shrimp and ginger; cook 5 to 6 minutes or until shrimp are opaque throughout, stirring occasionally.

3. Stir in soy, lime, basil, and remaining sesame oil; remove from heat. Serve over rice.

Anti-Aging BOOSTER

Green salad Mix 8 c. greens; 1¼ c. grape tomatoes; 1 avocado, sliced; and ¼ c. low-fat balsamic vinaigrette. Serves 4.

Salad for one Mix 2 c. greens; 5 grape tomatoes; ¼ avocado, sliced; and 1 Tbsp. low-fat balsamic vinaigrette.

Ambrosia Mix 1⅓ c. nonfat Greek yogurt with 2 tsp. honey and ½ tsp. vanilla extract. Place 2½ Tbsp. unsweetened coconut flakes; 3 c. strawberries, sliced; and ½ c. mini marshmallows on top. Serves 4.

Ambrosia for one Mix ⅓ c. nonfat Greek yogurt with ½ tsp. honey and ⅛ tsp. vanilla extract. Place 2 tsp. unsweetened coconut flakes; 5 strawberries, sliced; and 2 Tbsp. mini marsh-mallows on top.

Shrimp & Spicy Tomatoes

Total time 30 minutes · **Makes** 4 main-dish servings

2	large carrots, finely chopped
8	oz. green beans, cut into ½-inch pieces
1	c. whole wheat Israeli couscous
1	Tbsp. extra virgin olive oil
1	large onion (10 to 12 oz.), chopped
¼	tsp. crushed red pepper
1	can (14.5 oz.) no-salt-added fire-roasted diced tomatoes, undrained
1	lb. shrimp (16 to 20 count), peeled and deveined
	Salt

1. In large microwave-safe bowl, combine carrots, green beans, and 1 Tbsp. water. Cover with vented plastic wrap; microwave on High 5 minutes or until just tender.

2. Meanwhile, prepare couscous as label directs.

3. In 12-inch skillet, heat oil on medium-high. Add onion; cook 5 minutes or until golden, stirring. Add red pepper; cook 1 minute, stirring. Add carrot mixture and tomatoes. Heat to boiling; reduce heat to medium. Add shrimp; cook 5 minutes or until just opaque throughout, stirring occasionally. Stir in ½ tsp. salt. Serve over couscous.

Anti-Aging BOOSTER

Starter salad Toss 8 c. baby spinach; 4 packaged beets, cut into chunks; 4 oz. soft goat cheese; and ¼ c. toasted walnuts with ¼ c. reduced-fat balsamic vinaigrette. Serves 4.

Starter salad for one Toss 2 c. baby spinach; 1 packaged beet, cut into chunks; 1 oz. soft goat cheese; and 1 Tbsp. toasted walnuts with 1 Tbsp. reduced-fat balsamic vinaigrette.

Linguine with Carrot-Turkey Ragu

Active time 20 minutes · **Total time** 35 minutes · **Makes** 6 main-dish servings

	Salt and pepper	1	tsp. ground cinnamon
1	Tbsp. olive oil	2	cans (14.5 oz. each) no-salt-added diced tomatoes
1	large leek, white and light green parts only, sliced and well rinsed	1	lb. carrots
2	stalks celery, finely chopped	8	oz. whole wheat linguine
2	cloves garlic, finely chopped	1	Tbsp. chopped fresh parsley
1	lb. lean (93%) ground turkey		

1. Heat 5-quart saucepot of water to boiling on high. Add 2 tsp. salt.

2. In 12-inch skillet, heat oil on medium-high. Add leek, celery, garlic, and ⅛ tsp. each salt and freshly ground black pepper. Cook 5 minutes or until just tender, stirring occasionally.

3. Add turkey; cook 4 minutes or until meat loses its pink color, stirring and breaking into small pieces. Stir in cinnamon; cook 2 minutes. Stir in tomatoes. Heat to boiling, then reduce heat to simmer 15 minutes, stirring.

4. Meanwhile, with vegetable peeler, shave carrots into thin ribbons.

5. Add pasta to boiling water. Cook 1 minute less than label directs. Add carrots; cook along with pasta 1 minute. Drain and return to pot. Add turkey ragu, ¼ tsp. salt, and ½ tsp. pepper. Stir gently until well mixed. Top with parsley.

Garlicky spinach side Sauté a 6-oz. bag of baby spinach with 2 tsp. minced garlic in 1½ Tbsp. olive oil. Fold in ½ c. golden raisins. Serves 4.

Side for one Sauté 3 c. baby spinach and ½ tsp. minced garlic in 1½ tsp. olive oil. Fold in 2 Tbsp. golden raisins.

Anti-Aging BOOSTER

Pasta Primavera

Total time 30 minutes · **Makes** 4 main-dish servings

2	leeks (1¼ lbs.)	1	pint grape tomatoes, each cut in half
1	Tbsp. extra-virgin olive oil		
	Salt and pepper	¼	c. packed fresh flat-leaf parsley leaves, finely chopped
1	lb. thin asparagus		
1	pkg. (12 oz.) whole-grain spaghetti	¼	c. freshly grated Parmesan cheese
1	c. frozen peas		

1. Heat large covered saucepot of water to boiling on high. Meanwhile, trim and clean leeks, cutting leeks lengthwise in half, then crosswise into ¼-inch-wide slices.

2. In 12-inch skillet, heat oil on medium until hot. Add leeks and ¼ tsp. each salt and pepper; cook 9 to 10 minutes or until tender and golden, stirring occasionally. While leeks cook, trim asparagus and cut into 1½-inch-long pieces.

3. Add pasta to boiling water; cook as label directs. While pasta cooks, increase heat under skillet to medium-high. Add asparagus and ⅛ tsp. each salt and pepper; cook 1 minute or until bright green, stirring. Add peas, tomatoes, and ¼ tsp. each salt and pepper. Cook 2 minutes or until peas are bright green. From saucepot with pasta, scoop 1 c. water; pour into skillet with vegetables. Cook 5 minutes or until liquid has reduced and tomatoes have softened.

4. Drain pasta; transfer to large serving bowl. Add vegetable mixture. With tongs, toss until well combined. Divide among serving plates, and top with parsley and Parmesan.

Vegetable Lasagna Toss

Total Time 25 minutes · **Makes** 4 main-dish servings

(Vegetarians can use low-sodium vegetable broth)

8 oz. whole wheat lasagna noodles	3 large tomatoes, coarsely chopped
1 Tbsp. extra virgin olive oil	⅓ c. freshly grated Romano cheese,
2 cloves garlic, crushed with press	plus additional for serving
1 bag (12 oz.) broccoli florets	
1 c. low-sodium chicken broth	
1 can (15 to 19 oz.) white kidney beans (cannellini), drained and rinsed	

1. Heat 5- to 6-quart covered saucepot of salted water to boiling over high heat. Add noodles and cook until just tender, about 2 minutes longer than label directs.

2. Meanwhile, in nonstick 12-inch skillet, heat oil over medium heat; add garlic and broccoli and cook 1 minute, stirring frequently. Add broth; cover and cook 8 minutes. Stir in beans; cover and cook 2 to 3 minutes longer or until broccoli is very tender. Stir in tomatoes; remove from heat.

3. Drain lasagna noodles; add to broccoli mixture in skillet and sprinkle with Romano. Toss to coat noodles. Serve with additional Romano if you like.

Anti-Aging BOOSTER

Honeyed apricot dessert Mix 20 dried apricot halves in a bowl with ½ tsp. honey. In a glass ramekin, microwave 1 Tbsp. slivered almonds approximately 1½ minutes on High, shaking every 30 seconds. Top apricot mixture with "toasted" almonds. Serves 4.

Dessert for one Mix 5 dried apricot halves in a bowl with ⅛ tsp. honey. In a glass ramekin, microwave 1 tsp. slivered almonds for about 45 seconds on High, shaking after 20 seconds. Top apricot mixture with "toasted" almonds.

Whole Wheat Penne with Broccoli & Sausage

Total time 25 minutes · **Makes** 4 main-dish servings

12 oz. whole wheat penne pasta	½ c. loosely packed fresh basil leaves, chopped
1 large bunch broccoli, cut into florets	¼ c. freshly grated Pecorino Romano cheese
12 oz. hot Italian turkey sausage	
1 pt. grape tomatoes, each cut in half	

1. Heat large saucepot of salted water to boiling on high. Add pasta and cook as label directs, adding broccoli when 3 minutes of cooking time remain. Reserve ½ c. cooking water; drain pasta and broccoli.

2. Meanwhile, thinly slice sausage on the diagonal. In 12-inch nonstick skillet, cook sausage on medium 7 to 8 minutes or until it begins to brown, stirring occasionally. Add tomatoes and cook 5 minutes longer, stirring.

3. Stir pasta, broccoli, and ¼ c. pasta cooking water into sausage mixture in skillet; heat through, adding additional cooking water if needed. Remove from heat; stir in basil and cheese.

7 Ideas for Whole Wheat Pasta

Each of the weeknight-friendly recipes below calls for 12 ounces of whole wheat pasta and up to five pantry and already-prepared ingredients, not including salt or pepper. With a minimum of chopping, you'll have a healthy dinner—no more than 515 calories per serving, low in saturated fat, and with plenty of fill-you-up fiber—on the table in 30 minutes or less. If you have a whole wheat pasta of a similar shape in your cabinet, feel free to swap it in.

Creamy Peas & Ham Pasta

Cook penne as label directs; reserve ½ c. pasta water. Drain pasta; return to pot. Stir in 10 oz. frozen peas, thawed; 2 c. baby spinach; 1 c. part-skim ricotta cheese; 4 oz. thinly sliced low-sodium deli ham; reserved pasta water; and ¼ tsp. each salt and freshly ground black pepper. Serves 4.

Fall Sausage & Veggie Favorite Pasta

Heat 12-in. skillet with 1 Tbsp. olive oil on medium-high. Add 1 pkg. (20 oz.) peeled and cut butternut squash; 2 links low-fat precooked chicken sausage, sliced; and 4 cloves garlic, crushed with press. Cook 4 minutes or until browned, stirring occasionally. Reduce heat to medium. Add 1 c. water, cover, and cook 8 minutes or until squash is tender. Cook spaghetti as label directs; reserve ½ c. pasta water. Drain and add to squash mixture, along with 1 pkg. (10 oz.) frozen chopped spinach, thawed, reserved pasta water, and ¼ tsp. freshly ground black pepper. Toss until well mixed. Serves 4.

Italian Tuna Pasta

Cook penne as label directs. In 3-qt. saucepan, heat 1 Tbsp. olive oil on medium-high; add 8 oz. sliced cremini mushrooms and cook on medium 7 minutes or until mushrooms have softened, stirring occasionally. Stir in 2 cans (5 oz. each) chunk light tuna in water, drained; 1 c. marinara sauce; 2 Tbsp. capers, rinsed and drained; and ⅛ tsp. pepper; heat through. Reserve ¼ c. pasta water. Drain pasta; return to pot, along with tuna mixture and reserved pasta water. Stir until well coated. Serves 4.

Mac & Cheese Pasta

In 5-quart saucepan, whisk 2½ c. low-fat (1%) milk into 2 Tbsp. cornstarch. Heat to boiling on medium, whisking, and cook 2 minutes to thicken. Reduce heat to low; stir in 5 oz. shredded reduced-fat (50%) Cheddar cheese until melted. Meanwhile, cook penne 2 minutes less than label directs. To pasta in pot, add 1 pkg. (1 lb.) frozen broccoli-cauliflower mix; cook 2 minutes. Drain; stir into cheese mixture along with ¼ tsp. freshly ground black pepper. Serves 4.

Mediterranean Feta & Tomato Pasta

Cook spaghetti 2 minutes less than label directs. To pasta in pot, add 1 can (14.5 oz.) lower-sodium white (cannellini) beans, rinsed and drained, and 1 pint grape tomatoes; cook 2 minutes. Reserve ¼ c. pasta water; drain and immediately transfer to large bowl. Toss with 9 c. (5-oz. bag) baby arugula, ¾ c. crumbled feta cheese, reserved pasta water, and ¼ tsp. freshly ground black pepper. Serves 4.

Spring Shrimp Pasta

From 1 lemon, grate 1 Tbsp. peel and squeeze 2 Tbsp. juice. Cook spaghetti 4 minutes less than label directs. To pasta in pot, add 2 lbs. asparagus, trimmed and cut into 2-inch lengths, and 12 oz. shelled, deveined shrimp; cook 4 minutes or until pasta is cooked. Reserve ¼ c. pasta water. Drain pasta; return to pot. Stir in 2 Tbsp. extra virgin olive oil, reserved lemon peel and juice, reserved pasta water, and ¼ tsp. each salt and freshly ground black pepper. Serves 4.

Tofu Lo Mein

Cook spaghetti 1 minute less than label directs. To pasta in pot, add 1 pkg. (14 oz.) coleslaw mix and 1 pkg. (8 oz.) stringless snap peas; cook 1 minute. Drain and immediately transfer to large bowl. Toss with 1 box (14 oz.) firm tofu, drained and cut up; ⅓ c. lower-sodium teriyaki sauce; 1 Tbsp. toasted sesame oil; and ¼ tsp. freshly ground black pepper. Serves 4.

Grilled Veggie Pizza

Total time 30 minutes · **Makes** 4 main-dish servings

2	medium portobello mushroom caps, sliced		Salt and pepper
1	small red onion (4 to 6 oz.), sliced into rounds	1	lb. whole wheat pizza dough
		2	plum tomatoes, thinly sliced
1	small yellow summer squash, sliced	½	c. shredded smoked mozzarella (2 oz.)
1	Tbsp. olive oil	¼	c. packed fresh basil leaves, sliced

1. Preheat grill on medium. Brush mushrooms, onion, and squash with oil; sprinkle with ¼ tsp. each salt and pepper.

2. Grill vegetables, covered, 6 minutes or until tender and browned, turning once. Remove from grill and separate onion rings; set aside. Reduce heat on grill to medium-low.

3. Cover large cookie sheet with foil; spray with cooking spray. Stretch dough into 10" by 14" rectangle. Place on cookie sheet.

4. Lift dough and foil; place, dough side down, on grill, gently peeling off foil. Cover; cook 3 minutes or until bottom is crisp. Turn crust over. Quickly top with tomatoes, vegetables, and cheese. Cover; cook 2 minutes longer or until bottom is crisp. Slide onto cutting board; garnish with basil.

Caprese side salad Slice 4 tomatoes and lay slices on a plate. Top tomatoes with 4 oz. part-skim mozzarella, sliced, and ¼ c. fresh basil leaves, chopped. Drizzle 2 tsp. olive oil and 1 Tbsp. plus 1 tsp. balsamic vinegar over salad. Serves 4.

Salad for one Slice 1 tomato and lay slices on a plate. Top tomato slices with 1 oz. part-skim mozzarella, sliced, and 1 Tbsp. fresh basil leaves, chopped. Drizzle ½ tsp. olive oil and 1 tsp. balsamic vinegar over salad.

Red Lentil & Vegetable Soup

Total time 30 minutes · **Makes** 4 main-dish servings

1	Tbsp. olive oil	1	can (14 to 14.5 oz.) vegetable
4	medium carrots, chopped		broth (1³/₄ c.)
1	small onion, chopped	1	c. dried red lentils
1	tsp. ground cumin		Salt and pepper
1	can (14.5 oz.) diced tomatoes	1	bag (5 oz.) baby spinach

1. In 4-quart saucepan, heat oil on medium until hot. Add carrots and onion and cook 6 to 8 minutes or until lightly browned and tender. Stir in cumin; cook 1 minute.

2. Add tomatoes, broth, lentils, 2 c. water, ¼ tsp. salt, and ⅛ tsp. ground black pepper; cover and heat to boiling on high. Reduce heat to low and simmer, covered, 8 to 10 minutes or until lentils are tender. Stir in spinach. Makes about 7½ cups.

Dinner-roll side 1 per person, about 75 calories each.

Coconut-cream dessert Mix 1 c. part-skim ricotta with 2 tsp. vanilla extract, 1 Tbsp. honey, and 2 Tbsp. shredded unsweetened coconut. Top with 1 Tbsp. sliced almonds. Serves 4.

Dessert for one Mix ¼ c. part-skim ricotta with ½ tsp. vanilla extract, 1 tsp. honey, and 2 tsp. shredded unsweetened coconut. Top with 1 tsp. sliced almonds.

Grilled Portobello Burgers

Total time 20 minutes · **Makes** 4 main-dish servings

2	pkg. (6 oz. each) portobello mushroom caps (4 large)
3	Tbsp. bottled balsamic vinaigrette
⅓	c. light mayonnaise
¼	c. drained jarred roasted red peppers
4	whole wheat hamburger buns, split
1	large tomato, thinly sliced
4	Boston lettuce leaves
2	large carrots, sliced diagonally

1. Heat ridged grill pan on medium-high until hot. Place mushrooms, stem sides down, in pan. Brush with half of vinaigrette and grill 5 minutes. Turn mushrooms over; brush with remaining vinaigrette and grill 5 to 8 minutes longer or until very tender.

2. Meanwhile, place mayonnaise and red peppers in blender. Pulse until red peppers are chopped but not pureed, turning off blender and scraping down sides several times. Toast hamburger buns.

3. To serve, spread red pepper mayonnaise on cut sides of bottom buns. Place mushrooms on buns and top with tomato slices, lettuce, then bun tops. Serve carrot slices and chips with burgers.

Anti-Aging BOOSTER

Bean and pepper side salad Combine 1⅓ c. garbanzo beans; 2 red peppers, diced; 1 Tbsp. rice vinegar; 1 tsp. sesame oil; and 2 tsp. sesame seeds. Serve with 32 Food Should Taste Good Multigrain Chips (8 per person). Serves 4.

Bean and pepper salad for one Combine ⅓ c. garbanzo beans; ½ red pepper, diced; ¾ tsp. rice vinegar; ¼ tsp. sesame oil; and ½ tsp. sesame seeds. Serve with 8 Food Should Taste Good Multigrain Chips.

Stuffed Portobellos

Total time 30 minutes · **Makes** 4 main-dish servings

½ c. quinoa, rinsed	1 tsp. fresh thyme leaves
1¼ pounds Brussels sprouts	⅔ c. frozen corn
4 tsp. extra virgin olive oil	3 oz. crumbled feta cheese (¾ c.)
Salt and pepper	½ tsp. ground cumin
4 large portobello mushroom caps	

1. Preheat oven to 450°F. In 2-quart saucepan, combine quinoa and ¾ c. water. Heat to boiling on high; reduce heat to medium-low. Cover and cook 15 minutes or until liquid is absorbed.

2. Meanwhile, trim and halve sprouts. In 18" by 12" jelly-roll pan, toss sprouts, 2 tsp. oil, and ¼ tsp. each salt and freshly ground black pepper to evenly coat. Roast 10 minutes.

3. While sprouts cook, brush mushrooms with remaining 2 tsp. oil and sprinkle with ⅛ tsp. salt. Finely chop thyme and add to medium bowl along with corn, feta, cumin, and cooked quinoa.

4. When sprouts have roasted 10 minutes, push to one side of pan and arrange mushrooms, gill side up, on other side. Divide quinoa mixture among mushrooms; roast 10 minutes or until mushrooms are tender.

Anti-Aging BOOSTER

Bean salad side Combine 1 c. black beans; 1⅓ c. dark red kidney beans; 1 red pepper, diced; 2½ Tbsp. diced red onion; ½ c. canned corn; 1 Tbsp. plus 1 tsp. olive oil; and 2½ Tbsp. white wine vinegar. Serves 4.

Bean salad for one Combine ¼ c. black beans; ⅓ c. dark red kidney beans; ¼ red pepper, diced; 2 tsp. diced red onion; 2 Tbsp. canned corn; 1 tsp. olive oil; and 2 tsp. white wine vinegar.

For even more great recipes, download our free special report, Eat to Look *& Feel Younger, at 7yearsyounger.com/eattolookyoung.*

Look and Feel
7 Years Younger...

Chapter Eleven

...Forever

Congratulations on completing the 7 Years Younger program! You've learned to follow smart, healthy steps to look and feel younger again, and made a very important investment in yourself. Finding the time and energy to devote to their own well-being is something many women, pulled by many different responsibilities, find challenging. Our 7 Years Younger test panelists told us that this was the first time in a very long while that they'd focused on themselves, and that it felt great to take stock and make some positive changes. Hopefully, your own eight-week journey has left you feeling equally gratified—and motivated to continue your new skin- and hair-care, makeup, exercise, and diet routines; all designed to help you express your vitality and youthfulness for as long as you like.

In other words, this finish line is also your starting gate: the entrée to a lifetime of healthier, youth-enhancing habits. If you've ever lost weight before, you know that maintenance—making sure the lost pounds don't creep back on—can be the hardest part. And here you're planning to hold your weight steady while keeping up your other improvements, too—rejuvenated skin, lusher hair, stronger muscles, renewed energy, and more. We're betting that you entered into this endeavor with enthusiasm, so there's no reason you can't stay motivated and continue reaping the rewards of this program. The truth about any good habits and resolutions is that sometimes they get broken. Part of achieving ongoing success is simply realizing that there will be ups and downs, and not letting the downs derail you. Research shows that slipping back into old habits is commonplace—an expected part of change. And it takes time and persistence to develop new habits—the eight weeks you spent on this program are just the beginning. So be patient with yourself, but also stay focused on your goal of looking and feeling 7 years younger. As psychologist James Prochaska, Ph.D., who has been studying change for over 20 years, summarizes: "Change is a process, not an event."

THE SECRETS TO CHANGE THAT LASTS

It's easy to fall back into old habits, and so we purposely built a lot of safeguards into this plan. Stress, a crazy schedule, and fatigue are common reasons people give for reverting to their old ways, but now you have the tools to address them. Referring back to the sections on sleep (see page 238), meditation (see page 246), and multitasking (see page 214) will help you sidestep these common relapse risks. When you need to, find support from outside sources, friends, and family (see pages 250 and 256) who can offer advice and encouragement and help boost your ongoing determination. More tips to keep you on track:

Prevent Slipups

Honor your routine When asked to describe in one word the secret to living a healthy life, the Dalai Lama replied, "Routines." The eight weeks you spent following our prescribed program gave you a very structured foundation of routines, and while you can loosen up in some respects, it's still important to adhere to a regular schedule of anti-aging activities. The more habitually you practice the strategies that make you look and feel younger, the less you'll have to think about them. They'll just become a natural part of everyday life, like brushing your teeth.

Be flexible Life is anything but static. Schedules fluctuate, interests wax and wane, responsibilities rise and fall. Don't let this knock you off course. Sit down with your journal or a calendar and be strategic about adjusting your anti-aging agenda to whatever new circumstances have arisen. Recalibrate, cope; repeat as necessary.

Refocus your point of view Change can seem easier if you reframe the way you think about it. Instead of seeing it as a process of giving up things you love or have done for years, think of change as an exciting means of discovering new things and gaining the physical, psychological, or emotional benefits.

Root out obstacles You were following the program to a T...then, suddenly, you weren't. To get back on track, you need to discover the reasons for your derailment. So take it step by step. Ask yourself what's preventing you from exercising, getting your omega-3s, or sleeping eight hours. Be honest so that you can find the right fix. You find walking boring? OK, it's not a crime! Treat yourself to a new bike or find an elliptical trainer on eBay.

The same goes for omega-3s: Perhaps no one else in your family likes fish. Assess your other options. Tuna at lunch? An omega-3 supplement? And even in matters where the plan seems inflexible—like getting enough hours of sleep—you can be more mindful of the activities that conflict with getting your nightly rest. Perhaps you need to consider limiting casual Internet use or TV time in order to be in bed by 11 P.M. Make this program your own, and congratulate yourself on your creative solutions!

Get Right Back on Track

Forgive yourself and move on Hiccups in your new routine are bound to happen. Whatever the problem, the best thing you can do is forgive yourself. If you get upset, you may be more likely to experience what psychologists call the abstinence-violation effect: You get so angry at yourself for violating a rule that you punish yourself by abandoning self-control, or by deciding to give up because you've already messed up, and it becomes a vicious cycle. Instead, cut yourself some slack and remember that you can make a different choice right away. Your next meal can be lean and full of disease-fighting nutrients—and tomorrow morning you can go for that long, invigorating walk. As philosopher-historian Will Durant counseled, "Forget past mistakes. Forget failures. Forget everything except what you are going to do now and do it."

Applaud any positive steps Reward yourself for maintaining your new behaviors, and give yourself a pat on the back if you successfully avoided a relapse or a temptation. Reinforcement for *any* positive step is crucial in establishing new habits.

Rediscover your resolve You've had a bad day or even a bad week, and most of your anti-aging habits have gone out the window. Take a moment and consider what behavior specialist M.J. Ryan calls the Four A's:

1. Assess the current situation.
2. Adjust what needs to be done.

3. Admire yourself for being strong enough to start again.

4. Act quickly to implement your new course of action.

"The most important of the four *A*'s are the last two," says Ryan. "Self-admiration helps you stay positive and avoid spiraling into negativity—'See, I'm not capable of doing this right. This mess-up proves it.' It turns a mishap into an esteem boost when you remind yourself that it takes great courage and persistence to not give up. Acting quickly is also crucial. Otherwise, you'll lose the momentum of your commitment and slide back into bad old behaviors."

Keep Moving Forward

Look long-term You started this plan with the commitment to follow it for eight weeks. Going forward, you need to set additional, ongoing structured goals. Vague intentions of sticking to the program may bog down your progress. Instead, be specific: Plan to run or walk a 3K in three months, meditate three times a week in the course of a month, lose another few pounds by your college reunion. You don't have to improve everything at once; just pick a few goals to keep you focused.

Reflect on your progress Periodically take the time to review your motivations, resources, and progress in order to refresh your commitment and belief in your abilities to continue your new healthy behaviors.

Shift Into Maintenance: How to Keep the Pounds Off

Every strategy above can help you maintain the weight you lost on the 7 Years Younger program. But switching from a diet to a maintenance plan also has unique challenges. GHRI Nutrition Director Samantha B. Cassetty, M.S., R.D., has a set of maintenance principles she urges dieters to live by. Here's her 7-point plan for keeping pounds from creeping back on.

1 **Follow our plan in spirit** You may not continue eating exactly the same meals and snacks as you did on the plan, but whatever you choose should be built on the same foundation of lean, nutrient-rich foods eaten in moderate portions. Picture in your mind what our meals look like, then follow suit. And don't forget how important it is that you get pleasure from what you eat. Choose healthy foods you love so you're not tempted to veer off the path.

2 **Moderate your calories** Although not overly restricted, the calories on our plan were meant to shift you into weight-loss mode. If you've got more pounds to shed, then definitely stay with the same calorie count that we calculated for 7 Years Younger menus: 300 calories for breakfast, 400 for lunch, and 500 for dinner, along with two 125-calorie snacks. If you're moving into maintenance, however, you will have to keep an eye on calories as you eat meals that are not on the plan. Initially, you'll need to increase your intake slightly; an easy way to bump up calories a little is to eat more at breakfast or have another snack like the ones we provided on the plan.

3 **Boost your intake of foods with extra benefits** Calories are important, but so is the quality of the food you're eating. Choose foods with a bonus, value-added quality—ones that provide more than sustenance and serve a purpose greater than keeping your calories in check. A great example is all the fresh produce on the plan; fruits and vegetables add protective, anti-aging nutrients and/ or fill-you-up fiber to your diet, so that you don't overeat. Two other examples are the nuts and fish, which supply vital omega-3s and muscle-building, fat-burning lean protein.

4 **Weigh the costs and benefits** When you choose to indulge, ask yourself if it's something you really want or if it's something you're choosing simply because it's available. And remind yourself that this is not the last piece of cake or ice cream cone you'll ever have.

Just by making certain that the treats you eat are really worth it to you, you'll eliminate a lot of diet-derailing calories.

5 **Step on the scale once a week** Weighing yourself regularly lets you see how well your maintenance-eating plan is working. Use your scale as an early-warning device: If you are gaining back weight, you'll be able to catch it and do something about it before the prospect of weight loss becomes overwhelming. Keep in mind that your weight will undoubtedly fluctuate a little; an extra-heavy meal or water retention can drive up the numbers on the scale a pound, or even three. But if you've put on more than three pounds, take prompt action to cut back and reverse the gain.

6 **Keep your food diary handy** You're trying to eat right, so why do your jeans feel snug? Going back to using your food diary can help you ferret out the reason. Maybe you're serving yourself too many nuts, you're eating off your kids' plates, or your portions of rice and pasta have bulked up. Try to write down *everything* you eat to find the culprit. Then make the needed adjustment right away.

7 **Return to the Jumpstart or 7-week plan** This program is always here to help you get back on track. Revisiting the plan is also a great way to "recover" from a vacation or simply a few days of eating gone wild. You may need just a week to get back into a healthy groove. Don't forget to check the 7 Years Younger Facebook page (facebook.com/7yearsyounger), where you'll find inspiring and motivating ideas from our community of readers cheering one another on. We'd like to hear from you, too!

Remember the Rewards of All Your Good Work

You may have been motivated to start this program when you caught sight of a few gray hairs in the mirror, or because you wanted to lose that "middle age" belly or hoped to diminish the lines in the corners of your eyes. Whatever your reasons, all the time and energy you've invested to address aging on the outside has also gone a long way toward improving your health on the inside at the cellular level—and that's the most important anti-aging step you can take! If your resolve to look younger ever starts to fade, just remember how good you felt and how rejuvenated you looked during the weeks you followed the 7 Years Younger program. There's no reason you can't look and feel that good all the time. The payoff for keeping it up is priceless: You'll continue to enjoy dewy skin, lustrous hair, a fit and healthy body, and a sharp mind, and you will delight in the compliments about how great you look—from your friends, your family, even strangers—for years to come. And when you look in the mirror, you'll see your best self smiling back at you!

If you aren't already a part of the 7 Years Younger community, now is a great time to get even more expert advice and support to keep building on your anti-aging success. Sign up for our free weekly e-newsletter, Your Anti-Aging Tip Sheet, *at 7yearsyounger.com/newsletter and join us at facebook.com/7yearsyounger.*

Appendix

NUTRITIONAL ANALYSES

Here are the nutritional analyses for every recipe in the book, snacks included. In addition to the nutritional information commonly provided (calories, fiber, fat, etc.), we've also listed the amounts of vitamin C, calcium, and omega-3s in every meal or serving, since they're important nutrients with potent anti-aging properties.

Breakfasts

Asparagus Omelet Each meal: About 285 calories, 24 g protein, 15 g carbohydrate, 16 g total fat (5 g saturated fat), 196 mg cholesterol, 361 mg sodium, 5 mg vitamin C, 267 mg calcium, 4 g fiber, 170 mg omega-3

Bagel Spread Each meal: About 296 calories, 15 g protein, 41 g carbohydrate, 11 g total fat (4 g saturated fat), 200 mg cholesterol, 346 mg sodium, 31 mg vitamin C, 97 mg calcium, 6 g fiber, 120 mg omega-3

Breakfast Bowl Each meal: About 307 calories, 15 g protein, 60 g carbohydrate, 4 g total fat (1 g saturated fat), 5 mg cholesterol, 107 mg sodium, 49 mg vitamin C, 337 mg calcium, 8 g fiber, 70 mg omega-3

California Breakfast Wrap Each meal: About 326 calories, 15 g protein, 29 g carbohydrate, 16 g total fat (4 g saturated fat), 216 mg cholesterol, 564 mg sodium, 11 mg vitamin C, 65 mg calcium, 6 g fiber, 190 mg omega-3

Cereal & More Each meal: About 287 calories, 19 g protein, 56 g carbohydrate, 3 g total fat (0 g saturated fat), 5 mg cholesterol, 169 mg sodium, 7 mg vitamin C, 366 mg calcium, 12 g fiber, 60 mg omega-3

Cereal-Yogurt Parfait Each meal: About 282 calories, 19 g protein, 54 g carbohydrate, 6 g total fat (1 g saturated fat), 0 mg cholesterol, 172 mg sodium, 20 mg vitamin C, 316 mg calcium, 18 g fiber, 780 mg omega-3

Cozy Oats Each meal: About 322 calories, 14 g protein, 43 g carbohydrate, 13 g total fat (2 g saturated fat), 4 mg cholesterol, 79 mg sodium, 21 mg vitamin C, 270 mg calcium, 6 g fiber, 1,350 mg omega-3

Egg Scramble Each meal: About 300 calories, 22 g protein, 29 g carbohydrate, 12 g total fat (4 g saturated fat), 220 mg cholesterol, 610 mg sodium, 4 mg vitamin C, 179 mg calcium, 5 g fiber, 220 mg omega-3

Grab & Go Each meal: About 335 calories, 19 g protein, 39 g carbohydrate, 11 g total fat (2 g saturated fat), 12 mg cholesterol, 185 mg sodium, 1 mg vitamin C, 557 mg calcium, 4 g fiber, 0 mg omega-3

English Muffin Stack Each meal: About 303 calories, 15 g protein, 46 g carbohydrate, 9 g total fat (2 g saturated fat), 6 mg cholesterol, 418 mg sodium, 68 mg vitamin C, 206 mg calcium, 9 g fiber, 60 mg omega-3

Mixed Fruit Smoothie with Whole-Grain Blueberry Muffin Each meal: About 310 calories, 9 g protein, 50 g carbohydrate, 10 g total fat (1 g saturated fat), 18 mg cholesterol, 294 mg sodium, 67 mg vitamin C, 150 mg calcium, 6 g fiber, 280 mg omega-3

Monte Cristo Each meal: About 298 calories, 21 g protein, 36 g carbohydrate, 10 g total fat (3 g saturated fat), 40 mg cholesterol, 704 mg sodium, 90 mg vitamin C, 272 mg calcium, 4 g fiber, 110 mg omega-3

New York Bagel Each meal: About 301 calories, 17 g protein, 29 g carbohydrate, 15 g total fat (8 g saturated fat), 48 mg cholesterol, 950 mg sodium, 11 mg vitamin C, 117 mg calcium, 6 g fiber, 220 mg omega-3

On the Road Each meal: About 305 calories, 19 g protein, 42 g carbohydrate, 11 g total fat (2 g saturated fat), 115 mg cholesterol, 540 mg sodium, 0 mg vitamin C, 485 mg calcium, 7 g fiber, 0 mg omega-3

PB&A Each meal: About 289 calories, 9 g protein, 48 g carbohydrate, 10 g total fat (2 g saturated fat), 0 mg cholesterol, 265 mg sodium, 8 mg vitamin C, 98 mg calcium, 7 g fiber, 30 mg omega-3

PB&J B'fast Each meal: About 296 calories, 16 g protein, 51 g carbohydrate, 4 g total fat (1 g saturated fat), 2 mg cholesterol, 244 mg sodium, 37 mg vitamin C, 234 mg calcium, 6 g fiber, 70 mg omega-3

Peaches & Cream Each meal: About 280 calories, 17 g protein, 29 g carbohydrate, 12 g total fat (6 g saturated fat), 38 mg cholesterol, 171 mg sodium, 15 mg vitamin C, 358 mg calcium, 4 g fiber, 90 mg omega-3

Pronto Plate Each meal: About 286 calories, 12 g protein, 44 g carbohydrate, 8 g total fat (3 g saturated fat), 30 mg cholesterol, 583 mg sodium, 23 mg vitamin C, 88 mg calcium, 8 g fiber, 40 mg omega-3

Sweet Stuffed Waffle Each meal: About 291 calories, 10 g protein, 40 g carbohydrate, 12 g total fat (4 g saturated fat), 19 mg cholesterol, 398 mg sodium, 0 mg vitamin C, 189 mg calcium, 6 g fiber, 40 mg omega-3

Trail Oats Each meal: About 302 calories, 8 g protein, 48 g carbohydrate, 10 g total fat (1 g saturated fat), 0 mg cholesterol, 0 mg sodium, 0 mg vitamin C, 44 mg calcium, 10 g fiber, 0 mg omega-3

Whole-Grain Pancakes Each meal: About 308 calories, 11 g protein, 53 g carbohydrate, 7 g total fat (1 g saturated fat), 48 mg cholesterol, 563 mg sodium, 17 mg vitamin C, 301 mg calcium, 7 g fiber, 410 mg omega-3

Lunches

Asian Bowl Each meal: About 386 calories, 16 g protein, 56 g carbohydrate, 10 g total fat (1 g saturated fat), 0 mg cholesterol, 410 mg sodium, 95 mg vitamin C, 85 mg calcium, 8 g fiber, 20 mg omega-3

Burger Day Each meal: About 411 calories, 26 g protein, 56 g carbohydrate, 13 g total fat (6 g saturated fat), 23 mg cholesterol, 845 mg sodium, 66 mg vitamin C, 361 mg calcium, 11 g fiber, 170 mg omega-3

Cheesy Chili Each meal: About 412 calories, 21 g protein, 53 g carbohydrate, 15 g total fat (5 g saturated fat), 21 mg cholesterol, 923 mg sodium, 8 mg vitamin C, 255 mg calcium, 11 g fiber, 10 mg omega-3

Deli Twist Each meal: About 382 calories, 23 g protein, 63 g carbohydrate, 6 g total fat (0 g saturated fat), 20 mg cholesterol, 1,072 mg sodium, 100 mg vitamin C, 112 mg calcium, 9 g fiber, 140 mg omega-3

Fast Fuel Each meal: About 402 calories, 27 g protein, 54 g carbohydrate, 9 g total fat (4 g saturated fat), 36 mg cholesterol, 872 mg sodium, 18 mg vitamin C, 411 mg calcium, 5 g fiber, 0 mg omega-3

Greek Feast Each meal: About 376 calories, 21 g protein, 64 g carbohydrate, 6 g total fat (2 g saturated fat), 5 mg cholesterol, 597 mg sodium, 14 mg vitamin C, 149 mg calcium, 13 g fiber, 70 mg omega-3

Hot Roast Beef Hero Each meal: About 400 calories, 23 g protein, 64 g carbohydrate, 9 g total fat (2 g saturated fat), 31 mg cholesterol, 1,078 mg sodium, 106 mg vitamin C, 98 mg calcium, 11 g fiber, 90 mg omega-3

Mediterranean Tuna Salad Each meal: About 393 calories, 24 g protein, 64 g carbohydrate, 8 g total fat (2 g saturated fat), 32 mg cholesterol, 968 mg sodium, 36 mg vitamin C, 144 mg calcium, 12 g fiber, 800 mg omega-3

Microwavable Meal Each meal: About 379 calories, 16 g protein, 55 g carbohydrate, 13 g total fat (4 g saturated fat), 14 mg cholesterol, 478 mg sodium, 43 mg vitamin C, 329 mg calcium, 11 g fiber, 140 mg omega-3

Pita Pizza Each meal: About 420 calories, 24 g protein, 49 g carbohydrate, 16 g total fat (8 g saturated fat), 32 mg cholesterol, 983 mg sodium, 20 mg vitamin C, 460 mg calcium, 8 g fiber, 180 mg omega-3

Protein Plate Each meal: About 412 calories, 18 g protein, 53 g carbohydrate, 17 g total fat (4 g saturated fat), 198 mg cholesterol, 585 mg sodium, 53 mg vitamin C, 215 mg calcium, 10 g fiber, 60 mg omega-3

Roast Beef Sammy Each meal: About 409 calories, 30 g protein, 57 g carbohydrate, 8 g total fat (4 g saturated fat), 46 mg cholesterol, 1,169 mg sodium, 18 mg vitamin C, 469 mg calcium, 9 g fiber, 80 mg omega-3

Souped-Up Soup Each meal: About 386 calories, 23 g protein, 64 g carbohydrate, 6 g total fat (0 g saturated fat), 0 mg cholesterol, 1,822 mg sodium, 7 mg vitamin C, 126 mg calcium, 19 g fiber, 0 mg omega-3

Spicy Butternut Squash Soup Each meal: About 404 calories, 11 g protein, 66 g carbohydrate, 13 g total fat (1 g saturated fat), 0 mg cholesterol, 1,412 mg sodium, 11 mg vitamin C, 132 mg calcium, 11 g fiber, 10 mg omega-3

Spinach Salad with Tuna & Avocado Each meal: About 421 calories, 24 g protein, 58 g carbohydrate, 14 g total fat (2 g saturated fat), 28 mg cholesterol, 867 mg sodium, 96 mg vitamin C, 153 mg calcium, 17 g fiber, 620 mg omega-3

Spring Salad Each meal: About 397 calories, 44 g protein, 29 g carbohydrate, 14 g total fat (4 g saturated fat), 77 mg cholesterol, 771 mg sodium, 28 mg vitamin C, 219 mg calcium, 7 g fiber, 1,070 mg omega-3

Stuffed Sweet Potato Each meal: About 413 calories, 15 g protein, 46 g carbohydrate, 21 g total fat (4 g saturated fat), 0 mg cholesterol, 252 mg sodium, 20 mg vitamin C, 85 mg calcium, 10 g fiber, 40 mg omega-3

Supermarket Sushi & Salad Bar Each meal: About 388 calories, 11 g protein, 62 g carbohydrate, 11 g total fat (1 g saturated fat), 5 mg cholesterol, 918 mg sodium, 21 mg vitamin C, 99 mg calcium, 9 g fiber, 10 mg omega-3

Turkey Wrap Each meal: About 386 calories, 25 g protein, 41 g carbohydrate, 14 g total fat (2 g saturated fat), 38 mg cholesterol, 1,159 mg sodium, 14 mg vitamin C, 164 mg calcium, 6 g fiber, 40 mg omega-3

Veggie Wrap Each meal: About 417 calories, 13 g protein, 55 g carbohydrate, 18 g total fat (5 g saturated fat), 13 mg cholesterol, 590 mg sodium, 43 mg vitamin C, 680 mg calcium, 7 g fiber, 100 mg omega-3

White Pizza Each meal: About 408 calories, 19 g protein, 58 g carbohydrate, 15 g total fat (5 g saturated fat), 24 mg cholesterol, 802 mg sodium, 70 mg vitamin C, 348 mg calcium, 13 g fiber, 770 mg omega-3

Snacks

Sweet Treats

Banana Pudding Each serving: About 121 calories, 2 g protein, 27 g carbohydrate, 2 g total fat (1 g saturated fat), 1 mg cholesterol, 202 mg sodium, 4 mg vitamin C, 5 mg calcium, 1 g fiber, 10 mg omega-3

Banana Split Each serving: About 119 calories, 2 g protein, 25 g carbohydrate, 2 g total fat (1 g saturated fat), 0 mg cholesterol, 14 mg sodium, 9 mg vitamin C, 9 mg calcium, 3 g fiber, 30 mg omega-3

Berries & Chocolate Each serving: About 115 calories, 10 g protein, 18 g carbohydrate, 0 g total fat (0 g saturated fat), 0 mg cholesterol, 55 mg sodium, 2 mg vitamin C, 102 mg calcium, 1 g fiber, 10 mg omega-3

Coffee Break Each serving: About 128 calories, 11 g protein, 19 g carbohydrate, 2 g total fat (1 g saturated fat), 5 mg cholesterol, 158 mg sodium, 3 mg vitamin C, 371 mg calcium, 0 g fiber, 0 mg omega-3

Greek Yogurt with Honey Each serving: About 112 calories, 15 g protein, 13 g carbohydrate, 0 g total fat (0 g saturated fat), 0 mg cholesterol, 64 mg sodium, 0 mg vitamin C, 114 mg calcium, 0 g fiber, 0 mg omega-3

Ice Cream Waffle Each serving: About 130 calories, 3 g protein, 22 g carbohydrate, 4 g total fat (1 g saturated fat), 10 mg cholesterol, 183 mg sodium, 0 mg vitamin C, 230 mg calcium, 1 g fiber, 0 mg omega-3

Kashi TLC Fruit & Grain Bar Each serving: About 120 calories, 4 g protein, 21 g carbohydrate, 4 g total fat (2 g saturated fat), 0 mg cholesterol, 50 mg sodium, 0 mg vitamin C, 0 mg calcium, 4 g fiber, 0 mg omega-3

Kettle Corn Each serving: About 120 calories, 3 g protein, 21 g carbohydrate, 4 g total fat (1 g saturated fat), 0 mg cholesterol, 140 mg sodium, 0 mg vitamin C, 0 mg calcium, 3 g fiber, 0 mg omega-3

Kind Mini Fruit & Nut Delight Bar with grapes Each serving: About 125 calories, 3 g protein, 16 g carbohydrate, 6 g total fat (1 g saturated fat), 0 mg cholesterol, 10 mg sodium, 3 mg vitamin C, 2 mg calcium, 2 g fiber, 0 mg omega-3

On the Run Each serving: About 110 calories, 6 g protein, 15 g carbohydrate, 3 g total fat (1 g saturated fat), 1 mg cholesterol, 88 mg sodium, 5 mg vitamin C, 233 mg calcium, 1 g fiber, 0 mg omega-3

Trail Mix Each serving: About 125 calories, 3 g protein, 10 g carbohydrate, 8 g total fat (1 g saturated fat), 0 mg cholesterol, 15 mg sodium, 0 mg vitamin C, 20 mg calcium, 2 g fiber, 0 mg omega-3

Vanilla Ice Cream with Strawberries Each serving: About 115 calories, 3 g protein, 19 g carbohydrate, 4 g total fat (2 g saturated fat), 20 mg cholesterol, 45 mg sodium, 28 mg vitamin C, 68 mg calcium, 1 g fiber, 30 mg omega-3

Watermelon Salad Each serving: About 113 calories, 6 g protein, 21 g carbohydrate, 3 g total fat (2 g saturated fat), 8 mg cholesterol, 360 mg sodium, 11 mg vitamin C, 90 mg calcium, 2 g fiber, 0 mg omega-3

100% Whole Grain Fig Newtons Each serving: About 110 calories, 1 g protein, 22 g carbohydrate, 2 g total fat (0 g saturated fat), 0 mg cholesterol, 115 mg sodium, 0 mg vitamin C, 20 mg calcium, 2 g fiber, 0 mg omega-3

Savory Selections

Asian App Each serving: About 120 calories, 10 g protein, 10 g carbohydrate, 4 g total fat (0 g saturated fat), 0 mg cholesterol, 70 mg sodium, 0 mg vitamin C, 80 mg calcium, 1 g fiber, 0 mg omega-3

Cheese Plate Each serving: About 121 calories, 6 g protein, 13 g carbohydrate, 6 g total fat (4 g saturated fat), 20 mg cholesterol, 1 mg sodium, 8 mg vitamin C, 7 mg calcium, 1 g fiber, 10 mg omega-3

Chips & Cheese Each serving: About 128 calories, 10 g protein, 11 g carbohydrate, 5 g total fat (1 g saturated fat), 5 mg cholesterol, 264 mg sodium, 0 mg vitamin C, 211 mg calcium, 2 g fiber, 0 mg omega-3

Chips & Salsa Each serving: About 117 calories, 2 g protein, 15 g carbohydrate, 5 g total fat (1 g saturated fat), 0 mg cholesterol, 335 mg sodium, 0 mg vitamin C, 31 mg calcium, 3 g fiber, 0 mg omega-3

Cottage Cheese with Melon Each serving: About 124 calories, 15 g protein, 13 g carbohydrate, 1 g total fat (1 g saturated fat), 5 mg cholesterol, 467 mg sodium, 19 mg vitamin C, 75 mg calcium, 1 g fiber, 30 mg omega-3

Endive Boats Each serving: About 110 calories, 6 g protein, 3 g carbohydrate, 9 g total fat (2 g saturated fat), 6 mg cholesterol, 157 mg sodium, 1 mg vitamin C, 31 mg calcium, 1 g fiber, 10 mg omega-3

Hard-Cooked Egg plus Veggie Juice Each serving: About 116 calories, 8 g protein, 8 g carbohydrate, 5 g total fat (2 g saturated fat), 187 mg cholesterol, 168 mg sodium, 54 mg vitamin C, 40 mg calcium, 1 g fiber, 40 mg omega-3

Mezze Each serving: About 112 calories, 5 g protein, 17 g carbohydrate, 4 g total fat (1 g saturated fat), 0 mg cholesterol, 127 mg sodium, 22 mg vitamin C, 29 mg calcium, 5 g fiber, 10 mg omega-3

Mini Babybel Light with Triscuits Each serving: About 130 calories, 8 g protein, 13 g carbohydrate, 6 g total fat (2 g saturated fat), 15 mg cholesterol, 280 mg sodium, 0 mg vitamin C, 200 mg calcium, 2 g fiber, 0 mg omega-3

Parm Plate Each serving: About 131 calories, 8 g protein, 13 g carbohydrate, 5 g total fat (3 g saturated fat), 14 mg cholesterol, 330 mg sodium, 1 mg vitamin C, 254 mg calcium, 2 g fiber, 60 mg omega-3

Pear with Cheese Each serving: About 121 calories, 3 g protein, 25 g carbohydrate, 2 g total fat (1 g saturated fat), 5 mg cholesterol, 231 mg sodium, 6 mg vitamin C, 73 mg calcium, 5 g fiber, 0 mg omega-3

Popcorn with Parmesan Each serving: About 115 calories, 5 g protein, 20 g carbohydrate, 2 g total fat (1 g saturated fat), 3 mg cholesterol, 53 mg sodium, 0 mg vitamin C, 39 mg calcium, 4 g fiber, 20 mg omega-3

Roast Beef Rolls Each serving: About 122 calories, 17 g protein, 5 g carbohydrate, 4 g total fat (2 g saturated fat), 35 mg cholesterol, 311 mg sodium, 30 mg vitamin C, 64 mg calcium, 1 g fiber, 0 mg omega-3

Soy Mix Each serving: About 129 calories, 8 g protein, 7 g carbohydrate, 6 g total fat (1 g saturated fat), 0 mg cholesterol, 0 mg sodium, 1 mg vitamin C, 26 mg calcium, 5 g fiber, 540 mg omega-3

Dinners

Chicken & Turkey

Almond-Crusted Chicken with Rainbow Slaw Each meal: About 487 calories, 33 g protein, 48 g carbohydrate, 21 g total fat (3 g saturated fat), 63 mg cholesterol, 591 mg sodium, 178 mg vitamin C, 141 mg calcium, 9 g fiber, 710 mg omega-3

Arugula & Cranberry Salad Each meal: About 461 calories, 49 g protein, 27 g carbohydrate, 19 g total fat (7 g saturated fat), 157 mg cholesterol, 1,291 mg sodium, 6 mg vitamin C, 388 mg calcium, 3 g fiber, 90 mg omega-3

BBQ Chicken Slaw Each meal: About 502 calories, 44 g protein, 56 g carbohydrate, 12 g total fat (3 g saturated fat), 137 mg cholesterol, 1,111 mg sodium, 32 mg vitamin C, 97 mg calcium, 9 g fiber, 50 mg omega-3

Black Bean Burritos Each meal: About 500 calories, 46 g protein, 45 g carbohydrate, 13 g total fat (3 g saturated fat), 137 mg cholesterol, 1,146 mg sodium, 44 mg vitamin C, 144 mg calcium, 7 g fiber, 0 mg omega-3

Chicken Bruschetta Each meal: About 522 calories, 48 g protein, 49 g carbohydrate, 16 g total fat (2 g saturated fat), 99 mg cholesterol, 359 mg sodium, 52 mg vitamin C, 35 mg calcium, 9 g fiber, 80 mg omega-3

Chicken in Lettuce Cups Each meal: About 487 calories, 44 g protein, 37 g carbohydrate, 19 g total fat (3 g saturated fat), 82 mg cholesterol, 675 mg sodium, 12 mg vitamin C, 37 mg calcium, 9 g fiber, 70 mg omega-3

Chicken Parm Casserole Each meal: About 504 calories, 49 g protein, 34 g carbohydrate, 19 g total fat (7 g saturated fat), 154 mg cholesterol, 1,166 mg sodium, 13 mg vitamin C, 307 mg calcium, 7 g fiber, 100 mg omega-3

Chicken Quesadillas with Avocado-Tomato Salsa Each meal: About 513 calories, 42 g protein, 48 g carbohydrate, 18 g total fat (5 g saturated fat), 86 mg cholesterol, 1,223 mg sodium, 94 mg vitamin C, 441 mg calcium, 6 g fiber, 280 mg omega-3

Herb-Grilled Turkey Each meal: About 470 calories, 38 g protein, 57 g carbohydrate, 13 g total fat (2 g saturated fat), 66 mg cholesterol, 452 mg sodium, 43 mg vitamin C, 51 mg calcium, 12 g fiber, 150 mg omega-3

Soba Salad Each meal: About 496 calories, 36 g protein, 77 g carbohydrate, 9 g total fat (1 g saturated fat), 52 mg cholesterol, 1,274 mg sodium, 3 mg vitamin C, 55 mg calcium, 3 g fiber, 10 mg omega-3

Spinach & Beet Salad Each meal: About 473 calories, 45 g protein, 38 g carbohydrate, 17 g total fat (4 g saturated fat), 142 mg cholesterol, 1,056 mg sodium, 7 mg vitamin C, 79 mg calcium, 5 g fiber, 30 mg omega-3

Stuffed Pitas Each meal: About 480 calories, 45 g protein, 46 g carbohydrate, 15 g total fat (3 g saturated fat), 137 mg cholesterol, 1,145 mg sodium, 5 mg vitamin C, 10 mg calcium, 7 g fiber, 30 mg omega-3

Turkey & White Bean Chili Each meal: About 511 calories, 37 g protein, 57 g carbohydrate, 18 g total fat (3 g saturated fat), 81 mg cholesterol, 1,115 mg sodium, 53 mg vitamin C, 46 mg calcium, 15 g fiber, 120 mg omega-3

Turkey Burgers Each meal: About 479 calories, 34 g protein, 52 g carbohydrate, 12 g total fat (4 g saturated fat), 75 mg cholesterol, 671 mg sodium, 82 mg vitamin C, 225 mg calcium, 9 g fiber, 70 mg omega-3

Pork

Balsamic Roasted Pork with Berry Salad Each meal: About 489 calories, 29 g protein, 53 g carbohydrate, 19 g total fat (3 g saturated fat), 74 mg cholesterol, 578 mg sodium, 94 mg vitamin C, 155 mg calcium, 12 g fiber, 820 mg omega-3

Pork Chops Marsala Each meal: About 473 calories, 35 g protein, 54 g carbohydrate, 13 g total fat (2 g saturated fat), 67 mg cholesterol, 1,290 mg sodium, 4 mg vitamin C, 70 mg calcium, 9 g fiber, 10 mg omega-3

Pork à l'Orange Each meal: About 473 calories, 41 g protein, 40 g carbohydrate, 17 g total fat (3 g saturated fat), 84 mg cholesterol, 317 mg sodium, 75 mg vitamin C, 42 mg calcium, 8 g fiber, 160 mg omega-3

Beef

Beef & Peppers Stir-Fry Each meal: About 474 calories, 29 g protein, 36 g carbohydrate, 25 g total fat (6 g saturated fat), 59 mg cholesterol, 580 mg sodium, 67 mg vitamin C, 47 mg calcium, 6 g fiber, 110 mg omega-3

Flank Steak with Red Wine & Oven Fries Each meal: About 512 calories, 37 g protein, 62 g carbohydrate, 14 g total fat (5 g saturated fat), 55 mg cholesterol, 460 mg sodium, 11 mg vitamin C, 20 mg calcium, 12 g fiber, 40 mg omega-3

Fish and Seafood

Cod Livornese with Couscous Each meal: About 489 calories, 47 g protein, 54 g carbohydrate, 11 g total fat (3 g saturated fat), 82 mg cholesterol, 582 mg sodium, 41 mg vitamin C, 241 mg calcium, 11 g fiber, 430 mg omega-3

Pomegranate-Glazed Salmon Each meal: About 480 calories, 37 g protein, 48 g carbohydrate, 16 g total fat (3 g saturated fat), 84 mg cholesterol, 122 mg sodium, 85 mg vitamin C, 110 mg calcium, 11 g fiber, 2,860 mg omega-3

Roasted Cod & Mushroom Ragout Each meal: About 500 calories, 37 g protein, 52 g carbohydrate, 18 g total fat (2 g saturated fat), 65 mg cholesterol, 490 mg sodium, 91 mg vitamin C, 152 mg calcium, 9 g fiber, 310 mg omega-3

Roasted Shrimp Scampi Each meal: About 500 calories, 37 g protein, 88 g carbohydrate, 3 g total fat (1 g saturated fat), 129 mg cholesterol, 304 mg sodium, 77 mg vitamin C, 166 mg calcium, 18 g fiber, 580 mg omega-3

Salmon with Gingery Cabbage Each meal: About 507 calories, 42 g protein, 38 g carbohydrate, 21 g total fat (3 g saturated fat), 94 mg cholesterol, 508 mg sodium, 44 mg vitamin C, 99 mg calcium, 8 g fiber, 3,000 mg omega-3

Scallops & Parsnip Puree Each meal: About 525 calories, 26 g protein, 81 g carbohydrate, 15 g total fat (3 g saturated fat), 42 mg cholesterol, 856 mg sodium, 10 mg vitamin C, 26 mg calcium, 18 g fiber, 30 mg omega-3

Shrimp & Asparagus Stir-Fry Each meal: About 483 calories, 40 g protein, 51 g carbohydrate, 16 g total fat (4 g saturated fat), 172 mg cholesterol, 708 mg sodium, 68 mg vitamin C, 134 mg calcium, 9 g fiber, 160 mg omega-3

Shrimp & Spicy Tomatoes Each meal: About 494 calories, 38 g protein, 52 g carbohydrate, 17 g total fat (6 g saturated fat), 185 mg cholesterol, 639 mg sodium, 38 mg vitamin C, 200 mg calcium, 12 g fiber, 1,170 mg omega-3

Pasta

Creamy Peas & Ham Pasta Each meal: About 494 calories, 27 g protein, 79 g carbohydrate, 8 g total fat (3 g saturated fat), 34 mg cholesterol, 557 mg sodium, 15 mg vitamin C, 224 mg calcium, 11 g fiber, 60 mg omega-3

Fall Sausage & Veggie Favorite Pasta Each meal: About 505 calories, 23 g protein, 85 g carbohydrate, 11 g total fat (2 g saturated fat), 40 mg cholesterol, 480 mg sodium, 32 mg vitamin C, 176 mg calcium, 15 g fiber, 90 mg omega-3

Italian Tuna Pasta Each meal: About 538 calories, 32 g protein, 75 g carbohydrate, 11 g total fat (1 g saturated fat), 45 mg cholesterol, 696 mg sodium, 1 mg vitamin C, 57 mg calcium, 10 g fiber, 80 mg omega-3

Linguine with Carrot-Turkey Ragu Each meal: About 487 calories, 25 g protein, 71 g carbohydrate, 14 g total fat (3 g saturated fat), 43 mg cholesterol, 443 mg sodium, 44 mg vitamin C, 147 mg calcium, 13 g fiber, 110 mg omega-3

Mac & Cheese Each meal: About 533 calories, 26 g protein, 82 g carbohydrate, 11 g total fat (5 g saturated fat), 33 mg cholesterol, 407 mg sodium, 36 mg vitamin C, 745 mg calcium, 10 g fiber, 10 mg omega-3

Mediterranean Feta & Tomato Pasta Each meal: About 472 calories, 23 g protein, 83 g carbohydrate, 8 g total fat (4 g saturated fat), 25 mg cholesterol, 366 mg sodium, 15 mg vitamin C, 268 mg calcium, 16 g fiber, 150 mg omega-3

Pasta Primavera Each meal: About 485 calories, 22 g protein, 90 g carbohydrate, 8 g total fat (2 g saturated fat), 5 mg cholesterol, 451 mg sodium, 31 mg vitamin C, 177 mg calcium, 19 g fiber, 10 mg omega-3

Spring Shrimp Pasta Each meal: About 529 calories, 35 g protein, 74 g carbohydrate, 13 g total fat (2 g saturated fat), 129 mg cholesterol, 283 mg sodium, 20 mg vitamin C, 136 mg calcium, 16 g fiber, 530 mg omega-3

Tofu Lo Mein Each meal: About 475 calories, 24 g protein, 79 g carbohydrate, 10 g total fat (1 g saturated fat), 0 mg cholesterol, 379 mg sodium, 63 mg vitamin C, 296 mg calcium, 15 g fiber, 20 mg omega-3

Vegetable Lasagna Toss Each meal: About 483 calories, 20 g protein, 83 g carbohydrate, 9 g total fat (2 g saturated fat), 8 mg cholesterol, 382 mg sodium, 0 mg vitamin C, 16 mg calcium, 12 g fiber, 0 mg omega-3

Whole Wheat Penne with Broccoli & Sausage Each meal: About 507 calories, 33 g protein, 72 g carbohydrate, 13 g total fat (5 g saturated fat), 61 mg cholesterol, 852 mg sodium, 77 mg vitamin C, 185 mg calcium, 10 g fiber, 130 mg omega-3

Vegetarian

Grilled Portobello Burgers Each meal: About 502 calories, 14 g protein, 68 g carbohydrate, 15 g total fat (1 g saturated fat), 7 mg cholesterol, 841 mg sodium, 85 mg vitamin C, 132 mg calcium, 13 g fiber, 70 mg omega-3

Grilled Veggie Pizza Each meal: About 502 calories, 21 g protein, 65 g carbohydrate, 19 g total fat (6 g saturated fat), 26 mg cholesterol, 913 mg sodium, 17 mg vitamin C, 218 mg calcium, 11 g fiber, 30 mg omega-3

Red Lentil & Vegetable Soup Each meal: About 490 calories, 26 g protein, 66 g carbohydrate, 15 g total fat (7 g saturated fat), 19 mg cholesterol, 836 mg sodium, 0 mg vitamin C, 204 mg calcium, 16 g fiber, 70 mg omega-3

Stuffed Portobellos Each meal: About 498 calories, 24 g protein, 69 g carbohydrate, 16 g total fat 5 g saturated fat), 19 mg cholesterol, 814 mg sodium, 172 mg vitamin C, 256 mg calcium, 18 g fiber, 390 mg omega-3

Binge Busters

Angel Berry Shortcake Each serving: About 125 calories, 2 g protein, 25 g carbohydrate, 2 g total fat (2 g saturated fat), 0 mg cholesterol, 213 mg sodium, 21 mg vitamin C, 45 mg calcium, 1 g fiber, 30 mg omega-3

Angel-Devil Cake Each serving: About 194 calories, 4 g protein, 31 g carbohydrate, 6 g total fat (3 g saturated fat), 21 mg cholesterol, 426 mg sodium, 1 mg vitamin C, 127 mg calcium, 1 g fiber, 70 mg omega-3

Buffalo Tenders Each serving: About 270 calories, 33 g protein, 15 g carbohydrate, 8 g total fat (0 g saturated fat), 83 mg cholesterol, 1,004 mg sodium, 12 mg vitamin C, 17 mg calcium, 2 g fiber, 430 mg omega-3

Chocolate Dream Ice Cream with chocolate wafers Each serving: About 172 calories, 4 g protein, 30 g carbohydrate, 4 g total fat (2 g saturated fat), 5 mg cholesterol, 115 mg sodium, 0 mg vitamin C, 104 mg calcium, 2 g fiber, 30 mg omega-3

Chocolate Dream Ice Cream with mini chocolate bar Each serving: About 157 calories, 4 g protein, 25 g carbohydrate, 4 g total fat (2 g saturated fat), 7 mg cholesterol, 51 mg sodium, 0 mg vitamin C, 113 mg calcium, 2 g fiber, 0 mg omega-3

Chocolate Dream Ice Cream with mini chocolate chips Each serving: About 172 calories, 3 g protein, 28 g carbohydrate, 5 g total fat (3 g saturated fat), 5 mg cholesterol, 46 mg sodium, 0 mg vitamin C, 103 mg calcium, 3 g fiber, 10 mg omega-3

Chocolate Dream Ice Cream with peppermint patty Each serving: About 203 calories, 3 g protein, 38 g carbohydrate, 4 g total fat (2 g saturated fat), 5 mg cholesterol, 51 mg sodium, 0 mg vitamin C, 102 mg calcium, 2 g fiber, 0 mg omega-3

Cinnamon Apple Delight Each serving: About 108 calories, 0 g protein, 28 g carbohydrate, 0 g total fat (0 g saturated fat), 0 mg cholesterol, 3 mg sodium, 8 mg vitamin C, 18 mg calcium, 4 g fiber, 20 mg omega-3

Faux French Cruller Each serving: About 95 calories, 2 g protein, 16 g carbohydrate, 3 g total fat (1 g saturated fat), 49 mg cholesterol, 32 mg sodium, 0 mg vitamin C, 17 mg calcium, 1 g fiber, 20 mg omega-3

Frozen Banana on a Stick Each serving: About 78 calories, 1 g protein, 18 g carbohydrate, 1 g total fat (0 g saturated fat), 0 mg cholesterol, 35 mg sodium, 5 mg vitamin C, 5 mg calcium, 2 g fiber, 30 mg omega-3

Ice Cream on Chocolate Wafers Each serving: About 105 calories, 2 g protein, 17 g carbohydrate, 3 g total fat (1 g saturated fat), 3 mg cholesterol, 84 mg sodium, 0 mg vitamin C, 29 mg calcium, 1 g fiber, 30 mg omega-3

Jelly-Jammed Ladyfinger Each serving: About 84 calories, 1 g protein, 17 g carbohydrate, 1 g total fat (0.5 g saturated fat), 29 mg cholesterol, 23 mg sodium, 1 mg vitamin C, 9 mg calcium, 0 g fiber, 10 mg omega-3

Light Lemon Square Each serving: About 81 calories, 0 g protein, 15 g carbohydrate, 1 g total fat (1 g saturated fat), 5 mg cholesterol, 30 mg sodium, 0 mg vitamin C, 13 mg calcium, 0 g fiber, 0 mg omega-3

Napoli Pita Pizza Each serving: About 196 calories, 12 g protein, 21 g carbohydrate, 8 g total fat (4 g saturated fat), 17 mg cholesterol, 347 mg sodium, 6 mg vitamin C, 239 mg calcium, 3 g fiber, 80 mg omega-3

Oven-Baked Fries Each serving: About 148 calories, 3 g protein, 24 g carbohydrate, 5 g total fat (0 g saturated fat), 0 mg cholesterol, 11 mg sodium, 11 mg vitamin C, 17 mg calcium, 3 g fiber, 440 mg omega-3

Quick Chips Each serving: About 16 calories, 0 g protein, 4 g carbohydrate, 0 g total fat (0 g saturated fat), 0 mg cholesterol, 583 mg sodium, 4 mg vitamin C, 3 mg calcium, 0 g fiber, 0 mg omega-3

Rice with Steamed Veggies Each serving: About 296 calories, 6 g protein, 51 g carbohydrate, 6 g total fat (1 g saturated fat), 0 mg cholesterol, 894 mg sodium, 27 mg vitamin C, 41 mg calcium, 5 g fiber, 40 mg omega-3

Vanilla Cream Bites Each serving: About 72 calories, 2 g protein, 13 g carbohydrate, 1 g total fat (0 g saturated fat), 24 mg cholesterol, 76 mg sodium, 0 mg vitamin C, 18 mg calcium, 0 g fiber, 10 mg omega-3

Veggie Burger Each serving: About 253 calories, 20 g protein, 41 g carbohydrate, 5 g total fat (1 g saturated fat), 1 mg cholesterol, 898 mg sodium, 4 mg vitamin C, 95 mg calcium, 7 g fiber, 50 mg omega-3

WORTH A SHOT?

Forget face-lifts. These days more people are looking to injectables—Botox and other noninvasive shots that relax wrinkles and fill lines. Injectables are not a replacement for a good daily-care routine, but they can deliver near-instant

The Shot	Best for	Downsides	Duration
Botulinum toxin type A (Botox, Dysport, Xeomin)	The toxin temporarily paralyzes muscles, helping to smooth brow wrinkles, forehead lines, crow's feet, sinewy-looking neck muscles, and corners of the mouth.	In untrained hands or if overused, injections could lead to freezing or drooping. Dysport spreads out more than Botox, says Anne Chapas, M.D., assistant professor of dermatology at New York University School of Medicine. You may need fewer shots if you have a large forehead, for example, but your doctor must take it into account to avoid treating unintended muscles.	Botox and Xeomin last up to four months; Dysport, the same amount of time or slightly longer.
Hyaluronic acid (Juvéderm, Restylane, Perlane, and Hydrelle)	Deep facial creases, nasolabial folds, forehead lines, and jaw contouring. Some doctors may also fill hollowed under-eye areas; Dr. Chapas warns that this thin-skinned area is prone to complications.	Swelling and bruising are common, usually lasting less than a week. Uneven or superficial injections can cause bumps. If you really don't like the results, ask about an injectable enzyme to dissolve the material.	One shot of Juvéderm lasts up to a year; the FDA OK'd a claim by Restylane makers that it persists for up to 18 months. You'll need a second injection after six months or so, but it's typically half the amount of your first shot.

gratification. They're also cheaper and involve less downtime than plastic surgery. Here's the crib sheet on what's available (prices can range anywhere from $400 to more than $1,000 per treatment depending on the injectable).

The Shot	Best for	Downsides	Duration
Synthetic fillers (Sculptra and Radiesse)	Both are most effective for filling in deep creases around the mouth or for bolstering severely hollowed cheeks.	Because you don't see results right away with Sculptra, the less-is-more rule applies to each doctor visit. There is also a tiny risk of hardened nodules, particularly if Radiesse is injected too superficially; avoid both around the thin-skinned eye area.	A year or more for Radiesse; up to two years for Sculptra.

Index

GENERAL INDEX

Abdominal fat, 140, 180
Abdominal muscles/exercises. *See* Belly-
flatteners; Core muscles
Acne, 36, 40–41, 42, 72
Activity, daily, 181–186. *See also* Exercising
Affirmations, 248–251, 293. *See also* Motivation
African-American skin and hair, 28–29, 82, 94
Age spots, 31–32, 56, 72
Alcohol, 63, 86, 150–151, 230, 338
Alpha hydroxy acids (AHAs), 26–27, 29
Alzheimer's disease
brain fitness as preventative, 214, 224–225.
See also Memory/brain fitness
caregivers and, 197
dental hygiene as preventative, 231
dietary choices and, 129, 232–233
high cholesterol link to, 230
smoking link to, 230
symptoms of, 216
turmeric spice as preventative, 129, 233
Alzheimer's Prevention Program, The (Small),
214
American Academy of Dermatology, 32
Anemia, 121
Anti-Aging Awards, 16, 17
Antioxidants, 27, 39–40, 128, 306
Aral, Birnur K.
biographical sketch, 14–15
on hair care, 98, 107
on skin care, 29, 55, 62
Arthritis
dietary choices and, 126, 129

exercise as preventative, 187
sleep as preventative, 238
Asian skin, 28–29, 40, 82
Ask the Expert topics
about: experts, 14–17. *See also* Aral, Birnur
K.; Cassetty, Samantha B.; Cook,
Jennifer; Judar, Nina; Westmoreland,
Susan
affirmations, 250
bronzers, 75
coffee creamers, 146
exercise, 188, 201, 209
exfoliators, 26
eye makeup application, 72, 74, 77, 80
fluid intake, 24, 148
foundation, 71
friendships, 258
hair care, 98, 102, 107, 115
juices, 131
lipsticks, 83
makeup bag essentials, 84
memory/brain fitness, 216, 219, 225, 229, 231
monitoring weight loss, 157
multivitamins, 144
night sweats, 242
nutritional requirements, 136–137
optimism and longevity, 250, 253
pulse rate monitoring, 198
skin-care product application, 30, 37, 55
skin sensitivities, 29
skin supplements, 62
sleep, 239, 240, 242
snacks, 163
sparkling and flavored water, 148

tooth sensitivity, 87
vegetarian options, 264

Balance exercises, 186
Ballet, 207
B-complex vitamins, 138, 232
Beans and lentils, 133, 134
Beer, 151, 338
Belly-flatteners, 133, 138, 151–152, 199–200, 201, 205, 274, 286, 293
Beverages, 148–151
Bleaching creams, 31
Bloating, 274. *See also* Belly-flatteners
Blood pressure, high
    chocolate as preventative, 153
    dietary choices and, 135, 138, 140–141, 145, 146
    exercise as preventative, 179–180, 187, 206
    memory problems and, 231
    salt intake and, 140
    sitting and, 185
    tea as preventative, 150
Blotchiness, 28–30. *See also* Redness, facial
Blueberries, 233
Blush, 74, 76, 84, 279
Bone health
    dietary choices and, 125–126, 128, 130, 144–145, 147
    exercise and, 180, 184, 187, 191
Botox injections. *See* Injectables
Brain fitness. *See* Memory/brain fitness
Breast cancer, 127, 133, 144, 146, 150, 242
Bronzer, 75, 76. *See also* Self-tanning
Brown spots, 27, 28, 54
Brow pencil, 76
Brow tweezers, 76
Brushes, makeup, 89
Brushing/flossing, 85–87, 91

Calluses, 57
Cancer
    alcohol as preventative, 150
    breast, 127, 133, 144, 146, 150, 242
    colon, 138, 145, 192
    dietary choices and, 126–127, 128–129, 133, 135, 138, 144–146
    exercise as preventative, 192
    sedentary lifestyle as risk factor, 184
    skin, 33, 37, 38, 50
    tea as preventative, 149
Cardiovascular disease. *See* Heart disease
Carotenoids, 64–65
Cassetty, Samantha B.
    biographical sketch, 15
    on diet and nutrition, 35, 131, 136–137, 144, 146
    on fluid intake, 24
    on meal plan, 163, 264, 321, 375–376
    on vegetarian options, 264

on weight loss and maintenance, 157, 163, 375–376
Cheater's Guide to Exercise, The 200
Chest, 54, 189–190
Chocolate, 153, 171
Cholesterol levels
    Alzheimer's disease link, 230
    chocolate as preventative, 153
    dietary choices and, 126–127, 129, 131, 133, 139
    exercise as preventative, 180, 184
    saturated fats and, 139
Circuit training, 196
Clarifying shampoos, 102
Clothing, 54
Cocoa, 233
Coffee, 24, 146, 149, 233, 300
Coleman, Kathy, 254–255, 300, 309, 310, 313
Collagen and elastin production, 44–45, 47, 61–62. *See also* Retinoids
Colon cancer, 138, 145, 192
Complexion, 27–32, 35. *See also* Redness, facial
Computers. *See also* Lifestyle
    before bedtime, 78–79, 238, 240, 244, 269
    for improving memory/brain fitness, 222, 225, 228
    for increasing laughter, 256
    for learning, 298–299
    multitasking and, 310
    posting motivational messages on, 293, 296
    sitting and, 184–185, 201
Concealer, 72–73, 74, 83, 84
Conditioner, 96–99, 104, 108–109, 116–117
Convenience foods, 164, 302–303, 329, 332–334, 347
Cook, Jennifer
    biographical sketch, 16
    on exercise, 188, 198, 201, 209
    on friendships, 258
    on memory/brain fitness, 216, 219, 225, 229, 231
    on optimism, 250, 253
    on sleep, 239, 240, 242
Core muscles, 199–200, 201–202, 207, 286
Cravings
    binge busters, 168–170, 388–389
    emotional hunger and, 171–173, 295
    managing, 164–167, 171, 175, 300
    smart swaps, 168–171, 281, 289, 300, 312–313, 318
    stress and, 160–161, 167, 171
Cross-training, 196–199
Crow's feet, 52, 59, 390

Daily checklist, 269–275
Dairy products, 144–148
Dancing, 181, 207
Dark circles, 52, 59, 72–73, 74

RECIPE INDEX

The information in this book is not meant to take the place of the advice of your doctor. Before embarking on a weight loss program, you are advised to seek your doctor's counsel to make sure that the weight loss plan you choose is right for your particular needs. Further, this book's mention of products made by various companies does not imply that those companies endorse this book.

Cover design by OCD
Book design by Joanna Williams
Photography Credits:
Expert Team Pictures: PHILIP FRIEDMAN/STUDIO D
Fitness Images pgs 189-202: PHILIP FRIEDMAN/STUDIO D
Test Subjects: BEFORE: CHRIS ECKERT/STUDIO D
                AFTER: ALEX BEAUCHESNE

Library of Congress Cataloging-in-Publication Data

7 years younger : the revolutionary 7-week anti-aging plan / by the editors of Good Housekeeping.
    p. cm.
  Includes index.
  ISBN 978-1-936297-63-4 (hardback)
  1. Longevity. 2. Rejuvenation. 3. Aging--Prevention. 4. Older people--Health and hygiene. 5. Exercise.
I. Good housekeeping (New York, N.Y.) II. Title: Seven years younger.
  RA776.75.S48 2012
  613.2--dc23
                        2012015060

10 9 8 7 6 5 4 3

Published by Hearst Magazines
300 West 57th Street
New York, NY 10019

Good Housekeeping is a registered trademark and 7YY is a trademark of Hearst Communications, Inc.

www.goodhousekeeping.com

www.7yearsyounger.com

Distributed to the trade by Hachette Book Group

All US and Canadian orders:
Hachette Book Group
Order Department
Three Center Plaza
Boston, MA 02108
Call toll free: 1-800-759-0190
Fax toll free: 1-800-286-9471

For information regarding discounts to corporations, organizations, non-book retailers and wholesalers; mail order catalogs; and premiums, contact:
Special Markets Department
Hachette Book Group
237 Park Avenue
New York, NY 10017
Call toll free: 1-800-222-6747
Fax toll free: 1-800-222-6902

For all international orders:
Hachette Book Group
237 Park Avenue
New York, NY 10017
Tel: 212-364-1325
Fax: 212-364-0933
international@hbgusa.com

Printed in the USA